Pharmaceutical Sciences: An Integrated Approach

Pharmaceutical Sciences: An Integrated Approach

Editor: Rodrik Ledger

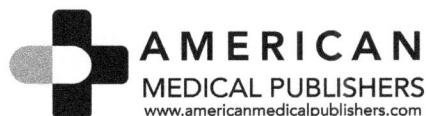

AMERICAN
MEDICAL PUBLISHERS
www.americanmedicalpublishers.com

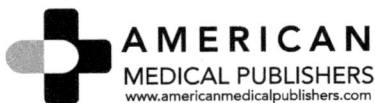

AMERICAN
MEDICAL PUBLISHERS
www.americanmedicalpublishers.com

Cataloging-in-Publication Data

Pharmaceutical sciences : an integrated approach / edited by Rodrik Ledger
    p. cm.
Includes bibliographical references and index.
ISBN 978-1-63927-546-5
1. Pharmacy. 2. Pharmacology. 3. Drugs. 4. Pharmaceutical chemistry. I. Ledger, Rodrik.
RS92 .P43 2022
615.1--dc23

© American Medical Publishers, 2022

American Medical Publishers,
41 Flatbush Avenue,
1st Floor, New York,
NY 11217, USA

ISBN 978-1-63927-546-5 (Hardback)

Contents

Preface...IX

Chapter 1   **Principles of Micellar Electrokinetic Capillary Chromatography Applied in Pharmaceutical Analysis** 1
Gabriel Hancu, Brigitta Simon, Aura Rusu, Eleonora Mircia and Árpád Gyéresi

Chapter 2   **Large Scale Generation and Characterization of Anti-Human CD34 Monoclonal Antibody in Ascetic Fluid of Balb/c Mice** 9
Leili Aghebati Maleki, Jafar Majidi, Behzad Baradaran, Jalal Abdolalizadeh, Tohid Kazemi, Ali Aghebati Maleki and Koushan Sineh sepehr

Chapter 3   **Multivariate Chemometric Assisted Analysis of Metformin Hydrochloride, Gliclazide and Pioglitazone Hydrochloride in Bulk Drug and Dosage Forms** 15
Radhika Bhaskar, Rahul Bhaskar, Mahendra K. Sagar and Vipin Saini

Chapter 4   **Comparison of *in Vitro* Activity of Doripenem versus Old Carbapenems against *Pseudomonas Aeruginosa* Clinical Isolates from both CF and Burn Patients** 21
Zoya Hojabri, Mohammad Ahangarzadeh Rezaee, Mohammad Reza Nahaei, Mohammad Hossein Soroush, Morteza Ghojazadeh, Tahereh Pirzadeh, Mostafa Davodi, Mona Ghazi, Reza Bigverdi, Omid Pajand and Mohammad Aghazadeh

Chapter 5   **High Performance Liquid Chromatographic Analysis of Almotriptan Malate in Bulk and Tablets** 26
Petikam lavudu, Avula Prameela Rani, Chepuri Divya and Chandra Bala Sekaran

Chapter 6   **Affinity Purification of Tumor Necrosis Factor-α Expressed in Raji Cells by Produced scFv Antibody Coupled CNBr-Activated Sepharose** 32
Jalal Abdolalizadeh, Jafar Majidi Zolbanin, Mohammad Nouri, Behzad Baradaran, AliAkbar Movassaghpour, Safar Farajnia and Yadollah Omidi

Chapter 7   **Synthesis and Antimicrobial Evaluation of Certain Novel Thiazoles**....................................... 37
Meesaraganda Sreedevi, Aluru Raghavendra Guru Prasad, Yadati Narasimha Spoorthy and Lakshmana Rao Krishna Rao Ravindranath

Chapter 8   **Thermoanalytical Investigation of Terazosin Hydrochloride**... 41
Ali Kamal Attia and Mona Mohamed Abdel-Moety

Chapter 9   **Extractive Spectrophotometric Determination of Ambrisentan** 46
Namasani Santhosh Kumar, Avula Prameela Rani, Telu Visalakshi and Chandra Bala Sekaran

Chapter 10   **Toxicity Effect of *Nigella Sativa* on the Liver Function of Rats**... 53
Mohammad Aziz Dollah, Saadat Parhizkar, Latiffah Abdul Latiff and Mohamad Hafanizam Bin Hassan

Chapter 11   **Analgesic Activity of Some 1,2,4-Triazole Heterocycles Clubbed with Pyrazole, Tetrazole, Isoxazole and Pyrimidine** 59
Shantaram Gajanan Khanage, Appala Raju, Popat Baban Mohite and
Ramdas Bhanudas Pandhare

Chapter 12   **Formulation, Characterization and Physicochemical Evaluation of Ranitidine Effervescent Tablets** 65
Abolfazl Aslani and Hajar Jahangiri

Chapter 13   **Mass-Production and Characterization of Anti-CD20 Monoclonal Antibody in Peritoneum of Balb/c Mice** 73
Koushan Sineh Sepehr, Behzad Baradaran, Jafar Majidi, Jalal Abdolalizadeh,
Leili Aghebati and Fatemeh Zare Shahneh

Chapter 14   **Design and Characterization of Microemulsion Systems for Naproxen** 78
Eskandar Moghimipour, Anayatollah Salimi and Soroosh Eftekhari

Chapter 15   **Targeted Fluoromagnetic Nanoparticles for Imaging of Breast Cancer MCF-7 Cells** 87
Mostafa Heidari Majd, Jaleh Barar, Davoud Asgari, Hadi Valizadeh,
Mohammad Reza Rashidi, Vala Kafil, Javid Shahbazi and Yadollah Omidi

Chapter 16   **Comparison of Cytotoxic Activity of L778123 as a Farnesyltranferase Inhibitor and Doxorubicin against A549 and HT-29 Cell Lines** 94
Saeed Ghasemi, Soodabeh Davaran, Simin Sharifi, Davoud Asgari, Ali Abdollahi and
Javid Shahbazi Mojarrad

Chapter 17   **A Unique Report: Development of Super Anti-Human IgG Monoclone with Optical Density Over Than 3** 99
Leili Aghebati Maleki, Behzad Baradaran, Jalal Abdolalizadeh,
Fatemeh Ezzatifar and Jafar Majidi

Chapter 18   **Simultaneous Determination of Loratadine, Desloratadine and Cetirizine by Capillary Zone Electrophoresis** 104
Gabriel Hancu, Camelia Câmpian, Aura Rusu, Eleonora Mircia and Hajnal Kelemen

Chapter 19   **Thermal Analysis of Some Antidiabetic Pharmaceutical Compounds** 109
Ali Kamal Attia, Magda Mohamed Ibrahim and Mohamed Abdel Nabi El-Ries

Chapter 20   **Impact of Caffeine on Weight Changes Due to Ketotifen Administration** 115
Bohlool Habibi Asl, Haleh Vaez, Turan Imankhah and Samin Hamidi

Chapter 21   **Microwave Assisted Synthesis of 1-[5-(Substituted Aryl)-1H-Pyrazol-3-yl]-3,5-Diphenyl-1H-1,2,4-Triazole as Antinociceptive and Antimicrobial Agents** 122
Shantaram Gajanan Khanage, Popat Baban Mohite, Ramdas Bhanudas Pandhare and
S. Appala Raju

Chapter 22   **Thin Layer Chromatographic Analysis of Beta-Lactam Antibiotics** 130
Gabriel Hancu, Brigitta Simon, Hajnal Kelemen, Aura Rusu, Eleonora Mircia and
Árpád Gyéresi

Chapter 23   **Application of Liquisolid Technology for Enhancing Solubility and Dissolution of Rosuvastatin** 135
Pavan Ram Kamble, Karimunnisa Sameer Shaikh and Pravin Digambar Chaudhari

Chapter 24   **Synthesis, Characterization and Antioxidant Property of Quercetin-Tb(III) Complex**..................143
Jafar Ezzati Nazhad Dolatabadi, Ahad Mokhtarzadeh, Seyed Morteza Ghareghoran and Gholamreza Dehghan

Chapter 25   **Modifications to the Conventional Nanoprecipitation Technique: an Approach to Fabricate Narrow Sized Polymeric Nanoparticles**.....................147
Moorthi Chidambaram and Kathiresan Krishnasamy

Chapter 26   **Preparation, Physicochemical Characterization and Performance Evaluation of Gold Nanoparticles in Radiotherapy**.....................151
Ali Kamiar, Reza Ghotaslou and Hadi Valizadeh

Chapter 27   **Electrochemical Studies for the Determination of Quetiapine Fumarate and Olanzapine Antipsychotic Drugs**.....................155
Manal A. El-Shal

Chapter 28   **Chiral Separation of Indapamide Enantiomers by Capillary Electrophoresis**.....................161
Amelia Tero-Vescan, Gabriel Hancu, Mihaela Oroian and Anca Cârje

Chapter 29   **Development and Validation of UV-Visible Spectrophotometric Method for Simultaneous Determination of Eperisone and Paracetamol in Solid Dosage Form**.....................167
Shantaram Gajanan Khanage, Popat Baban Mohite and Sandeep Jadhav

Chapter 30   **Influence of Foreign DNA Introduction and Periplasmic Expression of Recombinant Human Interleukin-2 on Hydrogen Peroxide Quantity and Catalase Activity in *Escherichia coli***.....................172
Lena Mahmoudi Azar, Elnaz Mehdizadeh Aghdam, Farrokh Karimi, Babak Haghshenas, Abolfazl Barzegari, Parichehr Yaghmaei and Mohammad Saeid Hejazi

Chapter 31   **Design Expert Assisted Formulation of Topical Bioadhesive Gel of Sertaconazole Nitrate**.....................180
Vishal Pande, Samir Patel, Vijay Patil and Raju Sonawane

Chapter 32   **A Novel Approach using Hydrotropic Solubalization Technique for Quantitative Estimation of Entacapone in Bulk Drug and Dosage Form**.....................189
Ruchi Jain, Nilesh Jain, Deepak Kumar Jain and Surendra Kumar Jain

Chapter 33   **Thermal Analysis Study of Antihypertensive Drugs Telmisartan and Cilazapril**.....................194
Refaat Ahmed Saber, Ali Kamal Attia and Waheed Mohamed Salem

Permissions

List of Contributors

Index

Preface

This book aims to highlight the current researches and provides a platform to further the scope of innovations in this area. This book is a product of the combined efforts of many researchers and scientists, after going through thorough studies and analysis from different parts of the world. The objective of this book is to provide the readers with the latest information of the field.

The set of sciences which studies the design, action, delivery and disposition of drugs is known as pharmaceutical science. Its aim is to optimize the delivery of drugs to the body in order to use it to create better therapies against diseases in humans. They integrate the basic principles of organic and physical chemistry with biochemistry, biology and engineering. There are four main branches of pharmaceutical sciences - pharmacology, pharmaceutical chemistry, pharmaceutics, and pharmacognosy. The biochemical and physiological effects of drugs on humans are studied under pharmacology. Pharmaceutical chemistry studies the drug design to optimize pharmacokinetics and pharmacodynamics in order to synthesize new drug molecules. Pharmaceutics focuses on the study and design of drug formulation for optimum stability and delivery. Pharmacognosy is related to the study of medicines derived from natural sources. This book contains some path-breaking studies in the field of pharmaceutical sciences. It presents researches and studies performed by experts across the globe. Researchers and students in this field will be assisted by this book.

I would like to express my sincere thanks to the authors for their dedicated efforts in the completion of this book. I acknowledge the efforts of the publisher for providing constant support. Lastly, I would like to thank my family for their support in all academic endeavors.

Editor

Principles of Micellar Electrokinetic Capillary Chromatography Applied in Pharmaceutical Analysis

Gabriel Hancu[1]*, Brigitta Simon[1], Aura Rusu[1], Eleonora Mircia[2], Árpád Gyéresi[1]

[1] *Department of Pharmaceutical Chemistry, Faculty of Pharmacy, University of Medicine and Pharmacy, Târgu Mureş, Romania.*

[2] *Department of Organic Chemistry, Faculty of Pharmacy, University of Medicine and Pharmacy, Târgu Mureş, Romania.*

ARTICLE INFO

Keywords:
Capillary electrophoresis
Micellar electrokinetic
Capillary chromatography
Pharmaceutical analysis

ABSTRACT

Since its introduction capillary electrophoresis has shown great potential in areas where electrophoretic techniques have rarely been used before, including here the analysis of pharmaceutical substances. The large majority of pharmaceutical substances are neutral from electrophoretic point of view, consequently separations by the classic capillary zone electrophoresis; where separation is based on the differences between the own electrophoretic mobilities of the analytes; are hard to achieve. Micellar electrokinetic capillary chromatography, a hybrid method that combines chromatographic and electrophoretic separation principles, extends the applicability of capillary electrophoretic methods to neutral analytes. In micellar electrokinetic capillary chromatography, surfactants are added to the buffer solution in concentration above their critical micellar concentrations, consequently micelles are formed; micelles that undergo electrophoretic migration like any other charged particle. The separation is based on the differential partitioning of an analyte between the two-phase system: the mobile aqueous phase and micellar pseudostationary phase. The present paper aims to summarize the basic aspects regarding separation principles and practical applications of micellar electrokinetic capillary chromatography, with particular attention to those relevant in pharmaceutical analysis.

Introduction

Capillary electrophoresis (CE) is an instrumental evolution of traditional electrophoretic techniques, where separation occurs in fused-silica capillaries and involves application of high voltages across buffer filled capillaries in order to achieve separation. Due to its speed of analysis, high efficiency, automated analytical equipment, low reagents and sample consumption and rapid method development, CE has gained momentum in pharmaceutical analysis, being regarded today as an alternative and also a complementary technique to the more frequently used high performance liquid chromatography (HPLC).

CE is actually a range of separation techniques based on different separation principles: capillary zone electrophoresis–CZE (based on the differences between the electrohoretic mobilities of the analytes), micellar electrokinetic capillary chromatography–MEKC (separation of neutral compounds using surfactant micelles), capillary gel electrophoresis–CGE (filtration of analytes through a gel network), capillary isoelectric focusing–CIEF (separation of zwitterionic analytes within a pH gradient), capillary electrochromatography–CEC (separation of analytes in a capillary filled with a chromatographic stationary phase).[1-4]

Various CE techniques offer various possibilities for pharmaceutical analysis. Depending on the complexity of the sample, the nature of its components, on the intended application and the nature of the analytes, each of these techniques will provide various advantages for the separation and detection of different pharmaceutical substances.

Substances of pharmaceutical interest are usually neutral from electrophoretic point of view and also frequently the separation of substances with very similar structural and physico-chemical properties is required. Being based on differences between the electrophoretic mobilities of the analytes, the classic CZE method is not suited for the separation of neutral substances, which migrate towards the detector with the same velocity as the electro-osmotic flow (EOF). MEKC is an electrophoretic technique developed in the early 90 by Shigeru Terabe that extends the applicability of CE to neutral analytes, which cannot be separated using simple free solution CE.

The same instrumentation that is used for CZE is used for MEKC, which demonstrates the versatility and adaptability of the method. MEKC differs from CZE because it uses an ionic micellar solution instead of the simple buffer salt solution. MEKC can be used for the

*Corresponding author: Gabriel Hancu, Faculty of Pharmacy, University of Medicine and Pharmacy TârguMureş, GhMarinescu 38, 540000 TârguMureş, Romania. E-mail: g_hancu@yahoo.com

separation of both ionic and neutral substances while CZE typically separates only ionic substances. Thereby MEKC has a great advantage over CZE in the separation of mixture containing both ionic and neutral analytes.[1,2,5]

The separation principle of MEKC is based on the differential partition of the analytes between micelles and water while CZE is based on the differences between the own electrophoretic mobility of the analytes.

Separation Principle

MEKC is based on the addition to the buffer solution of a micellar "pseudostationary" phase, which interacts with the analytes according to partitioning mechanisms, just like in a chromatographic method. The "pseudostationary" phase is composed of a surfactant added to the buffer solution in a concentration above its critical micellar concentration (CMC). In this system, EOF acts like a chromatographic "mobile phase". From a "chromatographic point of view", the EOF's "plug-like" flow profile is almost ideal as it minimizes band broadening, which can occur during the separation process.[5-7]

The most commonly used surfactant sodium dodecyl sulfate (SDS), an anionic surfactant. The anionic SDS micelles are electrostatically attracted towards the anode. The EOF transports the bulk solution towards the negative electrode due to the negative charge on the internal surface of the silica capillaries. But the EOF is usually stronger than the electrophoretic migration of the micelles and therefore the micelles will migrate also toward the negative electrode with a retarded velocity (Figure 1).[5-8,10]

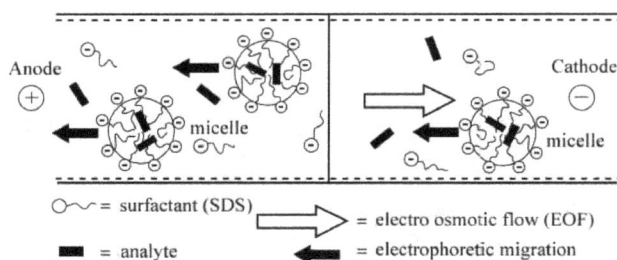

Figure 1. Schematic of the separation principle in MEKC[5]

When a neutral analyte is injected into the micellar solution, a fraction is incorporated into the micelle, while the remaining fraction of the analyte migrates with the electroosmotic velocity. Consequently, micelles decrease selectively the migration of neutral solutes they interact with (by partitioning mechanism), which otherwise would migrate with the same velocity as the EOF.

The separation depends on the individual partitioning equilibrium of the different analytes between the micellar and the aqueous phase. The greater percentage of analyte is distributed into the micelle, the slower it will migrate. Therefore, analytes that have greater

affinity for the micelles exhibit slower migration velocities compared with analytes that are mostly distributed in the bulk solution.[2,5,8,10,11]

With SDS micelles, the general migration order will be exactly the opposite as in ECZ: anions, neutral analytes and cations. Anions will remain mostly in the bulk solution due to electrostatic repulsions from the micelle; neutral molecules will be separated exclusively due to their hydrophobicity; while cations will migrate last due to the strong electrostatic attraction. This generalization regarding the migration order can be sometimes useful, but strong hydrophobic interaction between analytes and micelles can overcome repulsions and attractions. Likewise, the own electrophoretic mobilities of the analytes can also modify the migration order.[9,12]

Analytes which are highly retained by the micelle will have longer migration times, while analytes which have limited interactions with the micelle will have migration times close to the EOF (t_0). Very hydrophobic compounds may be totally included into the micelle and will migrate with the micelles velocity (t_{mc}). Methanol is not retained by the micelles and migrates with t_0 being used as marker for the EOF, while a dye Sudan III is totally included into the micelle and can be used as a micellar marker. The period between the migration time of the bulk solution and the migration time of the micelle is often referred to in the literature as migration time window (Figure 2).[5,8,13]

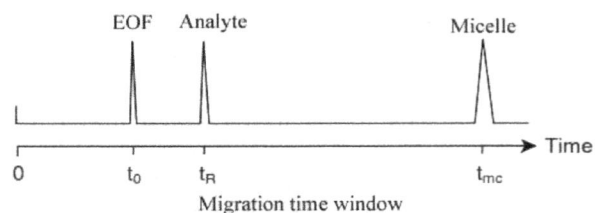

Figure 2. Migration time window in a MEKC separation[1]

A relatively recent development in MEKC has been to perform separations in the absence of EOF. This may be achieved using coated capillaries or at low pH values. This could be especially useful in the separation of acidic analytes, which would ionized at high pH values and would not interact with the negatively charged SDS micelle.[15]

Cationic surfactants can be used in MEKC to reverse the charge on the capillary wall, by absorption on the capillary wall surface through a mechanism involving electrostatic attraction between the positively charged ammonium moieties and the negatively charged Si-O- groups; when a reversal of the EOF takes place.[9]

Micelles and Surfactants

Surfactants are molecules with detergent properties, which are composed of a hydrophilic water-soluble head group and a hydrophobic water-insoluble hydrocarbon chain group.

Although a large number of surfactants are commercially available, a limited number are widely used in MEKC separations. The surfactants suitable for MEKC must be soluble in the buffer solution to form micelles and the micellar solution must be homogeneous, UV transparent and also have a low viscosity.

There are four major classes of surfactants: anionic, cationic, zwitterionic and nonionic (Table 1). Of these, ionic surfactants are generally used in MEKC. Every surfactant has a characteristic CMC and aggregation number (the number of surfactant molecules necessary to form a micelle). Another important parameter is the Kraft point, which represents the minimum temperature where the solubility of surfactants increases steeply due to the formation of micelles.[1,5,8,9]

Table 1. Surfactants classes and properties[1]

Surfactant	Type	CMC*	n
Sodium dodecyl sulphate (SDS)	anionic	8.1×10^{-3}	62
Sodium tetradecylsulphate (STS)	Anionic	2.1×10^{-3}	138
Sodium dodecanesulphate	anionic	7.2×10^{-3}	54
Sodium cholate	anionic	$13\text{-}15 \times 10^{-3}$	2-4
Cetyltrimethylammonium bromide (CTAB)	cationic	0.92×10^{-3}	61
Dodecyltrimethylammonium bromide	cationic	15×10^{-3}	56
Brij - 35	nonionic	0.1×10^{-3}	40
Sulfobetaine	zwitterionic	3.3×10^{-3}	55

Nonionic surfactants do not posses electrophoretic mobility and cannot be used, as "pseudostationary phase" in conventional MEKC, however can be useful for the separation of charged analytes. This technique using nonionic micelles can be classified as an extension of MEKC.[9,16]

Micelles are amphiphilic aggregates of surfactants. Above a specific surfactant concentration, the surfactant molecules begin to self-aggregate, forming micelles, spherical aggregates that exhibit electrophoretic migration like any other charged particle. Micelles are long chain molecules and are characterized as possessing a long hydrophobic tails and a hydrophilic head group. Generally micelles are formed in aqueous solution with the hydrophobic tails oriented towards the center of the aggregated molecules and the hydrophilic heads pointing outward into the aqueous solution.[6,9,10,12,14]

Micelle formation is a very dynamic process, as micelle disaggregate and reconstruct continuously, composing the "pseudostationary phase" which can include hydrophobic analytes.

Micellar solutions can solubilize hydrophobic compounds which otherwise would be insoluble in water. Micelles have the ability to interact with the analytes at molecular level based on hydrophobic and electrostatic interactions. Even neutral analytes can bind to micelles due to the very strong solubilization power of the hydrophobic core.[8,9]

The micelles used in MEKC are charged on the surface, so an analyte with the opposite charge will strongly interact with the micelle through electrostatic forces while an analyte with the same charge will interact weakly due to the electrostatic repulsion. Therefore the use of a cationic or an anionic surfactant will result in an entirely different result.

The micellar phase can be modified by adding two different surfactants to form a mixed micelle; addition of an ionic and a nonionic surfactant can provide different selectivity in separation. A mixed micelle has a lower surface charge and a larger size; consequently its electrophoretic mobility will be lower than the one of a simple ionic micelle.[8,9,12]

Some surfactants like bile salts are chiral and can be used for enantiomers separation.[16]

Buffer Additives

Since MEKC is often applied in the separation of analytes with very similar hydrophobicities and chemical characteristics, sometimes is useful to extend the concept of using a "mobile phase" and a "pseudostationary phase" to the use of buffer additives such as organic modifiers and cyclodextrines.

Organic solvents (methanol, acetonitrile) are used in CZE in order to increase solubility of the analytes, but their role in MEKC is more complex and profound. Organic solvents reduce EOF, consequently increase the migration times and migration time window of the analytes. Also, organic additives reduce the hydrophobic interactions between the micelle and the analyte and can be useful in the separation of analytes which otherwise are almost completely incorporated in micelles. The addition of organic solvents will increase the migration velocity of these hydrophobic analytes, by reducing the partition coefficient between the micelle and the bulk solution. However high concentration of organic solvents may break down the micellar structure, consequently concentrations above 25-30% should be avoided.[1,5,6,8,11,13]

Cyclodextrines (CD) are cyclic oligosaccharides with truncated cylindrical molecular shapes, having an external hydrophilic surface and an internal hydrophobic cavity, in which they can include other compounds by hydrophobic interactions. The inclusion mechanism is sterically selective, because analytes must fit the size of the cavity, the diameter of which depends on the number of glucose units in the CD structure.[17]

There is a wide range of both natural and derivatised CD commercially available. The native CD, α-, β-, and γ-CD possess different numbers of glucose sub-units, six, seven and eight respectively. These surface hydroxyl groups can be chemically replaced with groups such as hydroxypropy and dimethyl groups. Ionic chargeable CD offers the possibility of separation of neutral drug enantiomers or enhanced separation of ionic drugs. Several CE specific derivatised CDs have been produced with amino, sulfate or carboxylic groups.[18]

Because of the chirality of the hydroxyls in the glucose molecules that form the rim of the CD cavity, the inclusion complex formation will be chirally selective. If the enantiomers of a compound have different binding constants, then chiral separation is possible by adding the proper CD in the buffer electrolyte.[16]

CDs are neutral from electrophoretic point of view, and are not incorporated in micelles, because of the hydrophilic nature of the outside surface of the molecules. Therefore, an analyte included in the CD will migrate with the same velocity as the EOF. The addition of cyclodextrines reduces the apparent distribution coefficient of the analytes between the two phases.

Hydrophobic analytes can become incorporated into either the CD cavity or the micelle. Effectively the addition of the CD establishes two "pseudo stationary" phases in the electrolyte, which can reduce analysis times and offer the possibility of improved separation. CDs have advantages over organic solvents, as they are UV transparent and non-volatile. The schematic principle in cyclodextrin modified micellar electrokinetic chromatography is presented (CD-MEKC) (Figure 3).[1,5,16,17]

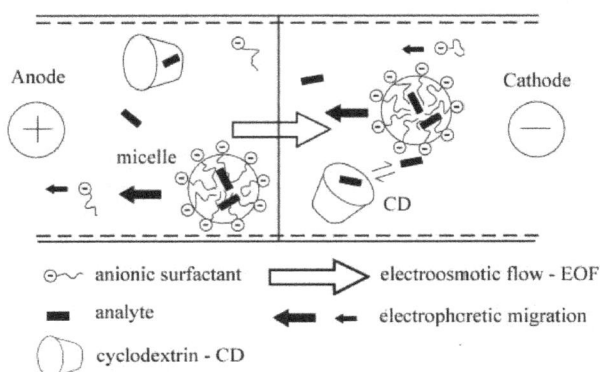

Figure 3. Schematic of the separation principle in CD – MEKC[5]

Theoretical Aspects

In MEKC we can define the capacity factor (k) similarly as in chromatography:[5]

$$k = n_{mc} / n_{aq}$$

where n_{mc} and n_{aq} are the amount of analyte incorporated into the micelle and in the aqueous respectively. It can be calculated from the migration time of the analyte (t_R), of the EOF (t_0) and of the micelle (t_{mc}):[5]

$$k = t_R - t_0 / t_0(1 - t_R/t_{mc})$$

When k = 0, the migration time of the analyte is equal to t_0, which means that the analyte does not interact with the micelle; and when k is infinity, the migration time of the analyte is equal to t_{mc}, which means that the analyte is totally incorporated into the micelle.

The capacity factor is a fundamental term in chromatography while the electrophoretic mobility is characteristic to the electrophoretic process. In ECZ the migration velocity (v) of the analyte is expressed as:[5,7,19]

$$v = (\mu_{eo} + \mu_a) E$$

where μ_{eo} and μ_a are the electrophoretic mobilities of the EOF and analyte respectively and E is the electric field strength. We can apply this equation to MEKC by defining the effective electrophoretic mobility of a neutral analyte (μ_{na}) as:[5,7,19]

$$\mu_{na} = \mu_{mc} k/1+k$$

where μ_{mc} is the electrophoretic mobility of the micelle and k/1+k represents the fraction of analyte incorporated into the micelle. Thus, the velocity of a neutral analyte in MEKC is given as:[5,7]

$$v = (\mu_{eo} + \mu_{na}) E$$

The capacity factor provides quantitative information about the analyte distribution between the two phases, while the electrophoretic mobility only gives qualitative information about it.

The resolution equation in MEKC can be given by the following equation:[1,5,19,20]

$$R_s = \frac{\sqrt{N}}{4} \left(\frac{\alpha - 1}{\alpha} \right) \left(\frac{k_2}{1 + k_2} \right) \left(\frac{1 - (t_0/t_{mc})}{1 + (t_0/t_{mc})k_1} \right)$$

where N is the theoretical plate number, α the separation factor between the two analytes and k_1 and k_2 their capacity factor.

The separation factor (α) is determined by the micellar solubilization process and is influenced by the chemical nature of both the micellar and aqueous phase. Various surfactant systems can be used as well as mixed micelles, possessing different solubilization characteristics, in order to control migration behavior of the analytes and optimize selectivity.

Method Development Guidelines

Micellar solutions exhibit a relatively high conductivity, so a capillary with small diameter could be the right choice to prevent excessive Joule heating. A longer capillary can be useful in the case of large amount sample solutions to obtain a better separation at the expense of time.[1]

The micellar solution is prepared by dissolving the surfactant in the buffer solution in a concentration above its CMC. Popular buffer solutions often used to prepare the micellar solution are phosphate, borate, or tris (hydroxymethyl) aminomethane (Tris). Concentrations between 25 and 100 mM are normally employed for both the surfactant and buffer. High concentrations will result in relatively high viscosities and high currents and should be avoided. It is essential that the pH of the buffer remains constant, being a critical parameter in the separation of ionizable analytes.[1,13]

It should be noted that the counter ion of the ionic surfactant is exchanged by the counter ion of the buffer electrolyte and, consequently, the character of the micelle may be changed.[1]

The sample solution can be prepared in any solvent; but water will be the first choice solvent if the analyte is soluble in it. When the sample contains high concentrations of an organic solvent, the peaks may be split due to incomplete mixing of the sample solution with the running solution.[1]

The applied voltage must be kept to a level that doesn't generate excessive current, the limit being determined by the capacity of the electrophoretic system to dissipate Joule heating. A compromise is, therefore, necessary between high Joule heating and fast separation time.[1]

It is also necessary to control the capillary temperature because MEKC methods are even more sensitive to temperature variation than CZE methods. The distribution coefficients are highly dependent on temperature; an increase in temperature will cause a decrease in the distribution coefficient of the analytes between the two phases. It is well known that an increase in temperature reduces viscosity of the buffer, which increases both electrophoretic and EOF velocities, reducing the migration time.[1,5,13]

When preliminary runs show unsatisfactory separation, several analytical parameters may need to be adjusted in order to optimize separation. It is useful to estimate the retention factors by measuring t_0 and t_{mc}. If problems occur in measuring t_{mc} due to the difficulty observing the micelle marker peak, it is advisable to simply assume that t_{mc} is four time longer than t_0. The optimum value of the capacity factor k can be estimated as being equal to $(t_{mc}/t_0)^{1/2}$.[1,5,8,13]

If optimum k values do not provide acceptable resolution, further tuning may be required; the use of additives such as organic solvents or CDs may be needed, or the use of alternate surfactants may prove effective. The selection of additives is extensive, but the first step is recommended to be the addition of an organic solvent in low concentration. If the analytes have closely related structures, addition of a CD derivative may prove effective. There are many different CD derivatives available, but initially ß-CD or

γ-CD can be tested. Further steps can be performed by selecting other CD derivatives if necessary. Another choice is the modification of the micelle by using mixed micelles, in particular, addition of a nonionic, adding cosurfactants, or by adding an organic counter ion.[1,5,8,13]

One of the issues that still remains unsolved in MEKC is the improvement in reproducibility in quantitative analysis, including migration time and peak height or peak area, a problem characteristic for every CE technique.[2,5]

MEKC Applications in the Analysis of Pharmaceutical Substances

In principle MEKC is used for the analysis of neutral compounds, or when analyzing mixtures of neutral and charged solutes. But MEKC conditions are also employed when selectivity requirements for a separation exceed the simple mobility differences obtainable in CZE.

MEKC can be especially useful for the determination of drugs in samples having a high protein content (clinical samples, biofluids) reducing the disadvantageous matrix effects caused by organic materials, while CZE through its simplicity and operation stability could be advantageous for pharmaceutical determinations. MEKC can be usually applied in simultaneous separation from complex mixtures of pharmaceutical substances with very similar structural and physico-chemical characteristics.

Many reports have been published detailing the use of MEKC for pharmaceutical applications; Table 2 presents briefly selected pharmaceutical applications and the description of the electrophoretic conditions.

Another application of MEKC is the chiral separation of optically active pharmaceutical substances. Enantiomer separation by MEKC involves the addition of a chiral agent such as chiral surfactants, crown ethers, or CDs to the background electrolyte with chiral/achiral micelles. Chiral MEKC with chiral surfactants is an important separation mode for chiral compounds, with chiral surfactants including also naturally occurring compounds such as bile salts, amino acids or glucose.[37]

Chiral separation in MEKC is affected by the affinity of the enantiomers toward the micelles, and the concentration of the micellar phase, which depends on the aggregation properties of the chiral surfactants.[1]

MEKC can be used for the separation of structural related impurities from the main active drug, and has been proven an alternative to HPLC for quantitation of compounds and the determination of drug-related impurities.[1]

The structurally related impurities of a drug will possess similar structural and physico-chemical characteristics to the main component, which makes their separation and determination a challenging task. The high separation efficiencies possible for CE often allows a small degree of selectivity to provide an acceptable resolution. The separation and determination of drug-related impurities using CE has been extensively studied, and the method performance and validation data obtained clearly shows that CE methods are successful applications in this area.

Table 2. Applications of MEKC in the analysis of different pharmaceutical substances

Pharmaceutical class	Substances	Electrophoretic conditions	Reference
Penicillins	Amoxicillin, Ampicillin, Benzylpenicillin, Phenoxymethypenicillin, Oxacillin, Cloxacilin	40 mM sodium tetraborate + 100 mM SDS, pH – 9.3 voltage: + 10kV, temperature: 20 ^{0}C, UV detection 210 nm	21
Penicillins	Amoxicillin, Ampicillin, Benzylpenicillin, Phenoxymethypenicillin, Oxacillin, Cloxacilin, Dicloxacillin, Nafcillin, Piperacillin	26 mM sodium tetraborate + 100 mM SDS, pH – 8.5 voltage: + 20kV, temperature: 30 ^{0}C, UV detection 220 nm	22
Cephalosporins	Cefazoline, Cefuroxime, Ceftriaxone, Cefoperazone, Ceftazidime	20 mM sodium tetraborate + 15 mM disodium hydrogenophosphate + 50 mM SDS pH – 6.5, voltage: + 18kV, temperature: 20^{0}C, UV detection 214 nm	23
Macrolides	Erythromycin, Tylosin and related substances	80 mM sodium phosphate + 20 mM sodium cholate + 7 mMcetyltrimethylammonium bromide, pH – 7.5, voltage: + 15kV, temperature: 25^{0}C, UV detection 280 nm	24
Aminoglycosides	Gentamicin, Sisomicin, Netilmicin, Kanamycin, Amikacin, Tobramycin	100 mM sodium tetraborate + 20 mM sodium deoxycholate + 15 mM beta-cyclodextrin, pH – 10 voltage: + 20kV, temperature: 25^{0}C	25
Tetracyclines	Tetracycline, Oxytetracicline, Democlocycline, Chlortetracycline, Doxycicline, Minocycline	15 mM ammonium acetate + 20 mM SDS, pH – 6.5, voltage: + 15kV, temperature: 25^{0}C	26
Sulfonamides	Sulfanilamide, Sulfathiazole, Sulfamethoxazole, Sulfaguanidine, Sulfadiazine	13.32 mM disodium hydrogen phosphate, 6.67 mM potassium dihydrogen phosphate + 40 mM SDS, pH – 7.5, voltage: + 21kV, temperature: 25^{0}C fluorescence detection	27
Sulfonamides	Sulfamethazine, Sulfamerazine, Sulfathiazole, Sulfachloropyridazine, Sulfamethoxazole, Sulfacarbamide, Sulfaguanidine	15 mM sodium tetraborate + 25 mM SDS + 20% methanol, pH – 9.3, voltage: + 20kV, temperature: 22^{0}C, UV detection 200 nm	28
Fluoroquinolones	Norfloxacin, Ciprofloxacin, Ofloxacin, Enrofloxacin, Danofloxacin	25 mM sodium carbonate + 100 mM SDS, pH – 9.2, voltage: + 20kV, temperature: 30^{0}C, UV detection 280 nm	29
Antifungal azoles	Fluconazole, Voriconazole, Itraconazole, Posaconazole	25 mM phosphoric acid + 100 mM SDS + 13 % acetonitrile + 13 % tetrahydrofuran, pH – 2.2	30
Barbiturates	Phenobarbital, Amobarbital, Pentobarbital, Secobarbital, Butabarbital	10 mM sodium tetraborate + 10 mM disodium hydrogenophosphate + 100 mM SDS + 15% acetonitrile. pH - 8.5, voltage: + 20 kV, UV detection 214 nm	31
Benzodiazepines	Flunitrazepam, Diazepam, Midazolam, Clonazepam, Bromazepam, Temazepam, Oxazepam, Lorazepam	25 mM phosphate/borate + 75 mM SDS, pH – 9.3	32
Benzodiazepines	Alprazolam, Bromazepam, Chlordiazepoxide, Diazepam, Flunitrazepam, Medazepam, Oxazepam, Nitrazepam	25 mM sodium tetraborate + 50 mM SDS + 12% methanol, pH – 9.3, voltage: + 25kV, temperature: 20 ^{0}C, UV detection 214 nm	33
Phenotiazines	Promethazino, Ethopropazine, Trimeprazine, Methoprimeprazine, Thioridazine	80 mM citric acid + 10 mMtetradecyltrimethylammonium bromide + 7 mM β-CD (9 mM HP β-CD), pH – 3.5, voltage: + 20kV, temperature: 25 ^{0}C, UV detection 254 nm enantiomer separation	34
Tricyclic antidepressants	Imipramine, Amitriptyline, Desipramine, Nortriptyline, Doxepin, Trimipramine	37.5 mM phosphate + 25 mMdodecyltrimethylammonium bromide + 2 M urea, pH – 8, voltage: + 25kV	35
Xanthines	Caffeine, Theobromine, Theophylline, Pentoxifylline	20 mM sodium tetraborate + 100 mM SDS, pH – 9.3, voltage: + 30kV, temperature: 25 ^{0}C, UV detection 274 nm	36

During the early phase and later phase of drug development, knowledge of physiochemical properties of pharmaceutical compounds is important in order to predict their bioavailability and blood-brain. Physicochemical properties such as acid dissociation constant (pKa), octanol–water partition-coefficient (logP), solubility, permeability, and protein binding are closely related to drug absorption, distribution, metabolism, and excretion. The pKa determination of acids and bases by CE is based on measuring the electrophoretic mobility of charged species associated with the acid–baseequilibria as a function of pH. CE techniques using "pseudostationary" phases in the background electrolyte, like MEKC, allow the measurement of log Pvalues because of the partitioning of solutes between the micellar and the aqueous phase. CE methods and especially MEKC has been applied successfully for physicochemical analysis of many pharmaceutical compounds and has many advantages over the traditional methods of log P and pKa determination.[38,39]

Concluding remarks

The use of CE methods in pharmaceutical analysis has become increasingly popular in recent years. The wide range of applications for which the use of this method has proved to be successful includes identification of pharmaceutical substances, assay of drugs, determination of drug-related impurities, physicochemical measurements of drug molecules or chiral separations.[11,19,20]

For pharmaceutical analysis, the range of applications for which CE can be used is extensive, possibly eclipsing the applications of the more frequently used HPLC. CE also offers a number of advantages over HPLC and other analytical techniques: the rapid development of the analysis method, its analysis speed, reduced consumable and solvent expenses, low sample amount, simplicity of operations, and a greater possibility of implementation of a single set of method conditions for the analysis of several different samples.[1]

MEKC is a branch of CE, which has become during the years one of the most popular techniques in CE due to its high resolving power and capability of separating both ionic and neutral analytes. MEKC is the most flexible of all CE techniques, offering the greatest selectivity to the widest range of compounds and can be considered the separation method of choice when performing CE analysis for pharmaceutical substances.

MEKC combines the separation mechanism of chromatography with the electrophoretic and electroosmotic movement of analytes and solutions for the separation of constituents in a sample.

In the last 10-15 years MEKC gained popularity among separation scientist as pointed out by the relatively large numbers of article published, therefore this papers main objective is to present the guiding principles regarding the full availability of the technique.

Conflict of Interest

There is no conflict of interest in this study.

References

1. Schmitt-Kopplin P. Capillary electrophoresis – Methods and Protocols. Totowa, NJ: Humana Press; 2008.
2. Altria KD. Analysis of pharmaceuticals by capillary electrophoresis.Chromatographia CE Series, Volume 2, Friedr. Braunschweig/Wiesbaden:Vieweg & Sohn Verlagsgesellschaft mbH; 1998.
3. European Pharmacopoeia. 7th ed. Strasbourg: Council of Europe; 2010.
4. British Pharmacopoeia. London: Her Majesty's Stationary Office; 2009.
5. Landers JP. Handbook of capillary and microchip electrophoresis and associated microtechniques. Boca Raton: CRC Press; 2008.
6. Altria KD. Overview of capillary electrophoresis and capillary electrochromatography. *J Chromatogr A* 1999; 856(1-2): 443-63.
7. Tagliaro F, Manetto G, Crivellente F, Smith FP. A brief introduction to capillary electrophoresis. *Forensic Sci Int* 1998; 98: 75-88.
8. Altria KD, McLean R. Development and optimisation of a generic micellar electrokinetic capillary chromatography method to support analysis of a wide range of pharmaceuticals and excipients. *J Pharm Biomed Anal* 1998; 18(4-5): 807-13.
9. Muijselaar PG, Otsuka K, Terabe S. Micelles as pseudo-stationary phases in micellar electrokinetic chromatography. *J Chromatogr A* 1997; 780: 41-61.
10. Rizvi SA, Do DP, Saleh AM. Fundamentals of micellar electrokinetic chromatography. *Eur J Chem* 2011; 2(2): 276-281.
11. Deyl Z, Miksik I, Tagliaro F. Advances in capillary electrophoresis. *Forensic Sci Int* 1998; 92(2-3): 89-124.
12. Riekkola ML, Wiedmer SK, Valko IE, Siren H. Selectivity in capillary electrophoresis in the presence of micelles, chiral selectors and non-aqueous media. *J Chromatogr A* 1997; 792(1-2): 13-35.
13. Ahuja S, Jimidar MI. Capillary electrophoresis methods for pharmaceutical analysis. London: Academic Press; 2008.
14. Bojiță M, Roman L, Săndulescu R, Oprean R. Analiza şi controlul medicamentelor, volume 2: *Metode instrumentale în analiza şi controlul medicamentelor*. Deva: Editura Intelcredo; 2003. pp. 240-88.
15. Altria KD. Enhanced pharmaceutical analysis by ce using dynamic surface coating system. *J Pharm Biomed Anal* 2003; 31(3): 447-53.
16. Otsuka K, Terabe S. Enantiomer separation of drugs by micellar electrokinetic chromatography using chiral surfactants. *J Chromatogr A* 2000; 875(1-2): 163-78.

17. Fanali S. Enantioselective determination by capillary electrophoresis with cyclodextrins as chiral selectors. *J Chromatogr A* 2000; 875(1-2): 89-122.
18. Gubitz G, Schmid MG. Chiral separation principles in capillary electrophoresis. *J Chromatogr A* 1997; 792: 179-225.
19. Altria KD, Kelly MA, Clark BJ. Current applications in the analysis of pharmaceuticals by capillary electrophoresis. I. *Trend Anal Chem* 1998; 17(4): 204-213.
20. Altria KD, Kelly MA, Clark BJ. Current applications in the analysis of pharmaceuticals by capillary electrophoresis.II. *Trend Anal Chem* 1998; 17(4): 214-26.
21. Nozal L, Arce L, Rios A, Valcarcel M. Development of a screening method for analytical control of antibiotic residues by micellar electrokinetic capillary chromatography. *Anal Chim Acta* 2004; 523(1): 21-8.
22. Perez MI, Rodriguez LC, Cruces-Blanco C. Analysis of different beta-lactams antibiotics in pharmaceutical preparations using micellar electrokinetic capillary chromatography. *J Pharm Biomed Anal* 2007; 43(2): 746-52.
23. Pajchel G, Tyski S. Adaptation of capillary electrophoresis to the determination of selected cephalosporins for injection. *J Chromatogr A* 2000; 895(1-2): 27-31.
24. Tobback K, Li YM, Pizarro NA, De Smedt I, Smeets T, Van Schepdael A, et al. Micellar electrokinetic capillary chromatography of macrolide antibiotics. Separation of tylosin, erythromycin and their related substances. *J Chromatogr A* 1999; 857(1-2): 313-20.
25. Wienen F, Holzgrabe U. A new micellar electrokinetic capillary chromatography method for separation of the components of the aminoglycoside antibiotics. *Electrophoresis* 2003;24(17):2948-57.
26. Chen YC, Lin CE. Migration behavior and separation of tetracycline antibiotics by micellar electrokinetic chromatography. *J Chromatogr A* 1998; 802(1): 95-105.
27. Lamba S, Sanghi SK, Asthana A, Shelke M. Rapid determination of sulfonamides in milk using micellar electrokinetic chromatography with fluorescence detection. *Anal Chim Acta* 2005; 552(1): 110-5.
28. Kowalski P, Plenis A, Oledzka I, Konieczna L. Optimization and validation of the micellar electrokinetic capillary chromatographic method for simultaneous determination of sulfonamide and amphenicol-type drugs in poultry tissue. *J Pharm Biomed Anal* 2011; 54(1): 160-7.
29. Schmitt-Kopplin P, Burhenne J, Freitag D, Spiteller M, Kettrup A. Development of capillary electrophoresis methods for the analysis of fluoroquinolones and application to the study of the influence of humic substances on their photodegradation in aqueous phase. *J Chromatogr A* 1999; 837(1): 253-65.
30. Lin SC, Liu HY, Lin SW, Yao M, Wu UI, Kuo HP, et al. Simultaneous determination of triazole antifungal drugs in human plasma by sweeping-micellar electrokinetic chromatography. *Anal Bioanal Chem* 2012; 404(1): 217-28.
31. Ferslew KE, Hagardorn AN, McCormick WF. Application of micellar electrokinetic capillary chromatography to forensic analysis of barbiturates in biological fluids. *J Forensic Sci* 1995; 40(2):245-9.
32. Schafroth M, Thormann W, Allemann D. Micellar electrokinetic capillary chromatography of benzodiazepines in human urine. *Electrophoresis* 1994; 15(1): 72-8.
33. Hancu G, Gaspar A, Gyeresi A. Separation of 1,4-benzodiazepines by micellar elektrokinetic capillary chromatography. *J Biochem Biophys Methods* 2007; 69(3): 251-9.
34. Lin CE, Chen KH, Hsiao YY, Liao WS, Chen CC. Enantioseparation of phenothiazines in cyclodextrin-modified micellar electrokinetic chromatography. *J Chromatogr A* 2002; 971(1-2): 261-6.
35. Lee KJ, Lee JJ, Moon DC. Determination of tricyclic antidepressants in human plasma by micellar electrokinetic capillary chromatography. *J Chromatogr* 1993; 616(1): 135-43.
36. Blanco M, Valverde I. Electrophoretic behaviour of pharmacologically active alkylxanthines. *J Chromatogr A* 2002; 950(1-2): 293-9.
37. Gubitz G, Schmid MG. Chiral separation by capillary electromigration techniques. *J Chromatogr A* 2008; 1204(2): 140-56.
38. Kibbey CE, Poole SK, Robinson B, Jackson JD, Durham D. An integrated process for measuring the physicochemical properties of drug candidates in a preclinical discovery environment. *J Pharm Sci* 2001; 90(8): 1164-75.
39. Jia ZJ. Physicochemical profiling by capillary electrophoresis. *Curr Pharm Anal* 2005; 1: 41-56.

Large Scale Generation and Characterization of Anti-Human CD34 Monoclonal Antibody in Ascetic Fluid of Balb/c Mice

Leili Aghebati Maleki[1,2,3], Jafar Majidi[1,3]*, Behzad Baradaran[1,3]*, Jalal Abdolalizadeh[1], Tohid Kazemi[1,3], Ali Aghebati Maleki[1], Koushan Sineh sepehr[1]

[1] Immunology Research Center, Tabriz University of Medical Sciences, Tabriz, Iran.

[2] Tabriz International University of Medical Sciences, Tabriz University of Medical Sciences, Tabriz, Iran.

[3] Department of Immunology, Faculty of Medicine, Tabriz University of Medical Sciences , Tabriz, Iran.

ARTICLE INFO

Keywords:
Monoclonal antibody
Large Scale generation
Ascetic fluid
Human CD34

ABSTRACT

Purpose: Monoclonal antibodies or specific antibodies are now an essential tool of biomedical research and are of great commercial and medical value. The purpose of this study was to produce large scale of monoclonal antibody against CD34 in order to diagnostic application in leukemia and purification of human hematopoietic stem/progenitor cells. ***Methods:*** For large scale production of monoclonal antibody, hybridoma cells that produce monoclonal antibody against human CD34 were injected into the peritoneum of the Balb/c mice which have previously been primed with 0.5 ml Pristane. 5 ml ascitic fluid was harvested from each mouse in two times. Evaluation of mAb titration was assessed by ELISA method. The ascitic fluid was examined for class and subclasses by ELISA mouse mAb isotyping Kit. mAb was purified from ascitic fluid by affinity chromatography on Protein A-Sepharose. Purity of monoclonal antibody was monitored by SDS -PAGE and the purified monoclonal antibody was conjugated with FITC. ***Results:*** Monoclonal antibodies with high specificity and sensitivity against human CD34 by hybridoma technology were prepared. The subclass of antibody was IgG1 and its light chain was kappa. ***Conclusion:*** The conjugated monoclonal antibody could be a useful tool for isolation, purification and characterization of human hematopoietic stem cells.

Introduction

Hybridomas are cells that have been engineered to produce a desired monoclonal antibody in large amounts.[1,2] Hybridoma technology is a well-known technique introduced to produce monoclonal antibodies in specialized cells.[3]

The CD34 antigen is a glycoprotein, expressed on all measurable hematopoietic stem cells and progenitor cells. The surface molecule CD34 is frequently used as a marker to identify hematopoietic progenitor cells with a molecular weight about 110 kDa.[4,5] CD34 has a heavily glycosylated type I transmembrane protein. There is a wide range of kinases such as Protein kinase C and Tyrosine kinases could be used to phosphorylate this transmembrane protein.[6,7]

The CD34 mAbs recognize different epitopes on the CD34 antigen. The classification of epitopes detected by different CD34 mAbs has aided the selection of appropriate antibodies for use in specific clinical and research laboratory settings.[8]

For mass- production of the monoclonal antibody, hybridoma cells must be grown by one of the following methods: in vivo method; Injection of requested clone into the abdominal cavity of a suitably prepared mouse or in vitro method; Culture of the cells in tissue culture flasks.[9]

Further processing of the mouse ascitic fluid and of the tissue culture supernatant are required to obtain mAb with the required purity and concentration. The mouse method is generally familiar, well understood, and widely available in many laboratories. The tissue-culture methods have been expensive and time-consuming and often failed to produce the required amount of antibody without considerable skilled manipulation. [9-12]

The aim of this study was to produce large scale of monoclonal antibody against CD34 in order to diagnostic application in leukemia and purification of human hematopoietic stem/progenitor cells.

Materials and Methods

Production of ascitic fluid in peritoneum of mouse

Balb/c female mice (4-6 weeks old) were provided from Pasteur institute of Iran. 0.5 ml Pristane (2, 6, 10, 14 tetra methyl pentadecane, Sigma) was injected

Corresponding author: Jafar Majidi and Behzad Baradaran, Immunology Research Center, Tabriz University of Medical Sciences, Tabriz, Iran.
Email: jmajidiz@yahoo.com and behzad_im@yahoo.com

intraperitoneally into each mouse. Ten days after priming with Pristane, the cells of a suitable mono clone in density of $1-2\times10^6$ cells/ 0.5 ml PBS were injected intraperitoneally into each mouse. The mice were surveyed daily for production of ascitic fluid after the injection of hybridoma cells. About ten days after the injection of cells, abdomen of the mice were completely enlarged and their skins were extended. Using 19 gage needles, their ascitic fluids were harvested.After 4 days, ascitic fluid of the mice were harvested again and centrifuged and the related supernatants were collected for characterization.[13]

Titration of antibody

The titer of monoclonal antibody was assessed by ELISA method. Wells of ELISA plate (Nunc, Germany) were coated with 100 μl of BSA-conjugated peptide (20 $\mu g/ml$ in PBS) overnight at 4 °C. Next day the plate was washed 3 times with PBS containing 0.05% Tween 20 (PBS-T) for 5 min. Non-specific sites of the plate were blocked with 2% BSA and incubated at 37°C for 90 minutes. Wells were then washed 3 times as above and ascitic fluid were added to the wells in two fold serial dilutions starting from 1:1000. The plate was incubated at 37 °C for 1.5 hr and washed again with PBS-T. At the next step, 100 μl of 1:4000 dilution of HRP-conjugated rabbit anti-mouse Ig (Sigma-Aldrich Co. Louis, USA) was added to the wells and incubation was continued for 1.5 hr at 37 °C. After washing, 100 ul of Tetramethylbenzidine (TMB) substrate was added to each well and the plate was incubated at room temperature in a dark place. After 20 min, the reaction was stopped by adding 100μl of stopping solution (0.16 M H2SO4) to each well. The Optical Density (OD) of the reactions was measured at 450 nm by an ELISA reader (STAT FAX 303+).[14]

Determination of mAb isotype

ELISA mouse mAb isotyping Kit (Thermo, USA) was used for determination the class and subclass of the mAbs. In this assay was used ELISA strip-well plates with individual wells pre-coated with anti-mouse heavy-chain capture antibody (anti-IgG1, IgG2a, IgG2b, IgG3, IgA and IgM) or anti-mouse light-chain capture antibody (kappa or lambda). First, Tris buffer saline (TBS) was used for 1/50000 dilution of the ascitic fluid and 50 μl of diluted antibody added to each well of the 8-well strip. Then 50 μl of the anti-mouse IgG + IgA+ IgM + HRP conjugated was added to each well of the 8-well strip and incubated for an hour at room temperature. After 3 times washing, 75 μl of TMB substrate was added to each well and the plate was incubated at room temperature in a dark place for10 min. At the next step, the reaction was stopped by 75μl of 5% solution of Sulfuric Acid. The absorbance of each well was read by ELISA Reader (STAT FAX 303+) at 450nm.

Antibody purification

The ascitic fluids were diluted two times with PBS and fractionated with 40% saturated ammonium sulfate. After several times of washing with 40% ammonium sulfate, the fraction was centrifuged for 15 minutes in 5000g. The precipitated fraction was dialyzed against 10 mM PBS, pH 7.4 and purified using Sepharose beads conjugated with Protein A column affinity chromatography equilibrated with 5-10 column volumes with the same buffer.

Mouse IgG1 was eluted with 0.1 M sodium phosphate buffer in pH 6.0. Confirmation of the purified fractions was monitored by SDS polyacrylamide gel electrophoresis. Finally, the purified fractions were kept for conjugation with fluorescein isothiocyanate.[15]

Confirmation of the mAb purity by SDS-PAGE

Purity of the monoclonal antibody was checked by SDS polyacrylamide gel electrophoresis in non-reducing condition and reducing form. 10 μg of purified mAb was mixed with 10 μl of sample buffer. The samples were boiled for 10 min at 100 °C .Electrophoresis was done in a 12.5% SDS-PAGE gel with a mini- PROTEAN electrophoresis instrument (Bio- Rad Laboratories, Hercules, CA, USA) 100 V for 1 hr. The gel was stained with Coomassie Brilliant Blue R-250 (Sigma).[13]

Conjugation of monoclonal antibody with fluorescein isothiocyanate (FITC)

For conjugation, 200 μl mAb (5mg/ml) was added in 800 μl Reaction Buffer (500 Mm Carbonate, pH=9.2) and dialyzed against PBS buffer in 24 hours. The antibody concentration was measured after buffer equilibration in 280 nm. 10 mg of FITC was dissolved in 1 mL anhydrous DMSO immediately before use. FITC (SIGMA, Germany) was added to give a ratio of 80 μg per mg of antibody and mixed immediately. The tubes were wrapping in foil then incubated and rotated at room temperature for 1 hour. The unreacted FITC was removed and exchanged the antibody into Storage Buffer (10mM Tris, 150mM Nacl, 0.1% NaH3, pH=8.2) by dialysis during overnight.[16]

Direct Immunofluorescence Staining

This technique was used for confirming the result of conjugation method and reactivity of fluorochrome-conjugated monoclonal antibody. First, human hematopoietic stem / progenitor cells as a positive control (CD34+) and SP2/0 as a negative control (CD34⁻) were prepared. Then 1/1000 dilution of FITC-conjugated monoclonal antibody was added. The mixture was incubated for 45 minutes at RT. Cells were washed two times with PBS buffer for 5 minutes. Cells were suspend in 200 μl of 3.7% formaldehyde solution for fixation of cells in 10 min at Room temperature. The washing was repeated then stained cells were examined by florescent microscope.[17]

Results

After priming of the mouse peritoneal with pristane, 1–2 millions cells related to the suitable mono clone (Figure 1) were suspended in 0.5 ml of sterile PBS and injected to each mouse. Approximately ten days later, 5 ml ascitic fluid collected from each mouse in two times (About 3.5 ml ascitic fluid was harvested from each mouse after ten day and about 1.5 ml ascitic fluid was harvested from their peritoneum for a second time, after 4 days).

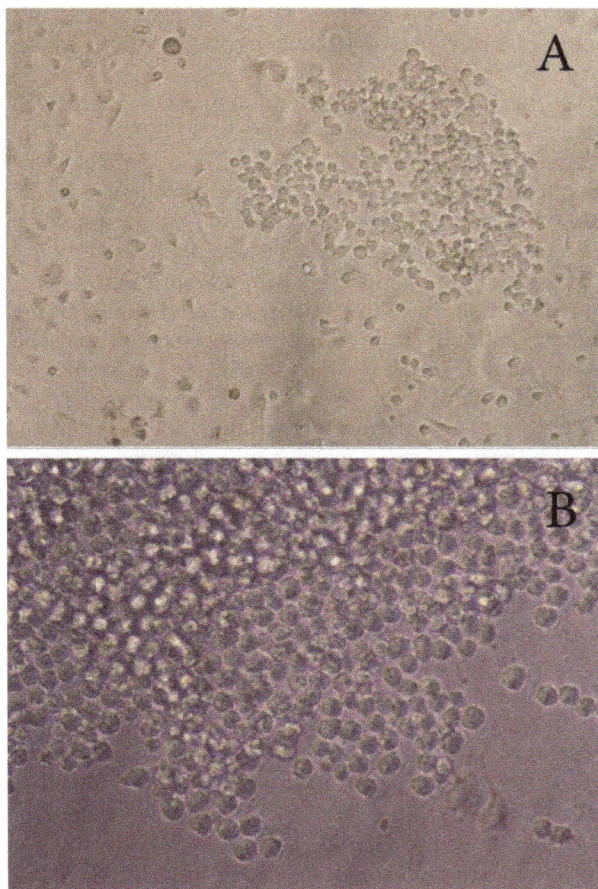

Figure 1. Proliferated suitable mono clone (Mag.10X) selected for injection into the peritoneum of mice. Monoclone in the growing form (A), Monoclone in the highly proliferated form (B)

The titer of monoclonal antibody in ascitic fluid was assessed by ELISA method. The mean absorbance of non-immune mouse serum, Immune mouse serum, and ascitic fluid was compared in Table 1 at 450 nm. The results showed that its 1/32000 dilution has high absorbance with CD34 antigen (above 1).

Table 1. Comparison of the mean absorbance of ascetic fluid at 450 nm

NC (SP/O)	NC* (Non-Immune mouse serum)	PC** (Immune mouse serum)	Ascetic fluid (1/32000 dilution)
0.09	0.13	1.18	1.03
* Negative Control with 1/8000 dilution			
** Positive Control with 1/8000 dilution			

Further characterization of this antibody showed that it is an IgG1 isotope with a kappa light chain. The product was precipitated by saturated ammonium sulfate and dialyzed against PBS. Concentration of the dialyzed product in assay with UV at 280 nm was about 35 mg. Purification by Protein-A-Sepharose column affinity chromatography yielded about 5.5 mg of monoclonal antibody.

The result of purification was confirmed with non-reducing SDS-PAGE and reducing SDS-PAGE. In reducing SDS-PAGE, two bands of 50 KD and 25 KD were appeared that demonstrator heavy and light chains. In non-reducing SDS-PAGE, only one 150 KD band was appeared that demonstrator of purified antibody (Figure 2).

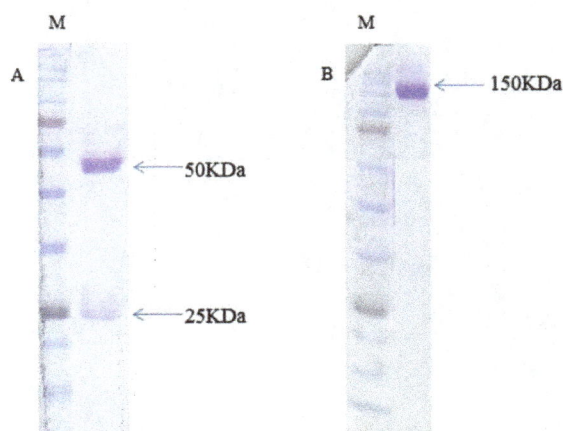

Figure 2. SDS-PAGE analysis of fraction from Protein-A affinity purification. Reducing SDS-PAGE (A) and non-reducing SDS-PAGE (B) of produced monoclonal antibody. In reduced form, two bands were seen in 50 & 25 kDa but in non-reducing SDS-PAGE condition, only one band was seen in about 150 kDa.

The purified monoclonal antibody was conjugated with fluorescein isothiocyanate (FITC) and used for direct staining of cell lines. To examine the specific attachment of purified mAb with CD34 antigen, cell lines were subjected to immunofluorescent staining (Figure 3).

Discussion

Monoclonal antibodies or specific antibodies are now an essential tool of biomedical research and are of great commercial and medical value. In recent century, after the first antibody-based therapy introduced, many researchers tried to use these molecules for diagnosis and treatment of several diseases.[18-20] Koehler and Milstein developed the basic methods of producing monoclonal antibodies in hybridoma cell of the mouse in 1975 which has changed slightly to date.[21]

The production of monoclonal antibody in the ascitic fluid is commercially useful for mass production. In this study, ascitic fluids were collected from the peritoneal cavity and the titer of monoclonal antibody was assessed by ELISA method. The results showed that 1/32000 dilution has high absorbance with CD34 antigen (above 1). Choice of procedure for antibody purification depends on the intended use of the antibodies, isotyping of antibodies and on the available resources.[22]

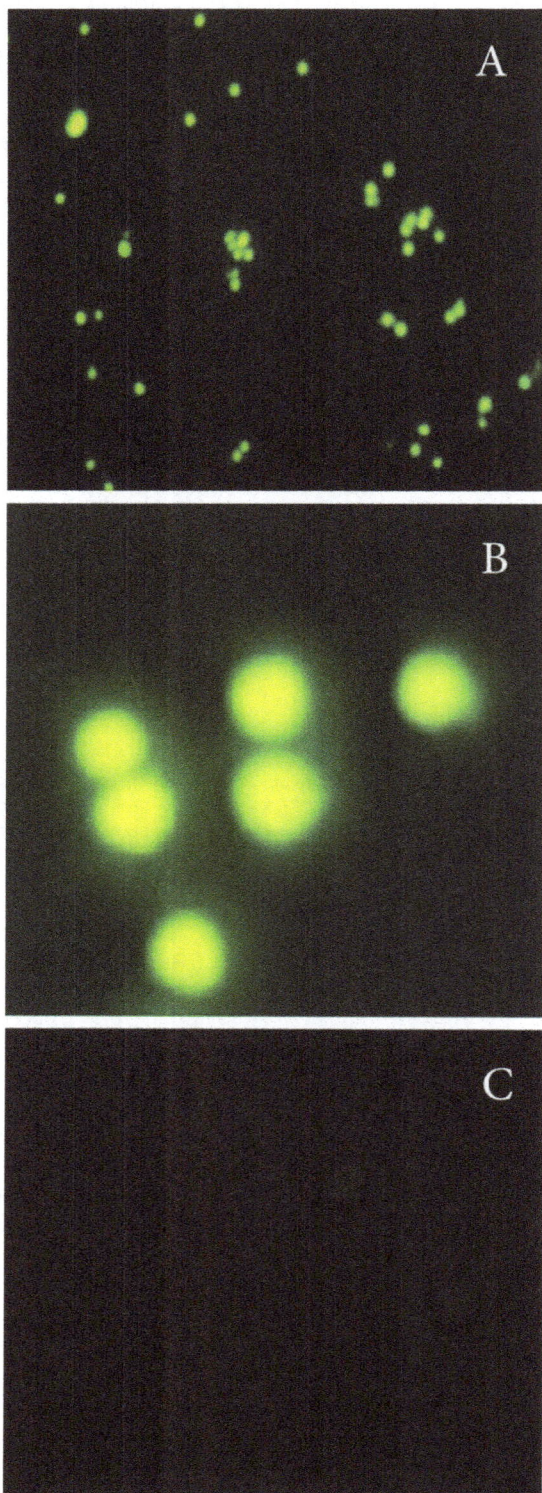

Figure 3. Direct Immunofluorescence Staining was used for confirming specific binding of purified mAb with CD34 antigen in the surface of Human hematopoietic stem / progenitor cells as a positive control (A&B Mag.10X, 40X respectively) and SP2/0 as a negative control (C).

The subclass of monoclonal antibody was IgG1 and its light chain was "kappa" type. The affinity chromatography method appears to be a simple, inexpensive, one-step and time-efficient approach in comparison with the other chromatography methods such as ion-exchange chromatography. Accordingly, we utilized this technique for purification of mAb produced.

The method of choice for determining purity is SDS-PAGE. Therefore, purity was evaluated by SDS-PAGE in non-reducing form and by SDS-PAGE in reducing condition. SDS-PAGE analysis showed that we obtained a protein with suitable purity after purification step.

The purified monoclonal antibody was conjugated with fluorescein isothiocyanate (FITC). Specific binding of purified mAb with CD34 antigen was monitored using immunofloresance techniques in the surface of human hematopoietic stem / progenitor cells. The results clearly showed that our antibody strongly reacts with CD34 antigen (shown in Figure 3).

Currently, we know two ways for production of the desired antibody: the mouse ascites method and the tissue-culture method which could be performed in vivo and in vitro.[23]

In vitro cell-culture method requires some expertise, requires special media, and can be expensive and time-consuming. Moreover, in this technique, unsuitable glycosylation may lead antibody to be unusable in in vivo experiments resulting from changes in immunogenicity, binding affinity, biologic functions, or clearance in vivo.[10,12]

In in vivo production method, at first, a primer such as pristane or Freud's incomplete adjuvant is injected to suppress the immune systems and then the multiplied hybridoma cells form antibody-rich ascitic fluid in the peritoneal cavity. The ascites technique has some advantages, mainly, high levels of antibody production ranges from 1 to 20 mg/ml. In addition, this technique is not excessively labour- intensive.[9] Briefly, ascitic fluid production enriched with mAb in mice is a rapid and economic method.

The amount of the injected pristane and the interval of priming with hybridoma cells are very important factors in ascitic fluid production. In addition it is important that side effects of tumor growth can be more severe due to incorrect i.p. injection of hybridoma cells as a result of insemination of hybridoma cells in abdominal organs, such as urinary bladder or intestines.[24] On the other hand the number of the cells injected to the peritoneum of mouse is highly effective on the acceleration of ascitic fluid production.[25]

During ascites development, animals should be observed at least three times per week for the first week and daily thereafter to monitor the degree of abdominal distention and signs of illness.[26] Peterson evaluated the effects on well-being of pristane injection and ascites production using factors such as wheel-running activity, food and water consumption, clinical observation, and plasma corticosterone concentration. No significant evidence of distress was obtained in the animals studied.[27] But, Mauch et al reported that elevation of the diaphragm due to ascites is associated with dyspnea, orthopnea, or tachypnea. It therefore seems reasonable to assume that mice with large accumulations of ascitic fluid experience discomfort and distress.[28]

In similar previous study, Baradaran et al used in vivo method for mass production of monoclonal antibody against EGFR in ascitic fluid efficiently and 10.4 mg antibody was purified with Ion exchange chromatography (IEC).[29]

In other study Brian Scott Hafley used in vivo method for development of monoclonal antibodies.[30] Moreover Mittal et al used the same in production of murine monoclonal antibodies against Haemophilus parasuis.[31] Furthermore Galen et al used in vivo method for mass production of monoclonal antibody against human rennin in ascitic fluid then the mAb with high purity was obtained by affinity chromatography.[32]

In all these studies, the mouse ascites methods were preferred for its economical, efficient and high concentrations of mAbs produced.

On the other hand, Shu-Fen Chou et al used in the tissue- culture in flasks method for scale-up of anti-AFP mAbs. Then monoclonal antibodies were purified by affinity chromatography on protein A Sepharose.[33]

Based on documented evidence, analysis of mAb produced in tissue culture reveals that a desired antibody function is diminished or lost. Furthermore tissue culture might be maintained for long periods, and some mAb were denatured during concentration or purification.

Nevertheless, for several parameters, in vivo method has fallen into disfavor. The most important reasons relate to the following: significant pain and distress in mice; High-quality in vitro production systems are progressing; and contamination mAb with infectious agents, such as viruses and other microorganisms.[25] Although, based on various reports there is now consensus that ascites production should be the exception, requiring rigorous and well-documented justification. Special circumstances that might justify the use of ascites production include the following: emerging therapeutic applications; downstream concentration of mAb from in vitro; denaturation and decreased antibody activity in the tissue culture; and poor growth of hybridoma cells in vitro system.[9,12]

Based on the reasons described above, it is reasonable to conclude that new developments in in vitro mAb production gradually will limit the use of animals for this purpose.

In general, ascitic fluid production method seems to be a very useful, inexpensive and economic. Finally, we recommend that mAb generation by the mouse ascites method be permitted if scientifically justified and approved by the relevant Institutional Animal Care and Use Committee (IACUC).

Acknowledgements
We would like to thank for Immunology Research Center (IRC) and Tabriz International University of Medical Sciences (Aras) for kind assistance, respectively. This work was supported by a grant from Faculty of Medicine, Tabriz University of Medical Sciences.

Conflict of Interest
The authors report no conflicts of interest in this work.

References
1. Pandey SH. Hybridoma technology for production of monoclonal antibodies. *Int J Pharm Sci Rev Res* 2010;1(2): 88-94.
2. Hybridoma technology. [Online encyclopedia] USA: Wikipedia; [cited 2013 January]; Available from: http://en.wikipedia.org/wiki/Hybridoma_technology.
3. Kohler G, Milstein C. Continuous cultures of fused cells secreting antibody of predefined specificity. *Nature* 1975;256(5517):495-7.
4. Qian W, Wang L, Li B, Wang H, Hou S, Hong X, et al. Development of new versions of anti-human CD34 monoclonal antibodies with potentially reduced immunogenicity. *Biochem Biophys Res Commun* 2008;367(2):497-502.
5. Gunsilius E, Gastl G, Petzer AL. Hematopoietic stem cells. *Biomed Pharmacother* 2001;55(4):186-94.
6. Deterding LJ, Williams JG, Humble MM, Petrovich RM, Wei SJ, Trempus CS, et al. CD34 antigen: Determination of specific sites of phosphorylation in vitro and in vivo. *Int J Mass spectrom* 2011;301(1-3):12-21.
7. Krause DS, Fackler MJ, Civin CI, May WS. CD34: structure, biology, and clinical utility. *Blood* 1996;87(1):1-13.
8. Lanza F, Healy L, Sutherland DR. Structural and functional features of the CD34 antigen: an update. *J Biol Regul Homeost Agents* 2001;15(1):1-13.
9. Jackson LR, Trudel LJ, Fox JG, Lipman NS. Monoclonal antibody production in murine ascites. I. Clinical and pathologic features. *Lab Anim Sci* 1999;49(1):70-80.
10. Mc Ardle J. Alternatives to ascites production of monoclonal antibodies. *Ani Welf Inform Cent Newslett* 1998; 8: 3-4.
11. Lang AB, Schuerch U, Cryz SJ Jr. Optimization of growth and secretion of human monoclonal antibodies by hybridomas cultured in serum-free media. *Hybridoma* 1991;10(3):401-9.
12. Jackson LR, Trudel LJ, Fox JG, Lipman NS. Monoclonal antibody production in murine ascites. II. Production characteristics. *Lab Anim Sci* 1999;49(1):81-6.
13. Baradaran B, Majidi J, Hassan ZM, Abdolalizadeh J. Large scale production and characterization of anti- human IgG monoclonal antibody in peritoneum of Balb/c mice. *Am J Biochem Biotechnol* 2006;1(4):190-3.

14. Hadavi R, Zarnani AH, Ahmadvand N, Mahmoudi AR, Bayat AA, Mahmoudian J, et al. Production of Monoclonal Antibody against Human Nestin. *Avicenna J Med Biotech* 2010; 2(2): 69-76.

15. Thurston CF, Henle LF. New Protein Techniques. In: Walker JM, editor. Methods in Molecular Biology. Clifton NJ: The Humana Press Inc.; 1988. P. 149-58.

16. Harlow E, Lane D. Labeling antibodies with fluorochromes. *CSH protocols* 2006;2006(2).

17. Tabatabaei-Panah AS, Zarnani AH, Montaser-Kouhsar Sh, Chamankhah M, Ghods R, Bayat AA, et al. Production and Characterization of Anti-Her2 Monoclonal Antibodies. *Yakhteh Med J* 2008;10(2):109-20.

18. Robinson M, Weiner L, Adams G. Improving Monoclonal Antibodies for Cancer Therapy. Drug Dev Res 2004;61:172-87.

19. Schrama D, Reisfeld R, Becker J. Antibody targeted drugs as cancer therapeutics. *Annu Rev Med* 2006; 5: 174-90.

20. Enever C, Batuwangala T, Plummer C, Sepp A. Next generation immunotherapeutics--honing the magic bullet. *Curr Opin Biotechnol* 2009;20(4):405-11.

21. Modjtahedi H. Monoclonal Antibodies as Therapeutic Agents: Advances and Challenges. *Iran J Immunol* 2005;2(1):3-21.

22. Fitzgerald J, Leonard P, Darcy E, O'Kennedy R. Immunoaffinity chromatography. *Methods Mol Biol* 2011;681:35-59.

23. Peterson NC, Peavey JE. Comparison of in vitro monoclonal antibody production methods with an in vivo ascites production technique. *Contemp Top Lab Anim Sci* 1998;37(5):61-6.

24. Walvoort NC. Assessment of distress through pathological examination. In: Hendriksen CFM, Köeter HBWM, editors. *Replacement, Reduction and Refinement: Present Possibilities and Future Prospects*. Amsterdam: Elsevier; 1991. P. 265-73.

25. Leenaars M, Hendriksen CF. Critical steps in the production of polyclonal and monoclonal antibodies: evaluation and recommendations. *ILAR J* 2005;46(3):269-79.

26. Peterson NC. Advances in monoclonal antibody technology: genetic engineering of mice, cells, and immunoglobulins. *ILAR J* 2005;46(3):314-9.

27. Peterson NC. Behavioral, clinical, and physiologic analysis of mice used for ascites monoclonal antibody production. *Comp Med* 2000;50(5):516-26.

28. Mauch P, Ultmann. Treatment of malignant ascites. In: DeVita VT, Hellman S, Rosenberg SA, editors. *Cancer: Principles and Practice of Oncology*. Philadelphia: Lippincott; 1985. P. 2150-3.

29. Baradaran B, Hosseini AZ, Majidi J, Farajnia S, Barar J, Saraf ZH, et al. Development and characterization of monoclonal antibodies against human epidermal growth factor receptor in Balb/c mice. *Hum Antibodies* 2009;18(1-2):11-6.

30. Hafley BS. Development of Monoclonal Antibodies for a Multiple Antigen ELISA to Verify Safe Cooking End-Point Temperatures in Beef and Pork [PhD Dissertation]. USA: Texas A&M University; 2005.

31. Tadjine M, Mittal KR, Bourdon S, Gottschalk M. Production and characterization of murine monoclonal antibodies against Haemophilus parasuis and study of their protective role in mice. *Microbiology* 2004;150(Pt 12):3935-45.

32. Galen FX, Devaux C, Atlas S, Guyenne T, Menard J, Corvol P, et al. New monoclonal antibodies directed against human renin. Powerful tools for the investigation of the renin system. *J Clin Invest* 1984;74(3):723-35.

33. Chou SF, Hsu WL, Hwang JM, Chen CY. Production of monoclonal and polyclonal antibodies against human alphafetoprotein, a hepatocellular tumor marker. *Hybrid Hybridomics* 2002;21(4):301-5.

Multivariate Chemometric Assisted Analysis of Metformin Hydrochloride, Gliclazide and Pioglitazone Hydrochloride in Bulk Drug and Dosage Forms

Radhika Bhaskar, Rahul Bhaskar*, Mahendra K. Sagar, Vipin Saini

Department of Pharmacy, Mahatma Jyoti Rao Phoole University, Jaipur, India.

ARTICLE INFO

Keywords:
Partial least-squares
Spectroscopy
Metformin
Gliclazide
Pioglitazone

ABSTRACT

Purpose: In this work a numerical method, based on the use of spectrophotometric data coupled to partial least squares (PLS) regression and net analyte preprocessing combined with classical least square (NAP/CLS) multivariate calibration, is reported for the simultaneous determination of metformin hydrochloride (MET), gliclazide (GLZ) and pioglitazone hydrochloride (PIO) in synthetic samples and combined commercial tablets. ***Methods:*** Spectra of MET, GLZ and PIO were recorded at concentrations within their linear ranges (5-25 µg/ml, 0.5-8 µg/ml and 0.5-3 µg/ml respectively) and were used to compute a total of 25 synthetic mixtures involving 15 calibration and 10 validation sets between wavelength range of 200 and 400 nm in 0.1N HCl. The suitability of the models was decided on the basis of root mean square error (RMSE) values of calibration and validation data. ***Results:*** The analytical performances of these chemometric methods were characterized by relative prediction errors and recovery studies (%) and were compared with each other. These two methods were successfully applied to pharmaceutical formulation, tablet, with no interference with excipients as indicated by the recovery study results. Mean recoveries of the commercial formulation set together with the figures of merit (calibration sensitivity, selectivity, limit of detection, limit of quantification etc.) were estimated. ***Conclusion:*** The proposed methods are simple, rapid and can be easily used as an alternative analysis tool in the quality control of drugs and formulation.

Introduction

Oral ingestion has long been the most convenient and commonly employed route of drug delivery due to its ease of administration, least aseptic constraints and flexibility in the design of the dosage form. It is well known that modified release dosage forms may offer one or more advantages over immediate release formulations of the same drug. There are many ways to design modified release dosage forms for oral administration; from film coated pellets, tablets or capsules to more sophisticated and complicated delivery systems such as osmotically driven systems, systems controlled by ion exchange mechanism, systems using three dimensional printing technology and systems using electrostatic deposition technology. The design of modified release drug product is usually intended to optimize a therapeutic regimen by providing slow and continuous delivery of drug over the entire dosing interval whilst also providing greater patient compliance and convenience.[1]

MET, GLZ and PIO are active principles widely used and frequently combined in pharmaceutical preparation. All these three drugs are complimentary to each other. GLZ being an insulin secretagogue helps in insulin secretion from pancreas[2] whereas; insulin secreted under GLZ influence can be utilized by MET for its action. MET not only utilizes the insulin secreted under gliclazide influence but also converts from peripheral tissues.[3] Drawbacks associated with GLZ are weight gain and hypoglycemia.[4] This can easily be overcome by MET. PIO on the other hand is basically responsible for eliminating the problem of insulin resistance occurred on long term uses of sulphonyl ureas.[5]

For the treatment of diabetes mellitus the usual combination of drugs which are available in the market consists of MET and PIO and/or glipizide, or MET and GLZ but all the three drugs are not available in a single formulation. This addition seems to be aimed at improving the antidiabetic efficacy.

Pharmaceutical processing and formulation often introduce various interferants (chemicals other than drug/s under investigation) into the system. When performing quantification these interferants can disturb univariate analysis, but with multivariate analysis the

*Corresponding author: Rahul Bhaskar, Department of Pharmacy, Mahatma Jyoti Rao Phoole University, Jaipur, India.
Email: rahul.bhaskar03@gmail.com

quantification can still be performed. Several multivariate techniques of data analysis have been developed and used in the chemometric community by the researchers, out of which PLS and NAP/CLS methods are one of them.[6] PLS regression is a supervised multivariate method with which quantitative analysis of multiple solid forms can be performed even if the differences between the spectra are minor.[7] The method involves a calibration step in which the relation between spectra and component concentrations is estimated from a set of reference samples, and a prediction step in which the results of the calibration are used to estimate the component concentrations in an unknown sample spectrum.[8] NAP/CLS is one of the methods under net analyte signal preprocessing (NAS). The NAS is the part of the signal which is directly related to the concentration predicted by the calibration model. In mathematical terms, it is the part of a spectrum which is orthogonal to the space spanned by the spectra of all analytes except one.[9]

Materials and Methods

Instrument, reagents and softwares
Elico SL 191 double beam UV-Visible Spectrophotometer, with 1 cm path length was used for the absorbance measurement. All the chemicals used were of analytical grade. Pure MET was obtained from Abhilasha Pharma Pvt. Ltd., Gujarat, GLZ was obtained from Kwality Pharmaceuticals, Amritsar and PIO from GMH Laboratories, Baddi.
The design expert 8.0.4 software and Matlab 7.5 with MVC1 toolbox were used for construction of binary mixtures and the statistical treatment of the data along application of various multivariate methods.

Preparation of standards
1mg/ml MET, GLZ and PIO stock solutions were prepared by dissolving accurately weighed amounts of finely powdered pure MET, GLZ and PIO in small quantity of methanol and the final volumes were made respectively with 0.1N HCl. Suitably diluted samples from each stock were utilized for λ_{max} determination of individual component followed by serial dilution with 0.1N HCl to obtain the aliquots falling in linearity.

Standard solutions for multivariate calibration
The calibration and validation mixtures were prepared by mixing MET, GLZ and PIO solutions in different ratios varying in their individual linearity ranges viz. 0-25 µg/ml, 0-8 µg/ml, 0-3 µg/ml. The concentrations of combinations were decided by design expert 8.0.4 software under central composite design. Total 25 sets were prepared out of which 15 sets (Table 1) were utilized as calibration set whereas, the rest 10 served as validation sets (Table 2). All the mixtures were scanned at 220-299 nm range digitized at every 3 nm. The absorbance below 220 nm and above 299 nm was not taken under consideration due to too much of noise and diminished responses respectively.

Table 1. Calibration set composition

Runs	MET (µg/ml)	GLZ (µg/ml)	PIO (µg/ml)
C1	5	1	1
C2	25	6	0.75
C3	25	1	3
C4	5	6	3
C5	0	3.5	2
C6	25	3.5	2
C7	15	3	2
C8	15	6	2
C9	15	3.5	0
C10	15	3.5	3
C11	16	4	1
C12	19	0	1
C13	20	8	1
C14	20	4	1
C15	18.5	2	1.6

Table 2. Validation set composition

Runs	MET (µg/ml)	GLZ (µg/ml)	PIO (µg/ml)
V1	25	0	1.3
V2	4.5	2	1.5
V3	6	0.5	3
V4	25	7	2.5
V5	13	6	3
V6	10	8	0.5
V7	25	8	3
V8	5	8	3
V9	16	4	2
V10	10	6	1

Sample preparation
Commercial tablets of MET, GLZ and PIO were analyzed for accuracy. The tablets were processed by taking at least 10 tablets for each and finely crushed to powder in separate mortar-pestles. An equivalent amount of the obtained powder of each drug was weighed, dissolved in methanol, sonicated for 20 min, made up the volume with 0.1N HCl and filtered through a 0.5 µm membrane filter. The final concentrations and analyte ratios in each test solution lied within the corresponding calibration ranges. Each sample solution was prepared in triplicate and measured in random order.

Theory
PLS-1: To start working on PLS-1 using MATLAB, first a data matrix X and a concentration vector Y need to be identify against J sensors and I samples. Both X and Y is required for the calculation of singular value decomposition (SVD). On performing PLSSVD on X and Y matrix, the result will be further 3 matrixes i.e. the singular value matrix (S), the right singular value matrix (V), and the left singular value matrix (U). V matrix can also be termed as loading matrix which helps in the determination of score matrix (T), using the following equation:

$$X \times V = T \qquad\qquad \textbf{Eq.1}$$

Reconstruction of original data matrix X is computed by using the preselected numbers of factors as:

$$X_{(estimated)} = T \times V' \qquad \textbf{Eq.2}$$

The predicted value of y can be stated as:

$$y_{(estimated)} = x_{(estimated)} \times b \qquad \textbf{Eq. 3}$$

Where, b is regression vector.[10]

Before finalizing the calibration data, to avoid over fitting, the optimum number of latent variables or factors (A) (figure1) should be selected by applying the cross validation method, leaving one sample at a time.[11]

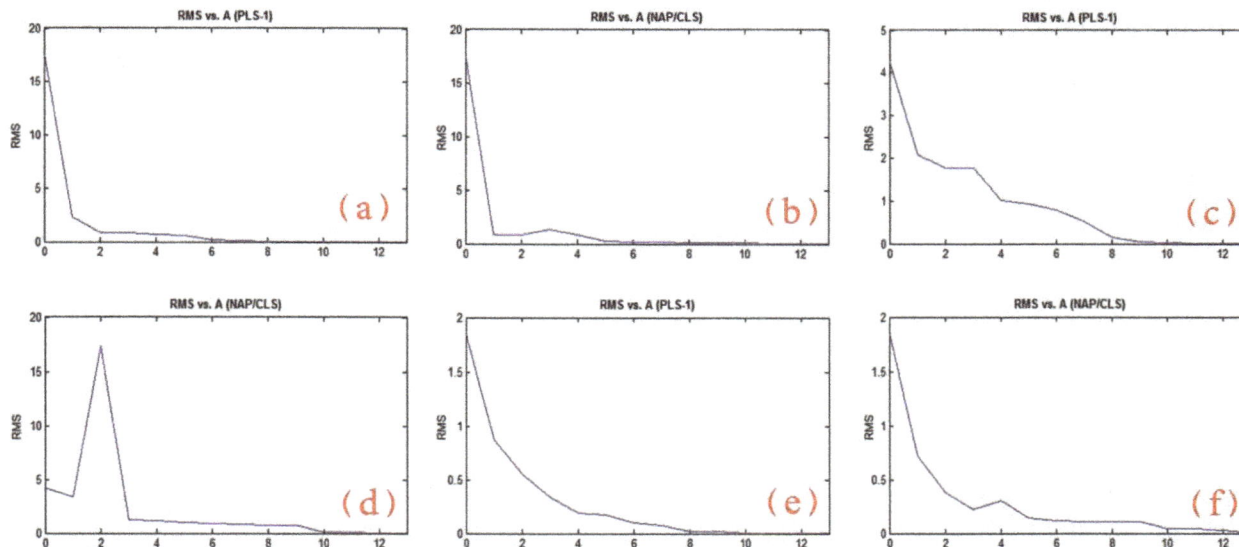

Figure 1. Plot of RMS(CV) vs factor number for calibration set prediction using cross validation of (a) MET PLS-1, (b) MET NAP/CLS, (c) GLZ PLS-1, (d) GLZ NAP/CLS, (e) PIO PLS-1, (f) PIO NAP/CLS

NAP/CLS[12]: In contrast to PLS-1, the concept of NAS based calibration utilizes the contribution of two types of analyte signals, Y_k i.e. the analyte of interest and Y_{-k}, signals developed by sources of variability. The virtual signals obtained are a sum of these two and can be presented as:

$$Y = Y_k + Y_{-k} \qquad \textbf{Eq.4}$$

For unit concentration of k the J×1 vector can be denoted as s_k hence

$$Y = x_k s_k' + Y_{-k} \qquad \textbf{Eq.5}$$

Both sides of equations when multiplied with an appropriate filtering or preprocessing J×J matrix, named, M_{NAP} which in turn is supposed to be orthogonal to Y_{-k}, the eq.5 get converted to:

$$YM_{NAP} = x_k s_k' M_{NAP} \qquad \textbf{Eq.6}$$

Eq.6 can also be presented as:

$$Y^\$ = x_k \left(s_k^\$\right)' \qquad \textbf{Eq. 7}$$

Where, $Y^\$$ is matrix of net analyte calibration spectra and $s_k^\$$ is net sensitivity for analyte k.

The filtering matrix in eq.6 as mentioned above is orthogonal to Y_k and can be calculated as

$$M_{NAP} = L - (Y_{-k})^p Y_{-k} \qquad \textbf{Eq. 8}$$

Where, L is J×J unitary matrix and $(Y_{-k})^p$ is pseudo-inverse of Y_{-k}. Pseudo-inverse of Y_{-k} can be calculated by applying singular value decomposition (SVD) at factor A:

$$M_{NAP} = [L - UU'] \qquad \textbf{Eq. 9}$$

The applied filter M_{NAP} removes all sources of variability except k. The new generated problem can be resolved by applying classical least square (CLS) method in combination with NAS and that leads to the generation of equation 10.

$$s_k^\$ = (Y_k^\$) \, x_k (x_k' x_k)^{-1} \qquad \textbf{Eq.10}$$

Hence unknown concentration x_k is determined by:

$$x_k = (s_k^{\$'} s_K^\$)^{-1} s_K^{\$'} y_k^\$ \qquad \textbf{Eq.11}$$

The usual statistical parameters giving an indication of the quality of fit of all data are the root mean square difference (RMSECV), square of the correlation coefficient (R^2) and relative error of prediction (REP%). The expressions of these parameters are:

$$RMSECV = \left[\frac{1}{m}\sum_1^m \left(c_{act} - c_{pred}\right)^2\right]^{1/2} \qquad \textbf{Eq. 12}$$

$$R^2 = 1 - \frac{\sum_1^m \left(c_{act} - c_{pred}\right)^2}{\sum_1^m \left(c_{act} - c\right)^2} \qquad \textbf{Eq.13}$$

$$REP\% = \frac{100}{c}\left[\frac{1}{m}\sum_1^m \left(c_{act} - c_{pred}\right)^2\right]^{1/2} \qquad \textbf{Eq.14}$$

$$Bias = \left[\frac{1}{m}\sum_1^m \left(c_{act} - c_{pred}\right)\right] \qquad \textbf{Eq.15}$$

Where c_{act} and c_{pred} are the actual and predicted concentrations during the cross validation process, m is number of samples used in cross validation and validation.[7] The goodness of data fit can be visualized in figure 2.

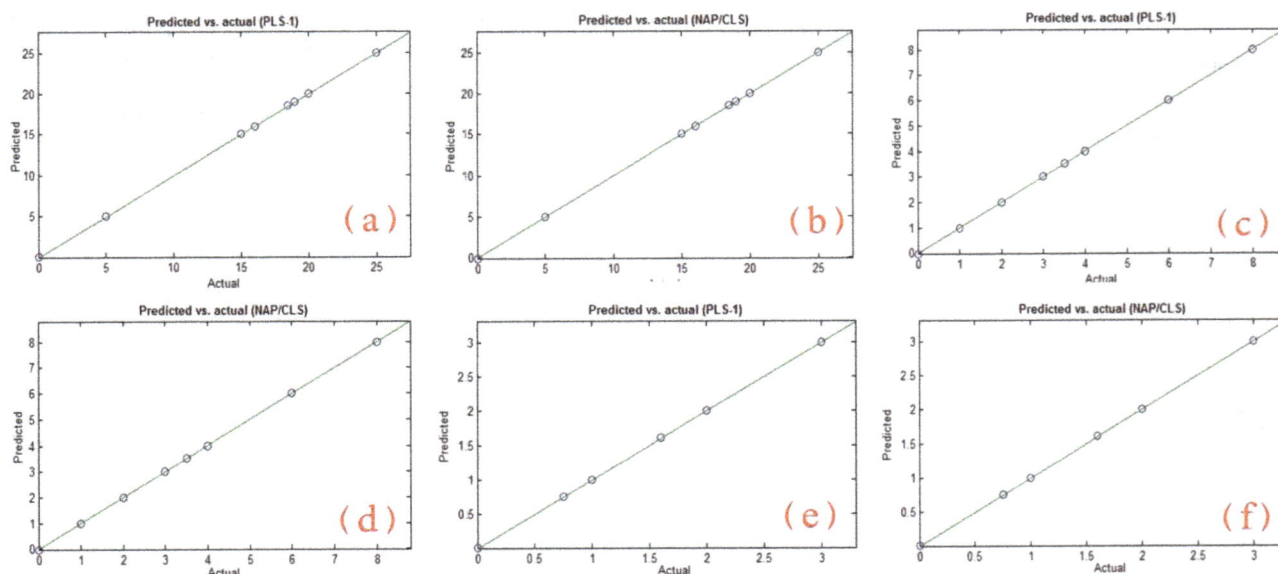

Figure 2. Plots of actual vs predicted values for (a) MET PLS-1, (b) MET NAP/CLS, (c) GLZ PLS-1, (d) GLZ NAP/CLS, (e) PIO PLS-1, (f) PIO NAP/CLS

Along with the above said statistical formulae, another preferred method for assessing the relative accuracy of the studied models is the linear regression analysis of actual verses predicted data by comparing the results of the estimated slope and intercept with their ideal value

of 1 and 0. If the point (1, 0) is inside the EJCR (elliptical joint confidence region) for cross validation data, it can be concluded that constant and proportional bias are absent (figure 3).

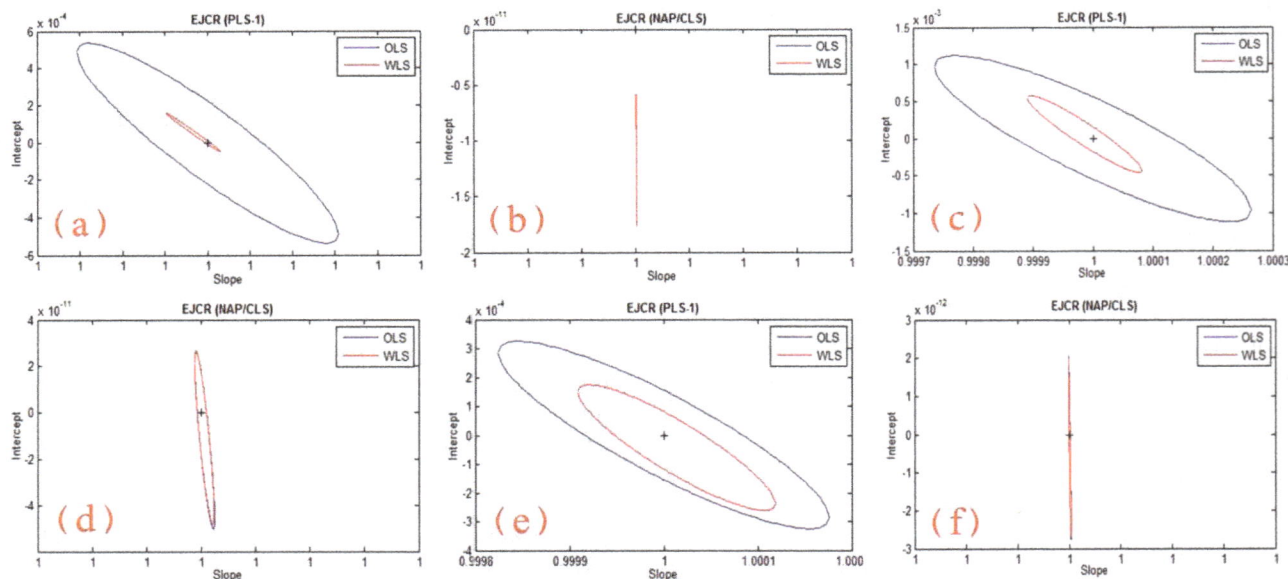

Figure 3. Ellipticle joint confident region for slope and intercept corresponding to regressions of the actual vs predicted concentrations of (a) MET PLS-1, (b) MET NAP/CLS, (c) GLZ PLS-1, (d) GLZ NAP/CLS, (e) PIO PLS-1, (f) PIO NAP/CLS

Results and Discussion

UV-Vis spectra of MET, GLZ, PIO and mixture

Figure 4 shows the individual absorption spectra of MET, GLZ and PIO along with their mixture in 0.1N HCl between 200 and 300 nm.

PLS-1 and NAP/CLS Results

The statistical parameters obtained after applying PLS-1 and NAP/CLS to the spectrophotometric data of cross validation and validation are shown in Table 3. The results suggest that the present method is accurate in concern to the validation samples, as suggested by the low RMSE and REP value for this validation set.

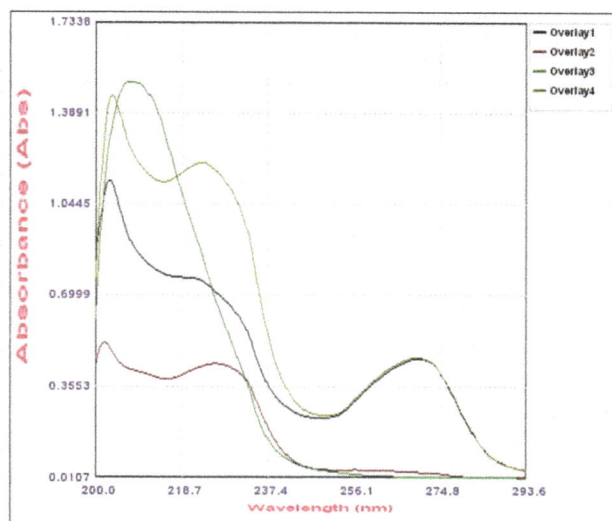

Figure 4. Overlay of MET, GLZ, PIO and Mixture.

Analysis of commercial sample

Commercial mixture products were analyzed using the proposed spectrophotometric methods. Results are summarized in Table 4. As can be seen, satisfactory results were obtained by the proposed methods.

Conclusion

A comparative study with the use of PLS-1 and NAP/CLS for the separation and simultaneous estimation of MET, GLZ and PIO in a binary mixture has been accomplished, showing that this spectrophotometric method provides a good example of the high resolving power of these techniques. In other words, almost comparable results were obtained for these three drugs in both synthetic and commercial mixture. The results obtained confirm the suitability of the proposed method for accurate analysis of MET, GLZ and PIO in pharmaceutical preparations. These methods were applied directly to the commercial mixture preparations without previous treatment. In addition the proposed methods are suitable for application without interference of the excipients as well.

Conflict of Interest

There is no conflict of interest in this study.

Table 3. Statistical parameters for the optimized models

Parameters		MET		GLZ		PIO	
		PLS-1	NAP/CLS	PLS-1	NAP/CLS	PLS-1	NAP/CLS
Calibration set results	No. of factors	6	6	9	11	8	10
	Press	0.6673	0.4725	0.0502	0.1022	0.0087	0.0273
	RMSE(µg/ml)	0.2110	0.1776	0.0579	0.0826	0.0241	0.0427
	REP%	1.3271	1.1172	1.5817	2.2535	1.4876	2.6345
	Slope	0.9996	1.0003	1.0000	1.0006	0.9987	0.9988
	R^2	0.9991	0.9994	0.9992	0.9984	0.9992	0.9976
	Bias	0.0000	0.0000	0.0000	0.0000	0.0000	0.0000
Validation set results	Press	0.5330	0.4973	0.1179	0.2057	0.0455	0.0904
	RMSE(µg/ml)	0.2309	0.2230	0.1086	0.1434	0.0674	0.0951
	REP%	1.6549	1.5986	2.1939	2.8977	3.2416	4.5721
	Slope	1.0010	1.0089	1.0018	1.0101	1.0193	0.9847
	R^2	0.9993	0.9993	0.9988	0.9979	0.9954	0.9884
	Bias	0.0677	0.0137	-0.0186	0.0141	0.0112	0.0121
Figure of merits	LOD(µg/ml)	0.1861	0.1564	0.0510	0.0727	0.0213	0.0377
	LOQ(µg/ml)	0.5639	0.4741	0.1546	0.2205	0.0646	0.1142
	SEM	0.0563	0.0474	0.0154	0.0221	0.0064	0.0114

Table 4. Prediction results on recovery samples

Commercial Sample (nominal content)	Metformin HCl*		Gliclazide*		Pioglitazone HCl*	
	PLS-1	NAP/CLS	PLS-1	NAP/CLS	PLS-I	NAP/CLS
MET-500mg, GLZ-30mg, PIO-15mg	500.33 (2.08) (100.06%)	501.33 (2.08) (100.26%)	30.33 (2.08) (101.11%)	29.00 (1.00) (96.66%)	14.33 (2.08) (95.55%)	16.66 (1.52) (111.11%)
MET-500mg, GLZ-30mg, PIO-45mg	500.33 (2.51) (100.06%)	496.66 (1.15) (99.33%)	31.00 (2.00) (103.33%)	29.33 (2.51) (97.77%)	45.33 (2.08) (100.74%)	45.00 (2.00) (100.00%)
MET-500mg, GLZ-80mg, PIO-15mg	496.66 (1.52) (99.33%)	500.00 (2.00) (100.00%)	79.00 (2.00) (98.75%)	82.66 (1.52) (103.33%)	15.00 (2.00) (100.00%)	14.33 (1.54) (95.55%)
MET-500mg, GLZ-80mg, PIO-45mg	498.66 (3.05) (99.73%)	498.33 (1.52) (99.66%)	82.00 (1.00) (102.50%)	79.33 (1.52) (99.19%)	46.00 (1.73) (102.22%)	44.33 (1.53) (98.51%)

*The results are averages of three replicates and are given in mg per sample. ±S.D. is in parenthesis.

References

1. Abdul S, Poddar SS. A flexible technology for modified release of drugs: multi layered tablets. *J Control Release* 2004; 97: 393– 405.

2. Campbellt DB, Laviellez R, Nathan C. The mode of action and clinical pharmacology of gliclazide: a review. *Diabetic Res Clin Pract* 1991; 14: S2l-36.

3. Dunn CJ, Peters DH. Metformin. A review of its pharmacological properties and therapeutic use in non-insulin-dependent diabetes mellitus. *Drugs* 1995; 49(5): 721-49.

4. Ziegler O, Drouin P. Hemobiological Properties of Gliclazide. *J Diab Gnnp* 1994; 8: 235-9.

5. Waugh J, Keating GM, Plosker GL, Easthope S, Robinson DM. Pioglitazone: A Review of its Use in Type 2 Diabetes Mellitus. *Drugs* 2006; 66(1): 85-109.

6. Olivieria AC, Goicoechea HC, Inon FA. MVC1: an integrated MatLab toolbox for first-order multivariate calibration. *Chemom Intell Lab Syst* 2004; 73:189-97.

7. Ni Y, Wang Y, Kokot S. Multicomponent kinetics spectrophotometric determination of pefloxacin and norfloxacine in pharmaceutical preparations and human plasma samples with the aid of chemometrics. *Spectrochim Acta A Mol Biomol Spectrosc* 2008;70(5):1049-59.

8. Culzoni MJ, Zan MMD, Robles JC, Mantovani VE, Goicoechea HC. Chemometrics-assisted UV-spectroscopic strategies for the determination of theophylline in syrup. *J Pharm Biomed Anal* 2005; 39(5):1068-74.

9. Goicoechea HC, Olivieria AC. A comparison of orthogonal signal correction and net analyte preprocessing methods.Theoretical and experimental studies. *Chemometr Intell Lab Syst* 2001; 56:73-81.

10. Mark H, Workman J. Chemometrics in spectroscopy. 1st ed. London: Academic Press; 2007.

11. Haaland DM, Thomas EV. Partial least square methods for spectral analyses: II. Application to simulated and glass spectral data. *Anal Chem* 1988; 60: 1193-202.

12. Goicoechea HC, Olivieria AC. MULTIVAR- A program for multivariate calibration incorporating net analyte signal calculations. *Trends Anal Chem* 2000; 19: 599-605.

Comparison of *in Vitro* Activity of Doripenem versus Old Carbapenems against *Pseudomonas Aeruginosa* Clinical Isolates from both CF and Burn Patients

Zoya Hojabri[1,2], Mohammad Ahangarzadeh Rezaee[1], Mohammad Reza Nahaei[1], Mohammad Hossein Soroush[1], Morteza Ghojazadeh[3], Tahereh Pirzadeh[1], Mostafa Davodi[1], Mona Ghazi[1], Reza Bigverdi[1], Omid Pajand[4], Mohammad Aghazadeh[1,2]*

[1] *Tabriz Research Center of Infectious and Tropical Diseases, Tabriz University of Medical Sciences, Tabriz, Iran.*

[2] *Microbiology Department, Faculty of Medicine, Tabriz University of Medical Sciences, Tabriz, Iran.*

[3] *Physiology department, Faculty of Medicine, Tabriz University of Medical Sciences, Tabriz, Iran.*

[4] *Student Research Committee, Tabriz University of Medical Sciences, Tabriz, Iran.*

ARTICLE INFO

Keywords:
Pseudomonas aeruginosa
Doripenem
Imipenem
Burn
Cystic fibrosis
Iran

ABSTRACT

Purpose: The antimicrobial activity of doripenem in comparison of imipenem, meropenem and ertapenem among *Pseudomonas aeruginosa* isolated from burn and Cystic Fibrosis (CF) patients were determined. *Methods:* Metallo-β-lactamase (MBL) genes in imipenem non susceptible *P. aeruginosa* isolates were detected using PCR method. The *in vitro* susceptibilities of doripenem, imipenem, meropenem and ertapenem were determined by Etests. MIC_{50} and MIC_{90} for corresponding antibiotics were determined individually in burn and CF isolates. *Results:* Among isolates which were resistant to imipenem, 16 isolates were positive for the *bla* $_{IMP}$ gene. All isolates had no *bla* $_{VIM}$ gene. All MBL producing isolates were excluded. MIC_{50}/MIC_{90} of doripenem in CF and burn isolates were 0.75/>32 and >32/>32 mg/L respectively. The corresponding values for imipenem in CF and burn isolates were 2/>32 and >32/>32 mg/L, respectively. *Conclusion:* The susceptibility rate of doripenem is higher than that of imipenem and meropenem among *P.aeruginosa* isolated from CF patients, whereas, there is no difference between the efficiency of doripenem and old carbapenems in non MBL producing *P.aeruginosa* isolates in burn patients.

Introduction

The synthesis of new carbapenem remain an area of intense research because of the broad-spectrum antibacterial activity of this chemical class.[1-3] Doripenem is a recently released antibiotic with significant potential for use in *Pseudomonas aeruginosa* infections occur in CF and burn patients.[4]

The *In vitro* antimicrobial activity of Doripenem, is generally comparable to that of meropenem and imipenem although it is more active against Gram-negative organisms than imipenem.[5] The activity of doripenem against *P. aeruginosa* isolates is slightly better than that of other carbapenems. However, development of carbapenem resistance may significantly compromise their efficacy.[6] Resistance to carbapenems including doripenem resulted from the complex interaction of several mechanisms including loss of the OprD porin, overexpression of efflux systems (MexAB-OprM, MexEF-OprN) and production of carbapenemase activity, usually a metallo-β-lactamase (MBL).[7-10] It should be noted that doripenem is no less susceptible to hydrolysis by MBL than are the other carbapenems and none of them is active against *P. aeruginosa* isolates harboring various MBL genes.[11] Since, there is no CLSI guideline for doripenem MIC breakpoint until now, so the results of MIC susceptibility pattern obtained from different geographical regions from different clinical isolates could be helpful in this regard.

Since, *P. aeruginosa* is one of the most frequently isolated pathogens from both CF and burn patients, we designed the study to determine susceptibility patterns of all the isolates and to compare the *in vitro* antibacterial activity of doripenem with that of imipenem, and meropenem among non MBL *P. aeruginosa* isolates from both CF and burn patients.

---

*Corresponding author: Mohammad Aghazadeh, Tabriz Research Center of Infectious and Tropical Diseases, Tabriz University of Medical Sciences, Tabriz, Iran. Email: aghazadehm@tbzmed.ac.ir

Materials and Methods
Bacterial Strains
From June to December 2011, a total number of 92 non repetitive *P. aeruginosa* isolates was enrolled in this study. Sixty three burns isolates were recovered from hospitalized patients in a level one burn care center and 29 isolates were collected from CF patients admitted to a children's medical center. This collection of bacteria was identified by conventional biochemical tests.

Antimicrobial Susceptibility Testing
The Kirby-Bauer disk diffusion method was employed to evaluate susceptibility of the following antimicrobial agents: piperacillin/tazobactam, aztreonam, ticarcillin, trimetoprime and tobramycin (MAST, UK). MIC values of the imipenem, meropenem, ertapenem (AB BIODISK, Solna, Sweden), doripenem, ceftazidime, cefepime, ciprofloxacin, amikacin, gentamicin (Liofilchem, Italy) were determined by Etests. Results were interpreted according to Clinical and Laboratory Standards Institute (CLSI) criteria, where applicable[12]. FDA interpretive criteria were applied to doripenem results (susceptible ≤ 2 mg/l for *P. aeruginosa*).[13] The results were examined to ensure that reported MICs were within acceptable standards set by CLSI based on a comparator agent and the following ATCC quality control strain, ATCC 25922 (*E. coli*).

Ethical Standards
Ethical approval to perform the study was obtained from the institutional review board of Tabriz University of Medical Sciences. Written informed consent was obtained from all patients included in the study.

MIC_{50} and MIC_{90} Calculation
The concentration of each antimicrobial agent, that inhibited 50% (MIC_{50}) and 90% (MIC_{90}) of the strains, was calculated for each of the antibiotics singly. The formula of geometric means was used as follows:[14]

$$MIC50 = (M < 50) + \frac{(n - X) \times [(M > 50) - (M < 50)]}{Y}$$

Where M < 50 is the MIC of the highest cumulative percentage below 50%, M > 50 is the MIC of the lowest cumulative percentage above 50%; n is 50% of the number of organisms tested, X is the number of organisms in the group at M <50, and Y is the number of organism in the group at M >50.

Screening for Metallo B-Lactamase (Mbl) Production
In order to identify MBL producing isolates, we detected non susceptible isolates against imipenem by Kirby-Bauer disk diffusion method using imipenem disk 10 mg/L. Imipenem non susceptible isolates were selected for detection of IMP and VIM metalloenzymes. Total genomic DNA of the isolates which were resistant to imipenem, was extracted as described previously.[15] Genes encoding class B carbapenemases were detected by PCR using specific primers for *bla*IMP and *bla*VIM metalloenzyme genes.

The sequences of primers were as follows: IMP-F1, (CATGGTTTGGTGGTTCTTGT), IMP-R1, (GTAAGTTTCAAGAGTGATGC), VIM-F1, (GTTTGGTCGCATATCGCAAC) and VIM-R1 (CTACTCGGCGACTGAGCGAT). The generated PCR products were 524 and 623 base pairs, respectively.

Results
Screening MBL Production
PCR Screening of isolates which were non susceptible to imipenem indicated the presence of 17 *P. aeruginosa* isolates harboring *bla*IMP gene. Only one isolate among CF and 16 isolates among burn patients were detected as MBL positive isolates. There was no *bla*VIM carrying isolate detected in our study. All MBL producing isolates were excluded to remove the effect of one of the most interfering factors involved in carbapenem resistance. To the best of our knowledge, our study was the first report of Iran that evaluated the *in vitro* activity of doripenem in comparison with that of previously FDA approved carbapenems.

Antimicrobial Susceptibility Testing
As shown in Table 1, the Kirby-Bauer disk diffusion method was performed in 75 non MBL *P. aeruginosa* which comprised of 47 burn and 28 CF isolates. Table 2, summarizes the MIC's of some antimicrobial agents other than those mentioned in Table 1. The tables showed that among the tested comparators, piperacillin/tazobactam (14.9% and 93.1% susceptible, respectively) provided the greatest activity in both burn and CF isolates, followed by tobramycin (12.8%) in burn isolates. The susceptibility rates of amikacin, imipenem, meropenem and doripenem were the same among burn isolates (10.6%). However, the susceptibility rate of doripenem among CF isolates was similar to that of amikacin (89.3%) and higher than that of old carbapenems (imipenem & meropenem). The greatest differences in the susceptibility rate between burn and CF strains were observed with doripenem (10.6% versus 89.3%), amikacin (10.6% versus 89.3%) and piperacillin/tazobactam (14.9 % versus 93.1%).

According to the Table 2, among CF isolates, at any given MIC concentration from ≤0.5 to 1.5 mg/L, doripenem (MIC_{50}, 0.75 mg/L) inhibited a slightly greater proportion of isolates than meropenem (MIC_{50}, 0.75 mg/L) and notably greater than imipenem (MIC_{50}, 2 mg/L). However, higher MIC levels of doripenem at 2 and 4 mg/L, provided the same coverage as meropenem, inhibiting 85.7% and 89.3% of isolates, respectively. Table 2 showed that ertapenem was the least efficacious carbapenem (susceptibility rate, 66.7%) that could inhibit only 25% of CF isolates at the MIC level of 4 mg/L.

On the other hand, among burn isolates, all carbapenems except ertapenem had the same activity (MIC_{50} and MIC_{90}, >32 mg/L). The proportion of isolates inhibited at MIC level ≥1 mg/L of doripenem and meropenem was similar (10.6%), however, the inhibition rates for doripenem at MIC levels of ≤0.5 and 0.75 mg/L were slightly higher than that of meropenem. At any given concentration from ≤ 0.5 to > 32 mg/L, doripenem inhibited a remarkably greater proportion of isolates than imipenem (Table 2). Similar to CF isolates, ertapenem identified as the least potent agent in burn isolates which inhibited 6.4% of burn isolates in comparison with 10.6% inhibition by other carbapenems.

Table 1. Results of disk diffusion method on non-MBL *P. aeruginosa* isolates.

Antibiotic	PTZ		ATM		TN		TM		TC	
Profile	S n(%)	NS n(%)	S n(%)	NS n(%)	S n(%)	NS n(%)	S n(%)	NS n(%)	S n(%)	NS n(%)
Burn(47)	7(14.9)	40(85.1)	4(8.5)	43(91.5)	6(12.8)	41(87.2)	0	47(100)	4(8.5)	43(91.5)
CF(28)	26(93.1)	2(6.9)	9(31)	19(69)	22(79.3)	6(20.7)	2(6.9)	26(93.1)	23(82.8)	5(17.2)
PTZ: piperacillin/tazobactam, ATM: aztronam, TN: tobramycin, TM: trimetoprime, TC: ticarcillin, S: susceptible, NS: non susceptible.										

According to the susceptibility rates, the MIC levels of imipenem, meropenem and doripenem were completely in line with each other except for 3 isolates; one burn and 2 CF isolates which showed the MIC level of imipenem of >32 mg/L but doripenem and meropenem MIC levels of ≤ 1 mg/L.

Table 2. *In vitro* activities of doripenem and comparators against non MBL *P. aeruginosa* isolates in burn and CF patients.

		MIC_{50}	MIC_{90}	Range (mg/L)	Susceptibility (%)	Cumuative % inhibited at MIC (mg/L)						
						≤0.5	0.75	1	1.5	2	4	>32
Amikacin	CF	5.5	>256	1->256	89.3	-	-	-	-	-	-	-
	Burn	256	256	3->256	10.6	-	-	-	-	-	-	-
Gentamicin	CF	6.83	>256		60.7	-	-	-	-	-	-	-
	Burn	128	>128	3->256	8.5	-	-	-	-	-	-	-
Cefepime	CF	12.25	>256	2->256	57.1	-	-	-	-	-	-	-
	Burn	256	256	0.75->256	6.4	-	-	-	-	-	-	-
Ceftazidime	CF	2	>256	0.5->256	75.0	-	-	-	-	-	-	-
	Burn	256	256	2->256	8.5	-	-	-	-	-	-	-
Ciprofloxacin	CF	0.19	6.25	0.047->32	78.6	-	-	-	-	-	-	-
	Burn	>32	>32	0.047->32	8.5	-	-	-	-	-	-	-
Imipenem	CF	2	>32	0.75->32	85.7	0	7.1	14.3	39.3	60.7	85.7	100
	Burn	>32	>32	0.75->32	10.6	0	2.2	2.2	6.5	8.7	8.7	100
Meropenem	CF	0.75	>32	0.125->32	85.7	28.6	50.0	78.6	82.1	85.7	89.3	100
	Burn	>32	>32	0.15->32	10.6	8.5	8.5	10.6	10.6	10.6	10.6	100
Doripenem	CF	0.75	>32	0.094->32	89.3	39.3	75.0	82.1	85.7	85.7	89.3	100
	Burn	>32	>32	0.125->32	10.6	10.6	10.6	10.6	10.6	10.6	10.6	100
Ertapenem	CF	32	>32	0.094->32	66.7	3.6	3.6	3.6	7.1	10.7	25.0	100
	Burn	>32	>32	3->32	6.4	0	0	0	0	0	8.5	100

Discussion

Infections caused by *P. aeruginosa* in burn and CF patients often treated with difficulty due to the emergence of resistance and lack of effective antibiotics.[16] Doripenem as a new carbapenem offers potentially enhanced carbapenem activity but does not expand the spectrum of activity of this class[4]. Like other carbapenems, doripenem has stability against many β-lactamases, but remains labile to class B enzymes, known as metallo-β-lactamases.[5] Therefore,

in the present work, we attempted to assess the *in vitro* activity of doripenem among non MBL *P. aeruginosa* isolated from CF and burn patients, in comparison with other carbapenems.

Despite the higher carbapenem MIC rates in our CF isolates as compared with similar studies,[15,16] it can be concluded that doripenem has much greater potency than imipenem. Although the MIC_{50} of both doripenem and meropenem was similar, the more inhibition rate of 25% of this recently approved carbapenem indicated that doripenem could be considered as a good alternative therapeutic agent in CF patients. In a recent similar study,[16] antibiotic susceptibility of *P. aeruginosa* isolated from CF patients, doripenem showed as the most active antibiotic in the absence of piperacillin/tazobactam. Totally, it seems that doripenem can be considered as the most potent carbapenems against *P. aeruginosa* infections in CF patients.

Since, MBLs were the most important mechanisms in high level of resistance against all carbapenems, we decided to exclude the MBL positive isolates to explore the probable difference in doripenem MIC's versus old carbapenems. Although the susceptibility rates against doripenem in burn isolates showed no superiority to old carbapenems, the greater population of isolates were inhibited at any concentration of doripenem as compared with imipenem and meropenem. Among burn isolates, all cabapenems have the same activity except for ertapenem which has the least efficiency.

We found 3 imipenem resistant isolates which were susceptible to meropenem and doripenem. This phenomenon occurred to those isolates with nonenzymatic resistance involving loss of porin OprD and up-regulation of efflux pumps[13] which we intend to explore in a further study. Conversely, other researchers declared that this could be the exception other than a rule with no reason.[17]

Although ertapenem is not a representative of carbapenems with the consideration of broad spectrum activity which can not be used to treat infections due to non-fermentative Gram-negative bacteria,[13] we intended to investigate the *in vitro* activity of this antimicrobial agent for the first time in Iran. Our results are consistent with the results of other investigators[18] which showed the lowest susceptibility rate among all used carbapenems in both burn and CF isolates (6.4% and 66.7%). Our results corroborated by the results of the study conducted by Quale *et al.* They found only 18% of *P. aeruginosa* isolates that were susceptible against ertapenem while imipenem and meropenem were more potent, inhibiting 55% and 64% of isolates compared to ertapenem.

Conclusion

Although doripenem is more active than imipenem and meropenem against *P. aeruginosa* isolated from CF patients, no superiority of doripenem is observed to old carbapenems in non MBL producer *P. aeruginosa* isolates in burn patients. In terms of MIC level of doripenem, this antibiotic is the most active but this advantage is partly offset by lower regulatory breakpoints. Ertapenem is the least potent agent against *P. aeruginosa* isolates.

Acknowledgments

We are grateful to Dr. Saber Yousefi from Department of Clinical Laboratory Medicine, Faculty of Paramedicine, Urmia University of Medical Sciences.

This work was supported fully by Tabriz Research Center of Infectious and Tropical Diseases (grant No.89/16), Tabriz University of Medical Sciences, Tabriz, Iran.

This is a report of a database from thesis entitled "Evaluation of MexAB-OprM and MexXY-OprM efflux systems, AmpC cephalosporinase and OprD protein expressions to investigate their association with resistance against carbapenemes in Pseudomonas aeruginosa isolated from clinical specimens" registered in Tabriz University of Medical Sciences.

Conflict of interest

There is no conflict of interest in this study.

References

1. Nomura S, Nagayama A. In vitro antibacterial activity of s-4661, a new parenteral carbapenem, against urological pathogens isolated from patients with complicated urinary tract infections. *J Chemother* 2002;14(2):155-60.

2. Ohba F, Nakamura-Kamijo M, Watanabe N, Katsu K. In vitro and in vivo antibacterial activities of er-35786, a new antipseudomonal carbapenem. *Antimicrob Agents Chemother* 1997;41(2):298-307.

3. Watanabe A, Takahashi H, Kikuchi T, Kobayashi T, Gomi K, Fujimura S, et al. Comparative in vitro activity of s-4661, a new parenteral carbapenem, and other antimicrobial agents against respiratory pathogens. *Chemotherapy* 2000;46(3):184-7.

4. Parkins MD, Elborn JS. Newer antibacterial agents and their potential role in cystic fibrosis pulmonary exacerbation management. *J Antimicrob Chemother* 2010;65(9):1853-61.

5. Lascols C, Legrand P, Merens A, Leclercq R, Armand-Lefevre L, Drugeon HB, et al. In vitro antibacterial activity of doripenem against clinical isolates from french teaching hospitals: Proposition of zone diameter breakpoints. *Eur J Clin Microbiol Infect Dis* 2011;30(4):475-82.

6. Rodriguez-Martinez JM, Poirel L, Nordmann P. Molecular epidemiology and mechanisms of carbapenem resistance in pseudomonas aeruginosa. *Antimicrob Agents Chemother* 2009;53(11):4783-8.

7. El Amin N, Giske CG, Jalal S, Keijser B, Kronvall G, Wretlind B. Carbapenem resistance mechanisms in pseudomonas aeruginosa: Alterations of porin oprd and efflux proteins do not fully explain resistance patterns observed in clinical isolates. *Acta Pathol Microbiol Immunol Scand* 2005;113(3):187-96.

8. Wolter DJ, Smith-Moland E, Goering RV, Hanson ND, Lister PD. Multidrug resistance associated with mexxy expression in clinical isolates of pseudomonas aeruginosa from a texas hospital. *Diagn Microbiol Infect Dis* 2004;50(1):43-50.

9. Pai H, Kim J, Lee JH, Choe KW, Gotoh N. Carbapenem resistance mechanisms in

pseudomonas aeruginosa clinical isolates. *Antimicrob Agents Chemother* 2001;45(2):480-4.

10. Livermore DM. Of pseudomonas, porins, pumps and carbapenems. *J Antimicrob Chemother* 2001;47(3):247-50.

11. Rice LB. Challenges in identifying new antimicrobial agents effective for treating infections with acinetobacter baumannii and pseudomonas aeruginosa. *Clin Infect Dis* 2006;43 Suppl 2:S100-5.

12. Clinical and Laboratory Standards Institute. Performance standards for antimicrobial susceptibility testing; 19th informational supplement. CLSI document M100-S19. Wayne PA: CLSI; 2009.

13. Castanheira M, Jones RN, Livermore DM. Antimicrobial activities of doripenem and other carbapenems against pseudomonas aeruginosa, other nonfermentative bacilli, and aeromonas spp. *Diagn Microbiol Infect Dis* 2009;63(4):426-33.

14. Smith JA, Henry D, Ngui-Yen J, Castell A, Coderre S. Comparison of agar dilution, microdilution, and disk elution methods for measuring the synergy of cefotaxime and its metabolite against anaerobes. *J Clin Microbiol* 1986;23(6):1104-8.

15. Bou G, Cervero G, Dominguez MA, Quereda C, Martinez-Beltran J. Pcr-based DNA fingerprinting (rep-pcr, ap-pcr) and pulsed-field gel electrophoresis characterization of a nosocomial outbreak caused by imipenem- and meropenem-resistant acinetobacter baumannii. *Clin Microbiol Infect* 2000;6(12):635-43.

16. Traczewski MM, Brown SD. In vitro activity of doripenem against pseudomonas aeruginosa and burkholderia cepacia isolates from both cystic fibrosis and non-cystic fibrosis patients. *Antimicrob Agents Chemother* 2006;50(2):819-21.

17. Paterson DL, Depestel DD. Doripenem. *Clin Infect Dis* 2009;49(2):291-8.

18. Quale J, Bratu S, Gupta J, Landman D. Interplay of efflux system, ampc, and oprd expression in carbapenem resistance of pseudomonas aeruginosa clinical isolates. *Antimicrob Agents Chemother* 2006;50(5):1633-41.

High Performance Liquid Chromatographic Analysis of Almotriptan Malate in Bulk and Tablets

Petikam lavudu[1], Avula Prameela Rani[2], Chepuri Divya[1], Chandra Bala Sekaran[3]*

[1] *Department of Pharmaceutical Biotechnology, Vishnu Institute of Pharmaceutical Education and Research, Narsapur, Andhra Pradesh-500072.*

[2] *University College of Pharmaceutical Sciences, Acharya Nagarjuna University, Guntur, Andhra Pradesh-522510.*

[3] *Department of Biotechnology, Jagarlamudi Kuppuswamy Choudary College, Guntur, Andhra Pradesh-522006.*

ARTICLE INFO

Keywords:
Almotriptan Malate
HPLC
Validation
Tablets
Analysis

ABSTRACT

Purpose: A simple RP-HPLC method has been developed and validated for the determination of almotriptan malate (ATM) in bulk and tablets. *Methods:* Chromatographic separation of ATM was achieved by using a Thermo Scientific C18 column. A Mobile phase containing a mixture of methanol, water and acetic acid (4:8:0.1 *v/v*) was pumped at the flow rate of 1 mL/min. Detection was performed at 227 nm. According to ICH guidelines, the method was validated. *Results:* The calibration curve was linear in the concentration range 5–60 µg/mL for the ATM with regression coefficient 0.9999. The method was precise with RSD <1.2%. Excellent recoveries of 99.60 - 100.80% proved the accuracy of the method. The limits of detection and quantification were found to be 0.025 and 0.075 µg/mL, respectively. *Conclusion:* The method was successfully applied for the quantification of ATM in tablets with acceptable accuracy and precision.

Introduction

Almotriptan malate (ATM) is a serotonin receptor agonist used in the acute treatment of migraine headache in adults and adolescents aged from 12 to 17 years with or without aura.[1-3] Chemically, ATM is known as 1-[[[3-[2-(Dimethylamino) ethyl]-1H-indol-5-yl] methyl] sulfonyl] pyrrolidine malate (1:1). ATM stimulates specific serotonin receptors in intracranial blood vessels and sensory trigeminal nerves, thereby promote vascular constriction and relieve migraine.

A thorough literature survey has revealed that only a few liquid chromatographic methods are available for the quantification of ATM in bulk, pharmaceutical formulations and biological fluids. Assay of almotriptan in pharmaceutical dosage forms by HPTLC has been reported by Suneetha and Syamasundar.[4] Ravikumar et al. have developed LC-MS method for the determination of almotriptan in human plasma.[5] Nageswara Rao et al. have reported a LC-MS method for determining invivo metabolites of almotriptan in rat plasma, urine & faeces.[6] Jansat et al. and Fleishaker et al. have reported HPLC method for the determination of almotriptan concentration in human plasma and urine, respectively.[7,8]

Only two HPLC methods with UV detection were reported in the literature for the assay of ATM in pharmaceutical dosage forms. In a method reported by Suneetha and Syamasundar, separation and quantification of ATM were conducted on Phenomenex Gemini C18 column using potassium dihydrogen phosphate buffer:acetonitrile (80:20) as a mobile phase. The UV detection was performed at 227 nm.[9] Phani kumar and Sunandamma have reported a HPLC method using a Kromosil C18 column with a mobile phase comprising of 1% Triethyl amine: acetonitrile: methanol (05:55:40) and UV detection at 230 nm.[10] The reported HPLC with UV detection methods suffer from the disadvantages such as narrow range of linear response,[9] longer runtime for a single sample,[9,10] preparation of buffer,[9] strict control of pH,[9] and less precise with RSD values greater than 1.5.[10]

The present paper deals with the development and validation of a RP-HPLC method with UV detection for the determination of ATM in bulk and tablet dosage forms.

Materials and Methods
Instrumentation
Reverse Phase-High Pressure Liquid Chromatography was performed with an isocratic High Pressure Liquid Chromatography system (Shimadzu HPLC class VP series, Shimadzu Corporation, Kyoto, Japan) with two LC-10 AT, VP pumps, variable wavelength programmable UV/Visible detector SPD-10A, VP, CTO-10AS VP column oven, SCL-10A, VP system

---

*Corresponding author: Chandra Bala Sekaran, Department of Biotechnology, Jagarlamudi Kuppuswamy Choudary College, Guntur, Andhra Pradesh-522006, Email: balumphil@gmail.com

controller. The monitoring software was "class VP series version 5.03" (Shimadzu). Separation of the ATM was achieved by using a 250 mm × 4.6 mm I.D., 5 μm particle size, Thermo Scientific C18 (Phenomenex, Torrance, CA, USA) column under reversed-phase chromatographic conditions.

Chemicals and Reagents

All the chemicals were of HPLC grade quality. Milli-Q-water was obtained from Merck Specialties Private Ltd, Hyderabad, India and used right throughout the process. Methanol and glacial acetic acid were obtained from Sd fine Chem Limited, Mumbai, India. Pharmaceutical grade ATM was obtained from Matrix laboratories, Hyderabad, India. Branded ATM products (Axert tablets, Ortho-McNeil-Janssen Pharmaceuticals, Inc. USA), labeled to contain 6.25 and 12.5 mg of ATM were purchased and used in the present study.

Preparation of Mobile Phase

The mobile phase was prepared by mixing methanol, water and glacial acetic acid in the ratio of 4:8:0.1 v/v.

Preparation of Standard Drug Solutions

For the stock standard solution (1 mg/mL), an exactly weighed 100 mg of ATM was dissolved and diluted to the volume with the mobile phase in a 100 mL volumetric flask. Working standard solutions equivalent to 5 to 60 μg/mL of ATM were prepared by appropriate dilution of the stock standard solution with the mobile phase.

Preparation of Tablet Extract

Twenty tablets were weighed and finely powdered. A precisely weighed portion of the powder equivalent to 100 mg of ATM was extracted with mobile phase. The extract was transferred to a 100 mL volumetric flask and made up to the mark with the mobile phase. The solution was filtered through a 0.45 μm membrane filter. The tablet extract was appropriately diluted with mobile phase to obtain a concentration of 60 μg/mL.

Chromatographic Conditions

The mobile phase [methanol, water and acetic acid (4:8:0.1 v/v)] was pumped at a flow rate of 1 mL/min. It was filtered through 0.45 μm membrane filter and degassed before using with a helium sparge for 15 min. The injection volume was 20 μL and the eluent was monitored at 227 nm. The column temperature was 25±1°C.

Calibration Curve

A series of working standard solutions prepared above were taken. Twenty μl aliquot of each solution was injected automatically into the column in triplicate. The peaks were determined at 227 nm. The mean peak are as versus concentrations of almotriptan were plotted to obtain the calibration curve. The seven concentrations of the working standard solution were subjected to regression analysis to calculate regression equation, slope, intercept and regression coefficient. The concentration of the drug was calculated from the calibration curve or the regression equation.

Assay in Tablet Dosage Forms

A 20 μl aliquot of tablet extract (60 μg/mL) was injected into the HPLC system in triplicate. The peaks were determined at 227 nm. The concentration of the drug in tablet dosage form was calculated from the calibration curve or the regression equation.

Method Validation

The proposed method was validated for system suitability, linearity, limit of detection, limit of quantification, precision, accuracy, selectivity, robustness, ruggedness and stability of drug.

System Suitability

The study of system suitability was done to validate the sufficiency of the reproducibility of chromatographic system for the analysis of ATM. This was carried out by five replicate analyses of the drug at a concentration of 60 μg/mL. The proposed method was evaluated by analyzing the parameters like retention time, peak asymmetry, theoretical plates, plates per meter and height equivalent to theoretical plate.

Linearity

For the assessment of linearity, determination of ATM was done at seven concentration levels (5, 10, 20, 30, 40, 50 and 60 μg/mL). Twenty μl aliquot of each concentration solution was injected automatically into the column in triplicate and the peak areas were recorded.

Limit of Detection (LOD) and Limit of Quantification (LOQ)

LOD and LOQ were calculated by using the following expressions:

$$LOD = 3.3s / S$$
$$LOQ = 10s / S$$

Where "s" is the standard deviation of the regression line and "S" is the slope of calibration curve.

Precision and Accuracy

The precision and accuracy of the proposed method was assessed by intra-day and inter-day variation studies using three different concentrations of ATM (5, 30 and 60 μg/mL). During intra-day studies, five sample solutions of each concentration were analyzed on the same day whereas inter-day studies were determined by analyzing five sample solutions of each concentration for three consecutive days.

Recovery Studies

Recovery studies were performed using the standard addition method. For this study, a known amount of pure drug was added to the preanalyzed sample solution. Mean percent recovery of the ATM was determined.

Selectivity
Selectivity was assessed by examining peak interferences from excipients present in the tablet dosage forms and components of mobile phase. This was done by comparing the chromatograms of blank and tablet extract with the pure drug.

Robustness
To verify the robustness of the method, three vital experimental variables such as composition of mobile phase, detection wavelength and flow rate were slightly varied. The analysis was performed at the deliberately varied experimental conditions by taking two different concentrations of ATM (5 and 60 µg/mL)

Ruggedness
The method's ruggedness was established by the determination of ATM at two different concentrations (5 and 60 µg/mL). This was performed by two different analysts.

Solution Stability
To assess the stability of ATM in mobile phase, the sample solutions (5 and 60 µg/mL) were prepared in the mobile phase and stored at room temperature for 48

hr. The sample solutions were assayed at an interval of every 12 hr for 48 hr.

Results and Discussion
The quantification of the drugs in pharmaceutical dosage forms and biological fluids is necessary during the studies of stability, metabolism, pharmacokinetics, toxicity and drug quality control. For all these investigations, an efficient and validated analytical method is very significantly required.

Method Development
A reversed-phase C18, 250 mm × 4.6 mm I.D., 5 µm particle size column maintained at ambient temperature was used for the separation of ATM. Regarding the mobile phase, a mixture of methanol, water and glacial acetic acid was used. In order to improve the separation and peak symmetry, the mobile phase composition was varied until optimum composition was chosen (4:8:0.1 v/v). Isocratic elution at the flow rate of 1.0 mL/min has been employed in the present proposed method. Wavelength of 227 nm was chosen to be used for the UV detection. The column is kept at room temperature during the procedure. After this optimization, this method has been used for the assay of ATM. A good separation with satisfactory resolution has been obtained (Figure 1).

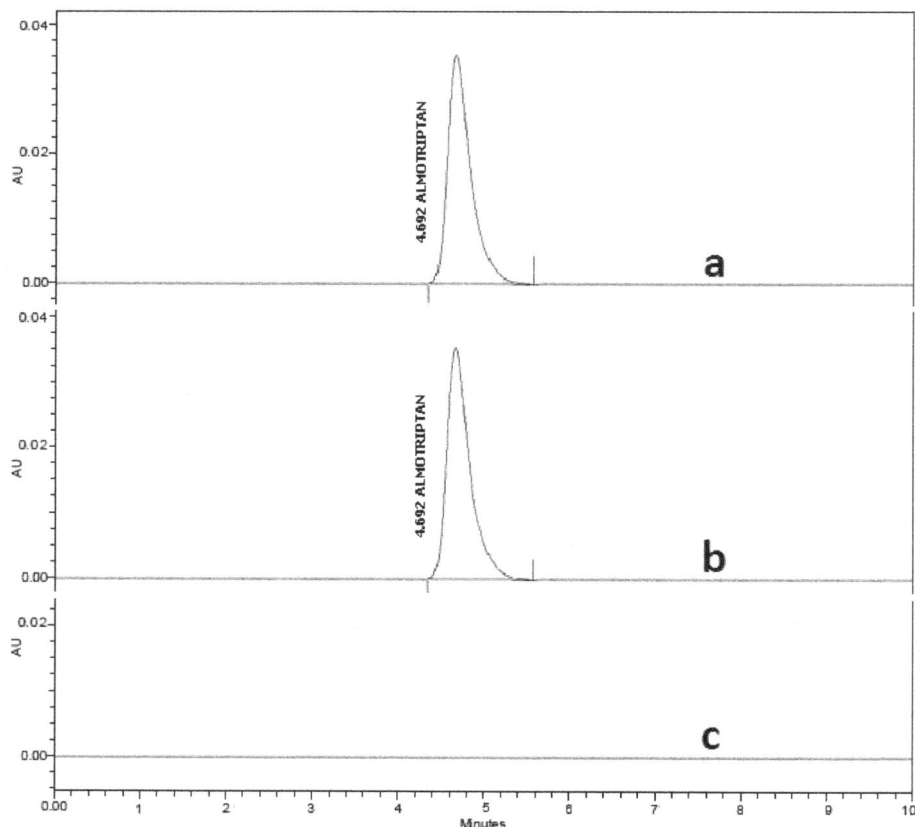

Figure 1. Representative chromatogram of pure ATM (a), tablet extract (b) and blank mobile phase.

Validation

System Suitability

The system suitability parameters, like retention time, peak asymmetry, theoretical plates, plates per meter and height equivalent to theoretical plate were calculated. From the results (Table 1), it was observed that all the values are within the limits.

Table 1. System suitability studies.

Parameter	Value	RSD (%)
Retention Time (t) (Min)	4.692	0.052
Theoretical Plates (n)	4832.82	1.06
Plates per Meter (N)	16100	1.113
Height equivalent to theoretical plate (HETP) (mm)	6.2×10^{-7}	1.021
Peak asymmetry	1.16	1.071
RSD: Relative standard deviation		

Linearity

Linear relationship was observed by plotting concentrations of the drug against peak areas. ATM exhibited linear response in the concentration range, 5 to 60 µg/mL. The corresponding linear regression equation was $y = 53532x + 39.216$ with regression coefficient (R^2) 0.9999.

The Llimit of Detection (LOD) and Limit of Quantification (LOQ)

LOD and LOQ of the proposed method were determined as s/S ratio 3.3 for LOD and 10 fold for LOQ. The low values of LOD and LOQ, that is, 0.025 and 0.075 µg/mL, respectively suggest the high sensitivity of the method.

Precision and Accuracy

The relative standard deviation for intra-day and inter-day analysis was in the range of 0.129 to 0.823 % and 0.822 to 1.170 %, respectively. Mean recovery of ATM using the proposed method was in the range of 99.60-100.30 (intra-day analysis) and 99.76–100.80 (inter-day analysis). The results point out the precision and accuracy of the method developed (Table 2).

Table 2. Precision and accuracy of the method.

Assay type	Concentration of ATM (µg/mL)		RSD (%)	Recovery (%)
	Taken	Recovered ± SD*		
Intra-day	5	4.98 ± 0.041	0.823	99.60
	30	30.09 ± 0.052	0.175	100.30
	60	60.04 ± 0.092	0.129	100.06
Inter-day	5	5.04 ± 0.059	1.170	100.80
	30	29.93 ± 0.298	0.995	99.76
	60	59.95 ± 0.493	0.822	99.91

*Average of five determinations; SD: Standard deviation; RSD: Relative standard deviation

Recovery Studies

Preanalyzed sample solution was spiked with pure ATM and then the total amount of ATM was determined by the proposed method. The results (Table 3) showed that the mean recovery and relative standard deviation were in the range of 99.97–100.09 % and 0.799-0.973%, respectively. From the recovery study it was apparent that the proposed method is very accurate for quantitative determination of ATM in tablet dosage form. The excipients and additives commonly present in the tablet dosage forms did not interfere in the assay.

Table 3. Results of recovery studies.

Concentration of ATM (mg)			RSD (%)	Recovery (%)
Tablet	Spiked	Recovered ± SD*		
6.25	3.0	9.248 ± 0.090	0.973	99.97
12.50	6.25	18.766± 0.150	0.799	100.09

* Average of five determinations , SD: Standard deviation, RSD: Relative standard deviation

Selectivity

The selectivity of the proposed method demonstrated that excipients in the tablet dosage forms and components of mobile phase did not interfere with the drug peak. In addition, the well shaped peaks also signify the selectivity of the proposed method (Figure 1).

Robustness

Robustness of the proposed method was assessed by making small changes in the composition of mobile phase, detection wavelength and flow rate. The small variations in any of the variables did not significantly affect the results (Table 4). The lower values of RSD (<1.3%) demonstrate the excellent robustness of the proposed method.

Table 4. Robustness of the method.

Experimental parameter	Concentration of ATM (µg/mL)		RSD (%)
	Taken	Recovered ± SD$	
Mobile phase*	5	5.05 ± 0.021	0.415
	60	59.97 ± 0.324	0.540
Detection wavelength**	5	5.02 ± 0.036	0.717
	60	59.90 ± 0.466	0.777
Flow rate***	5	4.96 ± 0.063	1.270
	60	60.01 ± 0.514	0.856

*Methanol, water and acetic acid ratios (v/v): 3.9:8.1:0.1, 4:8:0.1, 4.1:7.9:0.1
**Wavelength (nm) – 226,227 and 228
***Flow rate (mL/min) – 0.9, 1.0 and 1.1
$Average of three determinations
SD- Standard deviation
RSD- Relative standard deviation

Ruggedness
Ruggedness of the method was performed by analyzing 5 and 60 µg/mL of ATM by two different analysts keeping same experimental conditions. The results are presented in Table 5. The lower values of RSD (<1.0%) confirm the ruggedness of the proposed method.

Table 5. Ruggedness of the method

| Analyst | Concentration of ATM (µg/mL) | | SD** | RSD (%) |
	Taken	Recovered*		
I	5	4.96	±0.042	0.841
II	5	5.02		
I	60	59.90	±0.056	0.093
II	60	59.98		

* Average of five determinations, ** Standard deviation for two values, SD: Standard deviation, RSD: Relative standard deviation

Solution Stability
Relative standard deviation for assay of ATM during solution stability was <1.0% (Table 6). The results from solution stability experiments confirmed that ATM in the mobile phase was stable for up to 48 hr.

Table 6. Stability of ATM in mobile phase

| Time (hr) | Concentration of ATM (µg/mL) | | SD** | RSD (%) |
	Taken	Recovered*		
12	5	5.05	±0.044	0.880
24	5	5.02		
36	5	4.98		
48	5	4.95		
12	60	60.05	±0.062	0.103
24	60	59.95		
36	60	59.97		
48	60	59.90		

* Average of five determinations, ** Standard deviation for four values, SD: Standard deviation, RSD: Relative standard deviation

Application to Tablet Dosage Forms
The proposed method was effectively applied for the quantification of ATM in two different dosage forms. The results, shown in Table 7, are in good agreement with those obtained with the reference UV spectrophotometric method.[11]

Conclusion
The proposed HPLC method was found to be simple, precise, accurate and rapid for the estimation of ATM in bulk and in its dosage forms. The mobile phase is simple to prepare. The sample recoveries in all tablet dosage forms were in good agreement with their

respective labelled claim and suggested noninterference of tablet excipients in the estimation. Hence, this method can be easily and conveniently adopted for routine analysis of ATM in quality control laboratories.

Table 7. Results of analysis of ATM in tablets

| Formulation | Method | Concentration of ATM (mg) | |
		Tablet	Recovered ± SD**
Tablet*	Reference	6.25	6.246 ± 0.014 % R=99.93 % RSD=0.224
		12.50	12.504 ± 0.024 % R=100.09 % RSD=0.194
	Proposed HPLC method	6.25	6.249 ± 0.054 % R=99.98 % RSD=0.863 t Value$= 1.19 F value$$=3.29
		12.50	12.490 ± 0.120 % R=99.92 % RSD=0.960 t Value$= 1.11 F value$$=4.66

*Axert tablets, Ortho-McNeil-Janssen Pharmaceuticals, Inc. USA
** Average of five determinations
%R – Percentage recovery
% RSD – Percentage relative standard deviation
$ Tabulated t-value at 95% confidence level is 2.306
$$ Tabulated F- value at 95 % confidence level is 6.390

Acknowledgements
One of the authors, P. Lavudu, expresses his gratitude to the management of Vishnu Institute of Pharmaceutical Education & Research, Narsapur and Principal, University College of Pharmaceutical sciences, Acharya Nagarjuna University, Guntur for providing research facilities.

Conflict of Interest
The authors declare there is no Conflict of interest in the content of this study.

References
1. Chen LC, Ashcroft DM. Meta-analysis examining the efficacy and safety of almotriptan in the acute treatment of migraine. *Headache* 2007;47(8):1169-77.
2. Keam SJ, Goa KL, Figgitt DP. Spotlight on almotriptan in migraine. *CNS Drugs* 2002; 16(7):501-7.
3. Dodick DW. Oral almotriptan in the treatment of migraine: Safety and tolerability. *Headache* 2001; 41(5):449-55.
4. Suneetha A, Syamasundar B. Development and validation of HPTLC method for the estimation of almotriptan malate in tablet dosage form. *Indian J Pharm Sci* 2010; 72(5): 629-32.

5. Ravikumar K, Balasekhara Reddy C, Babu Rao C, Chandrasekhar KB. Method development and validation of almotriptan in human plasma by HPLC tandem mass spectrometry: Application to a Pharmacokinetic Study. *Sci Pharm* 2012;80(2):367-78.

6. Nageswara Rao R, Guruprasad K, Gangu Naidu C, Raju B, Srinivas R. LC-ESI-MS/MS determination of in vivo metabolites of almotriptan in rat plasma, urine and feces: Application to pharmacokinetics. *J Chromatogr B Analyt Technol Biomed Life Sci* 2012;891-892:44-51.

7. Jansat JM, Martinez-Tobed A, Garcia E, Cabarrocas X, Costa J. Effect of food intake on the bioavailability of almotriptan, an antimigraine compound, in healthy volunteers: An open, randomized, crossover, single-dose clinical trial. *Int J Clin Pharmacol Ther* 2006;44(4):185-90.

8. Fleishaker JC, Ryan KK, Jansat JM, Carel BJ, Bell DJ, Burke MT, et al. Effect of MAO-A inhibition on the pharmacokinetics of almotriptan, an antimigraine agent in humans. *Br J Clin Pharmacol* 2001;51(5):437-41.

9. Suneetha A, Syamasundar B. A Validated RP HPLC method for estimation of almotriptan malate in pharmaceutical dosage form. *J Chin Chem Soc-Taip* 2010;57(5A):1067-70.

10. Phani Kumar V, Sunandamma Y. New RP-HPLC method development and validation for analysis of almotriptan. *Int J Res Pharm Chem* 2011;1(3): 542-5.

11. Suneetha A, Syama sundar B. New simple UV Spectrophotometric method for estimation of almotriptan malate in bulk and pharmaceutical dosage forms. *Asian J Res Chem* 2010;3(1):142-5.

Affinity Purification of Tumor Necrosis Factor-α Expressed in Raji Cells by Produced scFv Antibody Coupled CNBr-Activated Sepharose

Jalal Abdolalizadeh[1,2], Jafar Majidi Zolbanin[3,4], Mohammad Nouri[5], Behzad Baradaran[4], AliAkbar Movassaghpour[6], Safar Farajnia[7], Yadollah Omidi[1,8]*

[1] Research Center for Pharmaceutical Nanotechnology, Tabriz University of Medical Sciences, Tabriz, Iran.

[2] Student' Research Committee, Tabriz University of Medical Sciences, Tabriz, Iran.

[3] Drug Applied Research Center, Tabriz University of Medical Sciences, Tabriz, Iran.

[4] Immunology Research Center, Tabriz University of Medical Sciences, Tabriz, Iran.

[5] Biochemistry Department, Medicine Faculty, Tabriz University of Medical Sciences, Tabriz, Iran.

[6] Hematology and Oncology Research Center, Tabriz University of Medical Sciences, Tabriz, Iran.

[7] Biotechnology Research Center, Tabriz University of Medical Sciences, Tabriz, Iran.

[8] Ovarian Cancer Research Center, Translational Research Center, University of Pennsylvania, Philadelphia, PA 19104, USA.

ARTICLE INFO

Keywords:
TNF-α expression
Affinity Purification
Monoclonal antibody
LPS

ABSTRACT

Purpose: Recombinant tumor necrosis factor-alpha (TNF-α) has been utilized as an antineoplastic agent for the treatment of patients with melanoma and sarcoma. It targets tumor cell antigens by impressing tumor-associated vessels. Protein purification with affinity chromatography has been widely used in the downstream processing of pharmaceutical-grade proteins. *Methods:* In this study, we examined the potential of our produced anti-TNF-α scFv fragments for purification of TNF-α produced by Raji cells. The Raji cells were induced by lipopolysaccharides (LPS) to express TNF-α. Western blotting and Fluorescence-activated cell sorting (FACS) flow cytometry analyses were used to evaluate the TNF-α expression. The anti-TNF-α scFv selected from antibody phage display library was coupled to CNBr-activated sepharose 4B beads used for affinity purification of expressed TNF-α and the purity of the protein was assessed by SDS-PAGE. *Results:* Western blot and FACS flow cytometry analyses showed the successful expression of TNF-α with Raji cells. SDS-PAGE analysis showed the performance of scFv for purification of TNF-α protein with purity over 95%. *Conclusion:* These findings confirm not only the potential of the produced scFv antibody fragments but also this highly pure recombinant TNF-α protein can be applied for various *in vitro* and *in vivo* applications.

Introduction

Cytokines, as low molecular-weight signaling molecules, are biologically functional in markedly low amounts. They play central roles upon the activity immune system, inflammation and cell growth. Of the cytokines, tumor necrosis factor alpha (TNF-α) possesses pleomorphic resulting in pivotal impacts on biological functions including inflammation, cell propagation, differentiation, immune regulation in addition to its ability to induce apoptosis within the tumor-associated endothelial cells.[1,2] It is mainly expressed by monocytes/macrophages,[3] even though other cells (T-lymphocytes, natural killer (NK) cells, astrocytes, fibroblasts, Kupffer cells, keratinocytes, smooth-muscle cells) as well as tumor cells can express

TNF-α.[4] The mature human TNF-α is a 157 amino acid (AA) protein (17 kDa) with an isoelectric point of 5.8, which contains one disulfide-bond (Cys69-Cys101). It is normally processed from a precursor form called transmembrane (a type II transmembrane protein with 26 kDa, 233 AA) revealing no glycosylation.[5]
Recombinant TNF-α has been harnessed as an antineoplastic agent alone or in combination with a conventional chemotherapy agent for the treatment of patients with melanoma and sarcoma.[6-8] It is able to induce apoptosis within the tumor-associated endothelial cells, resulting in complete eradication of the tumor vasculature.[8,9] Nevertheless, because of vasoplegia induction (also known as systemic

*Corresponding author: Yadollah Omidi, Ovarian Cancer Research Center, Perelman School of Medicine, University of Pennsylvania, Philadelphia, PA 19104, USA. E-mail: yomidi@mail.med.upenn.edu

inflammatory response), the therapeutic use of TNF in clinic was limited,[7] while most of clinical phases revealed that TNF alone cannot effectively suppress the growth of tumor. Besides, TNF has several *in vitro* applications such as Enzyme-linked immunosorbent assay (ELISA), biopanning and Western blotting.
We have previously produced anti-TNF-α scFv antibody fragments using phage display technology.[10] To examine the potential of these scFvs as ligate for affinity purification of expressed TNF-α, in the current study we stimulated Raji cells with lipopolysaccharide (LPS) that can elicit macrophages to produce TNF-α,[11,12] and exploit the scFvs for purification of the induced TNF-α. Figure 1 represents schematic illustration for upstream production of TNF in Raji cells and downstream affinity purification process for the expressed TNF molecules.

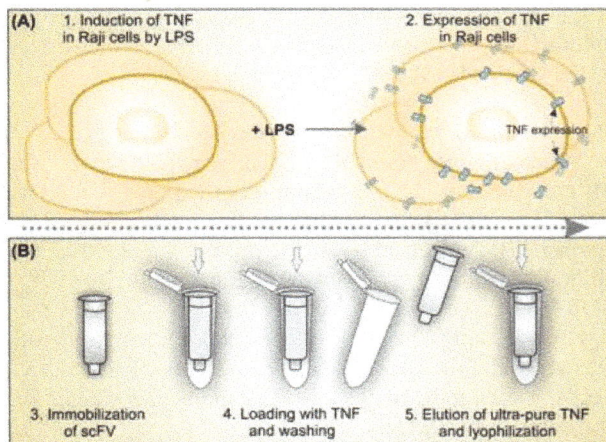

Figure 1. Schematic representation for upstream (A) and downstream (B) processing of TNF-α.

Materials and Methods

Culture of Raji Cell for induction of TNF expression
Human B-lymphoblastoid cells (Raji cell line)were cultured in T75 flasks and grown overnight in 18 ml RPMI-1640 medium supplemented with 10% heat-inactivated fetal bovine serum (FBS) in a tissue culture incubator humidified with a 5% CO2 at 37°C. Then, cells were induced to produce TNF-α by addition of 10 μg/mL LPS (Sigma Chem. Co., St. Louis, MO, USA). Cells were washed twice with cold PBS (pH 7.4) and incubated with the cell lysis buffer (PBS that contained 1% NP40, 0.5% sodium deoxycholate, 0.1% SDS, and 0.01% protease inhibitor cocktail) at 4°C for 1 h. After centrifugation, the supernatant was collected and TNF-α concentration was determined using Western blotting and Fluorescence-activated cell sorting (FACS) methods.

Western blotting analysis; assessment of TNF-α expression
Sodium dodecyl sulfate polyacrylamide gel electrophoresis (SDS-PAGE) analysis was conducted to determine the TNF-α expression in Raji cells. Cell lysates were mixed with sample buffer and separated by electrophoresis on reduced condition onto 12% gels. The protein profiles were electrically transferred on Polyvinylidene fluoride (PVDF) membrane (Millipore, Billerica, MA, USA) using transfer buffer (25 mM Tris, 193 mM glycine, and 20% methanol). The membrane was then blocked with the blocking solution and incubated with anti-TNF-α scFv monoclonal antibody (mAb), followed by incubation with anti-myc and HRP-conjugated anti-mouse IgG antibodies. After extensive washing, the protein bands were visualized by enhanced chemiluminescence (ECL; Amersham Biosciences, Freiburg, Germany) substrate.

Flow cytometry analysis using FITC conjugated scFv
For analysis of induced Raji cells for TNF-α expression, we harnessed the flow cytometry analysis using FITC conjugated scFv antibody fragments. To this end, we first purified scFv antibody fragments as described previously through antibody phage display technique[10] and then conjugated these scFvs with fluorescein isothiocyanate (FITC) (Sigma Chemical Co., St. Louis, MO, USA). Briefly, anti-TNF-α scFv was dialysed against 0.1 M sodium carbonate buffer, pH 9 overnight at 4°C.The FITC was dissolved in anhydrous DMSO (Sigma Chemical Co., St. Louis, MO, USA)at 1 mg/mL and added to1 mg/mL protein while gently and continuously stirring the protein solution and incubated in the dark for 8 h at 4°C. After addition of NH4Cl to a final concentration of 50 mM, the reaction incubated for 2 h at 4°C. Gel filtration was used to separate the unbound FITC from the FITC-conjugated scFvs.[13,14]
For FACS flow cytometry analysis, the LPS induced Raji cells were incubated with 1 mL of FITC labeled scFv at 1:1000 dilution for 1 h. After washing with PBS containing 10% FBS, to assess the fluorescence intensity, 10000 events were measured for each sample using FACSCalibur and analyzed with CellQuest Pro software (Becton Dickinson Biosciences, San Jose, CA, USA).

Preparation of scFv-coupled sepharose column
Affinity purified scFv was coupled to CNBr-activated sepharose 4B beads(Sigma Chemical Co., St. Louis, MO, USA) for preparation ofthe affinity column. Purified scFv antibodyfragments were dialyzed against coupling buffer (0.2 M NaHCO3, 0.5 M NaCl, pH 9.0) overnight at 4°C. Sepharose beads were then introduced to 1 mM HCl and washed with coupling buffer. ThescFv antibody fragments were added to resin, incubated overnight at 4°C and blocked withblocking buffer (200 mM Glycine, pH 8.0).[15] Antibody-coupled sepharose was transferred to column and washed (3×) with PBS.

Purification of TNF-α
TNF-αexpressed Raji cell lysates were dialyzed against PBS buffer (pH 7.4) and loaded on column. The bound

proteins were eluted using elution Buffer (100 mM Glycine, pH 2.5) and neutralized with 2 M Tris, pH 8.0. The purity was assessed by SDS-PAGE.

SDS-PAGE analysis of purified protein

SDS-PAGE analysis was performed for the purity assessment of the eluted protein. The collected protein fractions were subjected to electrophoresis in 12% SDS-PAGE on reduced condition.
Protein bands were visualized by Coomassie blue staining technique.

Results

Western blotting analysis for functional assessment of TNF-α expression

The Raji cell lysates were resolved by 12% SDS-PAGE on reducing condition and electrically transferred onto the PVDF membrane. The membrane was probed with anti-TNF-α scFv, anti-myc and HRP conjugated anti-mouse IgG antibodies. The ECL substrate was used for the visualization of protein bands. Figure 2 represents the Western blot analysis of the expressed TNF-α in Raji cells, showing the presence of a TNF-α protein band with a molecular weight of 17 KDa.

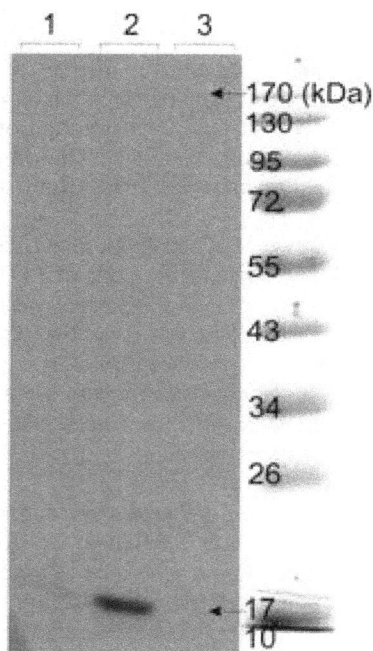

Figure 2. Western blot analysis of TNF-α in Raji cell lysates. Cultured human Raji cells were stimulated with 10 mg/mL LPS. SDS-PAGE was subjected onto cell lysates and blotted onto PVDF membrane. Lanes 1 and 3: Control. Lane 2: The detected band showing induction of the TNF-α.

FACS flow cytometry analysis for assessment of TNF-α expression

After induction of Raji cells with LPS for TNF-α expression, the cells were incubated with 1 mL of FITC labeled scFv at 1:1000 dilution for 1 h and washed with PBS containing 10% FBS. Figure 3 represents the fluorescence intensity of the TNF-α expressed by Raji cells and captured by FITC labeled scFvs.

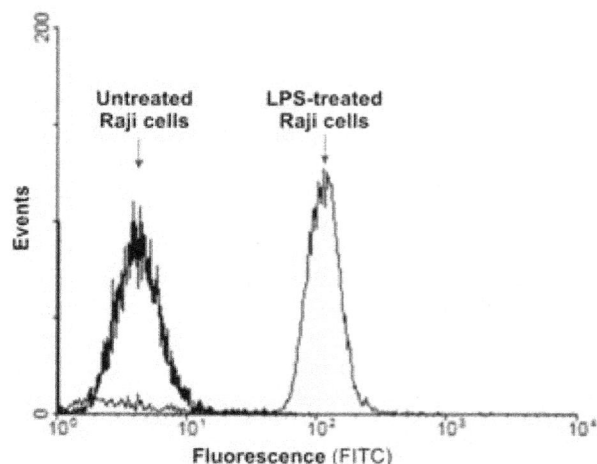

Figure 3. The fluorescence intensity of the TNF-α expressed by Raji cells and captured by FITC labeled scFvs.

Purification of TNF-α from crude protein extract

Purified scFv was coupled to CNBr-activated sepharose 4B beads and used for purification of expressed TNF-α from Raji cell lysates. After dialysis of cell lysates against PBS buffer, pH 7.4, the protein was loaded on column. The purity of eluted protein was analyzed by SDS-PAGE. The purity of protein was up to 95%. Figure 4 represents the electrophoretic pattern of purified TNF-α with CNBr-activated sepharose 4B beads, showing the major band at a molecular weight of approximately 17kDa.

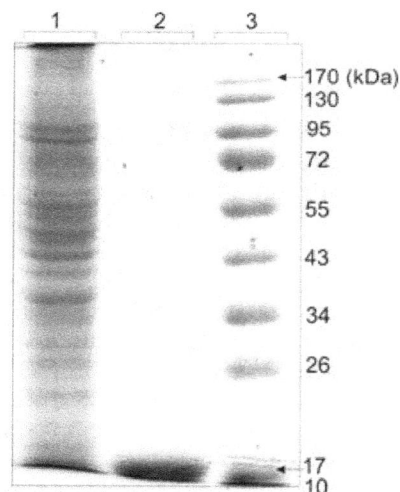

Figure 4. Electrophoretic pattern of purified TNF-α with CNBr-activated sepharose 4B beads. Expressed Raji cells lysates was dialyzed against PBS buffer, pH 7.4 and loaded on column containing coupled purified scFv-CNBr-activated sepharose 4B beads. The purity of eluted protein was analyzed by SDS-PAGE which was up to 95%. The major band at a molecular weight of approximately 17 kDa related to TNF-α protein was observed. Lane 1: Crude protein extract before chromatography, Lane 2: Pure elution fraction. Lane 3: Protein size marker. The gel was stained with Coomassie Blue R-25.

Discussion

Recombinant TNF-α has various applications in clinic as well as research studies. In clinic, it has been utilized as an antineoplastic agent either alone or in combination with chemotherapy for the treatment of patients with melanoma and sarcoma.[6-8] It targets tumor cells and suppress the tumor-associated microvasculature.[8,9] Nevertheless, it can induce vasoplegia that has some implications. Thus, its therapeutic use in clinic confined to administration through the limb perfusion.[7] In research, however it has been widely used for designing several tests such as ELISA, biopanning and Western blotting.

To produce ultra-pure TNF-α, in the current study, we have induced Raji cells with LPS to express the TNF-α. LPS simulate TNF expression through LPS dependent pathway.[16] The performance of such upstream bioprocessing (Figure 1) was further determined by Western blotting and FACS flow cytometry analysis. Western blot analysis of the TNF-α expression identified the prominent 17 kDa band as human TNF-α, representing the successful expression of TNF-α protein (Figure 2).

Having capitalized the phage display technology, we have previously produced a high affinity scFv antibody fragments against TNF-α.[10] We utilized these scFvs for detection and purification of TNF-α (Figure 1). The expression of the TNF-α in the Raji cells induced by LPS was confirmed by the FACS flow cytometry analysis through conjugation of the anti-TNF-α scFvs with FITC (Figure 3). Induction of TNF-α by LPS have been reported in different cells.[11,12,17,18]

Chromatography technology is the fundamental technique in all biopharmaceutical downstream processing. In fact, affinity chromatography has great impacts upon downstream processing of recombinant proteins that are used as effective modalities for different diseases particularly for the immunotherapy.[19-24] We harnessed the affinity chromatography using our previously produced scFvs for purification of expressed TNF-α in Raji cells. The produced scFvs through antibody phage display technology[10] was immobilized onto the CNBr-activated sepharose 4B and used for purification of expressed TNF-α. The immobilized scFvs onto the CNBr-Sepharose, as the immuno-adsorbent, can be used continuously for rapid purification of TNF-α from any biological sources. The SDS-PAGE analysis showed a high purity (over 95%) for the extracted protein in elution fraction (Figure 4).

In fact, for capturing proteins with high purity, the affinity chromatography method appears to be a simple, one-step and time-efficient approach in comparison with the other chromatography methods such as ion exchange chromatography and gel filtration.[25] We utilized this technique to produce highly pure recombinant TNF-α protein that can be applied successfully in clinic and different immunostaining methods. Thus, we propose this approach as basic technology for production of proteins therapeutics.

Conclusion

In conclusion, our results indicated that recombinant TNF-α protein successfully expressed in Raji cells and purified with the previously produced scFv, indicating that this scFv can be used effectively in affinity chromatography for production of ultra-pure recombinant TNF-α.

Acknowledgments

This study was supported by the Research Center for Pharmaceutical Nanotechnology, Tabriz University of Medical Sciences. These data are the result of Ph.D thesis registered No: 89007 in Tabriz University of Medical Sciences.

Conflict of interest

No conflict of interests to be declared.

References

1. Smyth MJ, Johnstone RW. Role of tnf in lymphocyte-mediated cytotoxicity. *Microsc Res Tech* 2000;50(3):196-208.
2. Ware CF. Network communications: Lymphotoxins, light, and tnf. *Annu Rev Immunol* 2005;23:787-819.
3. Pennica D, Nedwin GE, Hayflick JS, Seeburg PH, Derynck R, Palladino MA, et al. Human tumour necrosis factor: Precursor structure, expression and homology to lymphotoxin. *Nature* 1984;312(5996):724-9.
4. Mocellin S, Rossi CR, Pilati P, Nitti D. Tumor necrosis factor, cancer and anticancer therapy. *Cytokine Growth Factor Rev* 2005;16(1):35-53.
5. Rink L. Tumor Necrosis Factor-α. In: Delves PJ, Roitt IM, editors. Encyclopedia of Immunology. 2nd ed. Oxford: Elsevier; 1998. p. 2435-40.
6. Grunhagen DJ, de Wilt JH, ten Hagen TL, Eggermont AM. Technology insight: Utility of tnf-alpha-based isolated limb perfusion to avoid amputation of irresectable tumors of the extremities. *Nat Clin Pract Oncol* 2006;3(2):94-103.
7. Lejeune F, Ruegg C. Recombinant human tumor necrosis factor: An efficient agent for cancer treatment. *Bull Cancer* 2006;93(8):E90-100.
8. Lejeune FJ, Liénard D, Matter M, Ruegg C. Efficiency of recombinant human tnf in human cancer therapy. *Cancer Immun* 2006;6:6.
9. Corti A. Strategies for improving the anti-neoplastic activity of tnf by tumor targeting. *Methods Mol Med* 2004;98:247-64.
10. Abdolalizadeh J, Nouri M, Zolbanin JM, Baradaran B, Barzegari A, Omidi Y. Downstream characterization of anti-tnf-α single chain variable fragment antibodies. *Hum Antibodies* 2012;21(1):41-8.
11. Diya Z, Lili C, Shenglai L, Zhiyuan G, Jie Y. Lipopolysaccharide (lps) of porphyromonas

gingivalis induces il-1beta, tnf-alpha and il-6 production by thp-1 cells in a way different from that of escherichia coli lps. *Innate Immun* 2008;14(2):99-107.

12. He X, Shu J, Xu L, Lu C, Lu A. Inhibitory effect of astragalus polysaccharides on lipopolysaccharide-induced tnf-a and il-1β production in thp-1 cells. *Molecules* 2012;17(3):3155-64.

13. Harlow E, Lane D. Labeling antibodies with fluorochromes. *CSH protocols* 2006;2006(2).

14. Goding JW. Conjugation of antibodies with fluorochromes: Modifications to the standard methods. *J Immunol Methods* 1976;13(3-4):215.

15. Affinity Chromatography, Principles and Methods. Uppsala, Sweden: GE Healthcare Bio-Sciences AB; 2002.

16. Jiang C, Ting AT, Seed B. Ppar-γ agonists inhibit production of monocyte inflammatory cytokines. *Nature* 1998;391(6662):82-6.

17. Peng T, Shen E, Fan J, Zhang Y, Arnold JMO, Feng Q. Disruption of phospholipase cγ1 signalling attenuates cardiac tumor necrosis factor-α expression and improves myocardial function during endotoxemia. *Cardiovasc Res* 2008;78(1):90-7.

18. Chou YC, Sheu JR, Chung CL, Hsiao CJ, Hsueh PJ, Hsiao G. Hypertonicity-enhanced TNF-alpha release from activated human monocytic THP-1 cells requires ERK activation. *Biochim Biophys Acta* 2011;1810(4):475-84.

19. Cai R, Ye X. Preparation, purification and identification of the polyclonal antibody of phd finger protein 8. *Sheng Wu Gong Cheng Xue Bao*;26(3):393-7.

20. Loughran SaT, Loughran NB, Ryan BJ, D'Souza BN, Walls D. Modified his-tag fusion vector for enhanced protein purification by immobilized metal affinity chromatography. *Anal Biochem* 2006;355(1):148-50.

21. Steen J, Uhlen M, Hober S, Ottosson J. High-throughput protein purification using an automated set-up for high-yield affinity chromatography. *Protein Expression Purif* 2006;46(2):173-8.

22. Cass B, Pham PL, Kamen A, Durocher Y. Purification of recombinant proteins from mammalian cell culture using a generic double-affinity chromatography scheme. *Protein Expression Purif* 2005;40(1):77-85.

23. Chen C, Wang GR, Shi Q, Zhang BY, Mei GY, Li Y, et al. Preparations of the specific antibodies against exon 2 and exon 3 of human tau protein. *Zhonghua Shi Yan He Lin Chuang Bing Du Xue Za Zhi* 2009;23(2):146-8.

24. Bandehpour M, Khodabandeh M, Mosaffa N, Sharifnia Z, Ghazanfari T, Kazemi B. An efficient procedure for purification of recombinant human beta heat shock protein 90. *Daru* 2010;18(1):64-8.

25. Arnau J, Lauritzen C, Petersen GE, Pedersen J. Current strategies for the use of affinity tags and tag removal for the purification of recombinant proteins. *Protein Expression Purif* 2006;48(1):1-13.

Synthesis and Antimicrobial Evaluation of Certain Novel Thiazoles

Meesaraganda Sreedevi[1]*, Aluru Raghavendra Guru Prasad[2], Yadati Narasimha Spoorthy[1], Lakshmana Rao Krishna Rao Ravindranath[1]

[1] *Sri Krishnadevaraya Univerisity, Anantapur, Andhra Pradesh, India.*

[2] *ICFAI Foundation for Higher Education, Hyderabad, Andhra Pradesh, India.*

A R T I C L E I N F O

A B S T R A C T

Keywords:
Imidazole moiety
Thiazole moiety
Synthesis
Characterization
Antimicrobial activity

Purpose: This article makes an attempt to synthesize certain compounds containing thiazole and imidazole moieties and screen for the antimicrobial properties. *Methods*: The novel compounds synthesized were characterized by elemental analysis, IR and ¹HNMR spectral data. The antimicrobial activity of novel compounds was evaluated by cup plate method. *Results*: The compound *p*-t showed more antibacterial activity than that of the standard. *p*-hp and *p*-as showed considerable antibacterial activity. *p*-t demonstrated higher antifungal activity than that of the standard while *p*-hp and *p*-as showed considerable antifungal activity. *Conclusion*: The antimicrobial activity studies were conducted on certain selected bacteria and fungi. In each case antimicrobial activity of the compounds was compared with that of standards. *p*-t, *p*-hp, *p*-np, *p*-cp, *p*-ts and *p*-as showed considerable antimicrobial activity.

Introduction

The thiazole chemistry has been extensively developing because of their unique physiological properties. Thiazoles are stable, non-carcinogenic aromatic compounds with relatively small size. The reason being the susceptibility of reactive sites at 2-, 3- and 5-positions of the thiazole nucleus to biochemical attack during the metabolism involving reduction, hydrolysis, amination, decarboxylation of CO_2H group etc. Their wide variety of applications in medicinal chemistry has been encouraging and is reflected by the extensive literature available.[1-5] The potent medicinal significance of imidazoles is also well known.[6-9] In continuation of our effort[10] to incorporate multiple pharmacologically important moieties in a single entity, we herewith propose to synthesize novel compounds containing both imidazole and thiazole moieties.

Materials and Methods

The chemicals employed in the studies were of analytical reagent grade. Melting points were determined in open capillary tubes and were uncorrected. The infrared spectra were recorded on Perkin – Elmer KBr spectrometer. ν values were expressed in cm^{-1} ¹HNMR spectra were recorded on JEOL MODEL GSX 270 FT NMR Spectrometer and NMR 200 MHz Supercon machine, using CDCl₃ and DMSO – d₆ as solvents and TMS as an internal standard. Chemical shifts were expressed as δ values (ppm).

Results and Discussion

Synthesis and characterization of (2-methyl-5-nitro-4-phenylazo–imidazol-1-yl)-aceticacid N-(4-phenyl-thiazol-2-yl)-hydrazides 3

Phenyl aryl bromides and 3-(4ᴵ-substituted phenyl)-4-bromo acetyl sydnones were synthesized by the procedures reported in the literature.[10]

A mixture of (2-methyl-5-nitro -4-phenyl azo-imidazole-1-yl)-acetic acid hydrazide 1 (0.01 mole), potassium thiocyanate (0.02 mole), concentrated hydrochloric acid (1 mL), ethyl alcohol (10 mL) and water (20 mL) were refluxed for 3 hours. The cooled solution was filtered, the precipitate was washed with water, dried and recrystallized from ethanol-DMF mixture to yeild 2-methyl5-nitro-4-phenyl azo-imidazole-1-yl)-acete thiosemicarbazone 2. The structure of 2 was confirmed by IR and ¹HNMR spectral data.

Elemental analysis (Compound: Molecular Formula; Yield %; m.p (°C); found (cald) %.)
2: $C_{13}H_{14}N_8O_3S$; 68; 230 °C; C 43.58(43.09), H 3.67(3.89), N 31.24(30.92), O 13.46(13.25), S 8.34(8.85).

IR spectral details
The IR (KBr) spectrum of 2 showed absorption bands around 3220 cm^{-1} (NH-str), 2950 cm^{-1} (CH, str), 1679 cm^{-1} (C=O, str), 1540 cm^{-1} (C=N, str), 1610 cm^{-1} (N=N, str), 1500 cm^{-1} (asymmetric stretching, Nitro group), 1329 cm^{-1} (symmetric stretching, Nitro group).

*****Corresponding author:** Meesaraganda Sreedevi, Sri Krishnadevaraya Univerisity, Anantapur, Andhra Pradesh, India.
Email: sreedevisep@yahoo.in

¹HNMR spectral details

The ¹HNMR (200MHz) spectrum of 2 was recorded in CDCl₃+DMSO-d₆. The signals were noticed at δ 2.29 (s, 3H, CH₃), δ 4.80 (s, 2H, N-CH₂-CO), δ 3.33 (s, 2H, NH₂), δ 9.40 (s, 2H, CO-NH-NH), δ 7.4 – 7.6 (m, 5H, Ar-H).

A mixture of (2-methyl 5-nitro-4-phenyl azo-imidazole-1-yl)-acetyl thiosemicarbazone 2 (0.01 mole) in DMF (10 mL) and various bromoacetyl derivatives (0.01 mol) in ethanol (10 mL) was stirred at room temperature for 2 hours. The solid separated was filtered, dried and recrystallized from ethanol-DMF mixture. The compounds synthesized 3 have been characterized by means of IR and ¹HNMR spectral data.

The reaction sequence leading to the formation of these compounds is outlined in Scheme 1.

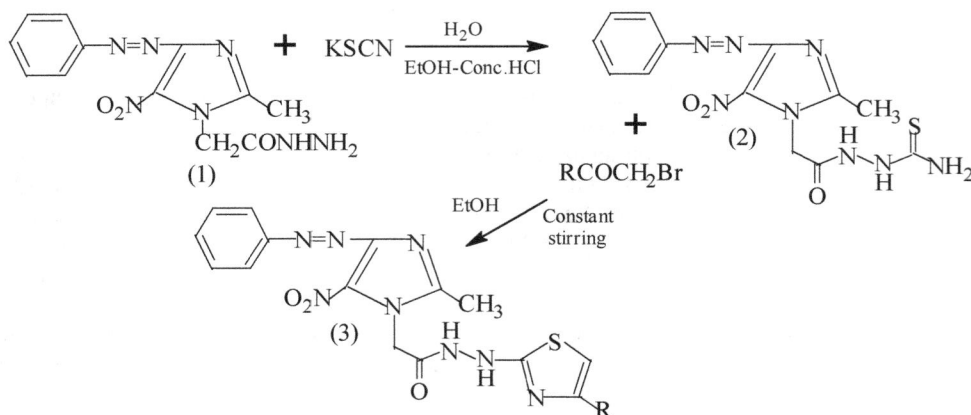

Scheme 1. *Synthesis and characterization of (2-methyl-5-nitro-4-phenylazo–imidazol-1-yl)- aceticacid-N-(4-phenyl-thiazol-2-yl)-hydrazide 3.* [R = phenyl (phe), p-tolyl (p-t), p-anisyl (p-a), p-hydroxy phenyl (p-hp), p-nitro phenyl (p-np), p-chloro phenyl (p-cp), p-bromo phenyl (p-bp), p-phenyl sydnonyl (p-ps), N-p-tolyl sydnonyl (p-ts), N-p-anisyl sydnonyl (p-as)]

Elemental analysis (Compound: R; Molecular Formula; Yield %; m.p (°C); found (cald) %.)

phe: phenyl; $C_{21}H_{18}N_8O_3S$; 66; 258; C 54.54(54.44), H 3.92(3.72), N 24.23(23.73), O 10.60 (10.39), S 6.47 (6.93).

p-t: *p*-tolyl; $C_{22}H_{20}N_8O_3S$; 45; 202; C 55.45(54.98), H 4.23(4.01), N 23.52(23.14), O 10.82 (10.08), S 6.57 (6.72).

p-a: *p*-anisyl; $C_{22}H_{20}N_8O_4S$; 54; 221; C 53.65(53.24), H 4.09(3.98), N 22.75(22.27), O 13.68 (13.01), S 6.89 (6.54).

p-hp: *p*-hydroxyphenyl; $C_{21}H_{18}N_8O_4S$; 50; 195; C 52.71(52.34), H 3.79(3.54), N 23.42(22.96), O 13.68 (13.39), S 6.49 (6.69).

p-np: *p*-nitro phenyl; $C_{21}H_{17}N_9O_5S$; 64; 232; C 49.70(49.27), H 3.38(3.16), N 24.84(24.40), O 16.47(15.78), S 6.21(6.31).

p-cp: *p*-chloro phenyl; $C_{21}H_{17}ClN_8O_3S$; 58; 193; C 50.76(50.31), H 3.45(3.23), N 22.55(22.10), O 10.65(10.22), S 6.21(82), Cl 7.99(7.55).

p-bp: *p*-bromo phenyl; $C_{21}H_{17}BrN_8O_3S$; 56; 204; C 46.59(46.13), H 3.17(2.95), N 20.70(20.31), O 9.24(8.87), S 6.31(5.92), Br 14.99(14.77).

p-ps: *p*-phenyl sydnonyl; $C_{23}H_{20}N_{10}O_5S$; 52; 197; C 50.36(49.84), H 3.68(3.43), N 25.53(25.06), O 00.00 (14.60), S 00.00 (5.84).

p-ts: *N*-*p*-tolyl sydnonyl; $C_{24}H_{22}N_{10}O_5S$; 57; 182; C 51.24(50.81), H 3.94(3.71), N 24.90(24.49), O 14.89(14.23), S 5.12(5.69).

p-as: N-*p*-anisyl sydnonyl; $C_{24}H_{22}N_{10}O_6S$; 43; 191; C 49.82 (49.45), H 3.83(3.69), N 24.21(23.78), O 17.21(16.61), S 5.12 (5.54).

IR spectral details

The IR (KBr) spectrum of (2-methyl-5-nitro-4-phenylazo–imidazol-1-yl) - aceticacid N-(4-phenyl-thiazol-2-yl)-hydrazide (phe) exhibited absorption bands at 3210 cm⁻¹ (C = O str), 1526 cm⁻¹ (C = N str). The data is given below.

IR spectral data (v in cm⁻¹):

phe: NH 3210, CH 2942, C=O 1672, C=N 1526, N=N 1612, N=O $\begin{bmatrix} 1500 \\ 1325 \end{bmatrix}$.

p-hp: NH 3230, CH 2956, C=O 1687, C=N 1546, N=N 1612, N=O $\begin{bmatrix} 1500 \\ 1329 \end{bmatrix}$.

p-np: NH 3240, CH 2960, C=O 1700, C=N 1540, N=N 1612, N=O $\begin{bmatrix} 1500 \\ 1325 \end{bmatrix}$.

p-cp: NH 3202, CH 2940, C=O 1667, C=N 1528, N=N 1612, N=O $\begin{bmatrix} 1500 \\ 1327 \end{bmatrix}$.

p-ps: NH 3256, CH 2921, C=O 1669, C=N 1539, N=N 1612, N=O $\begin{bmatrix} 1500 \\ 1325 \end{bmatrix}$, sydnone C=O str 1719.

¹HNMR spectral details
The ¹HNMR (200MHz) spectrum of (2-methyl-5-nitro-4-phenylazo–imidazol-1-yl) – acetic acid N-(4-phenyl-thiazol-2-yl)-hydrazide (phe) in $CDCl_3$ + DMSO-d_6 showed signals at δ2.30 (S, 3H, CH_3), δ7.1 (S, 1H, ArNH), δ6.5 – 6.70 (m, 5H, Ar-H), δ 7.12 – 7.36 (m, 5H, Ar-H), δ 9.2 (S, 1H, N-NH). The data is given below.
¹HNMR spectral data (δ ppm): phe: 2.30 (s, 3H, CH_3), 4.65 (s, 2H, N-CH_2-CO), 10.40 (s, 1H, CO - NH), 9.70 (s, 2H, NH-N-NH), 7.23 (s, 1H, thiazole-4H), 6.9 – 7.1 (m, 5H, Ar-H), 7.2 – 7.3 (m, 5H, Ar-H).

p-hp: 2.25 (s, 3H, CH_3), 7.90 (s, 1H, imidazole – 4H), 4.66 (s, 2H, N-CH_2-CO), 10.45 (s, 1H, CO-NH), 8.9 (s, 2H, NH – NH), 7.3 (s, 1H, thiazole – 4H), 6.9 – 7.10 (m, 5H, Ar – H), 7.3 (d, 2H, Ar – H), 7.4 (d, 2H, Ar – H), 4.3 (S, 1H, OH).

p-np: 2.30 (s, 3H, CH_3), 4.70 (s, 2H, N – CH_2 – CO), 10.35 (s, 1H, CO – NH), 9.8 (s, 2H, N – NH), 7.23 (s, 1H, thiazole – 4H), 6.9 – 7.1 (m, 5H, Ar – H), 7.3 (d, 2H, Ar – H), 7.45 (d, 2H, Ar – H).

p-cp: 2.38 (s, 3H, CH_3), 4.95 (s, 2H, NCH_2CO), 7.49 (d, 2H, *o*-protons of *p*-chlorophenyl), 7.70 (d, 2H, m-protons of *p*-chlorophenyl), 7.27 (s, 1H, thiazole – 4H), 9.69 (s, H, NH), 10.71 (s, H, CONH), 6.8-7.1 (m, 5H, Ar – H).

p-ps: 2.27 (s, 3H, CH_3), 4.66 (s, 2H, N-CH_2-CO), 7.61 – 7.81 (M, 5H, Ar – H), 7.26 (s, 1H, thiazole – 4H), 7.98 (s, 1H, imidazole – 4H), 9.85 (s, 1H, NH), 10.48 (s, 1H, CONH), 6.8 – 7.1 (m, 5H, Ar – H).

p-ts: 2.11 (s, 3H, CH_3), 2.25 (s, 3H, CH_3), 4.66 (s, 2H, N-CH_2-CO), 10.38 (s, 1H, CO-NH), 9.75 (s, 1H,N-NH) 7.25 (s, 1H, thiazole-4H), 6.8-7.1 (m, 5H, Ar-H), 7.2 (d, 2H, Ar-H), 7.4 (d, 2H, Ar-H), 7.94 (s, 1H, imidazole-4H).

Antibacterial Activity Studies
The antibacterial activity of the newly synthesized compounds was assessed by cup-plate method.[11]
The newly synthesized thiazole derivatives 3 were screened for antibacterial activity against *Escherichia coli, Pseudomonas aeruginosa, Klebsiella pneumonia and Staphylococcus aureus*. Among the compounds tested, the compound *p*-t showed more antibacterial activity than that of the standard. *p*-hp and *p*-as showed considerable antibacterial activity. The antifungal activity studies were carried out against *Candida albicans, Aspergillus flavus, Aspergillus fumigates and Trichophyton rubrum*. Among the compounds tested, *p*-t showed higher activity than that of the standard while *p*-hp and *p*-as showed considerable antifungal activity. The results are present in Table 1.

Table 1. *Details of antimicrobial studies of novel thiazoles 3.

Compound	Antibacterial activity (diameter of zone inhabitation in mm)				Antifungal activity (diameter of zone inhabitation in mm)			
	Escherichia coli	*Pseudomonas aeruginosa*	*Klebsiella pneumonia*	*Staphylococcus aureus*	*Candida albicans*	*Aspergillus flavus*	*Aspergillus fumigatus*	*Trichophyton rubrum*
p-t	23	25	25	26	22	26	24	22
p-hp	14	17	19	16	15	16	20	18
p-np	---	---	---	---	10	---	---	---
p-cp	---	14	---	---	---	12	---	09
p-ts	---	14	---	---	---	14	---	---
p-as	12	16	15	14	13	08	11	11
Ciprofloxacin (Std)	20	22	22	20	---	---	---	---
Ciclopiroxola-mine (Std)	---	---	---	---	20	22	22	20
Solvent control (DMF)	---	---	---	---	---	---	---	---

*'---' indicates that the compound is inactive.

Conclusion
The newly synthesized compounds containing thiazole and imidazole moieties 3 were characterized by elemental analysis and spectral analysis. The antimicrobial activity all compounds were evaluated and reported. Among the compounds tested, *p*-np, *p*-cp and *p*-ts showed antibacterial activity against certain microorganism only whereas *p*-t, *p*-hp and *p*-as showed considerable antibacterial activity against all the bacteria and fungi tested.

Conflict of Interest
The authors report no conflicts of interest in this work.

References
1. Luzina EL, Popov AV. Synthesis and anticancer activity of N-bis(trifluoromethyl)alkyl-N'-thiazolyl and N-bis(trifluoromethyl)alkyl-N'-benzothiazolyl ureas. *Eur J Med Chem* 2009;44(12):4944-53.

2. Wagle D, Vasan S, Egan JJ, inventors; Alteon Inc., assignee. Thiazole, imidazole and oxazole compounds and treatments of disorders associated with protein aging. USA patent 6960605. 2005 Nov 1.

3. Bharti SK, Nath G, Tilak R, Singh SK. Synthesis, anti-bacterial and anti-fungal activities of some

novel schiff bases containing 2,4-disubstituted thiazole ring. *Eur J Med Chem* 2010;45(2):651-60.

4. Rawal RK, Tripathi R, Katti SB, Pannecouque C, De Clercq E. Design, synthesis, and evaluation of 2-aryl-3-heteroaryl-1,3-thiazolidin-4-ones as anti-HIV agents. *Bioorg Med Chem* 2007;15(4):1725-31.

5. Dawane BS, Konda SG, Mandawad GG, Shaikh BM. Poly(ethylene glycol) (PEG-400) as an alternative reaction solvent for the synthesis of some new 1-(4-(4'-chlorophenyl)-2-thiazolyl)-3-aryl-5-(2-butyl-4-chloro-1H-imidazol-5yl)-2 - pyrazolines and their in vitro antimicrobial evaluation. *Eur J Med Chem* 2010;45(1):387-92.

6. Sharma D, Narasimhan B, Kumar P, Judge V, Narang R, De Clercq E, et al. Synthesis, antimicrobial and antiviral evaluation of substituted imidazole derivatives. *Eur J Med Chem* 2009;44(6):2347-53.

7. Krimer MZ, Makaev FZ, Styngach EP, Koretskii AG, Pogrebnoi SI, Kochug AI. Synthesis of substituted 2-amino-1-arylidenaminoimidazoles and 1-arylidenaminoimidazo[1,2-a]imidazoles. *Chem Heterocycl Compd* 1996; 32(9):1035-9.

8. Li WT, Hwang DR, Song JS, Chen CP, Chuu JJ, Hu CB, et al. Synthesis and biological activities of 2-amino-1-arylidenamino imidazoles as orally active anticancer agents. *J Med Chem* 2010;53(6):2409-17.

9. Ganguly S, Vithlani VV, Kesharwani AK, Kuhu R, Baskar L, Mitramazumder P, et al. Synthesis, antibacterial and potential anti-HIV activity of some novel imidazole analogs. *Acta Pharm* 2011;61(2):187-201.

10. Reddy MD, Guru Prasad AR, Spoorthy Y, Ravindranath L. Synthesis, characterization and antimicrobial activity of certain novel aryl hydrazone pyrazoline-5-ones containing thiazole moiety. *Adv Pharm Bull* 2013;3(1): 153-9.

11. Seelay HW, Van Demark PJ. Microbes in Action, A laboratory Manual in Microbiology. 2nd ed. Bombay: D.B. Taraporewala Sons and Co; 1975.

8

Thermoanalytical Investigation of Terazosin Hydrochloride

Ali Kamal Attia*, Mona Mohamed Abdel-Moety

National Organization for Drug Control and Research, P.O. Box 29, Cairo, Egypt.

A R T I C L E I N F O

Keywords:
Terazosin hydrochloride
Thermal analysis
Differential scanning calorimetry
Purity

A B S T R A C T

Purpose: Thermal analysis (TGA, DTG and DTA) and differential scanning calorimetry (DSC) have been used to study the thermal behavior of terazosin hydrochloride (TER). ***Methods:*** Thermogravimetric analysis (TGA/DTG), differential thermal analysis (DTA) and differential scanning calorimetry (DSC) were used to determine the thermal behavior and purity of the used drug. Thermodynamic parameters such as activation energy (E*), enthalpy (ΔH*), entropy (ΔS*) and Gibbs free energy change of the decomposition (ΔG*) were calculated using different kinetic models. ***Results:*** The purity of the used drug was determined by differential scanning calorimetry (99.97%) and specialized official method (99.85%) indicating to satisfactory values of the degree of purity. Thermal analysis technique gave satisfactory results to obtain quality control parameters such as melting point (273 °C), water content (7.49%) and ash content (zero) in comparison to what were obtained using official method: (272 °C), (8.0%) and (0.02%) for melting point, water content and ash content, respectively. ***Conclusion:*** Thermal analysis justifies its application in quality control of pharmaceutical compounds due to its simplicity, sensitivity and low operational costs. DSC data indicated that the degree of purity of terazosin hydrochloride is similar to that found by official method.

Introduction

Terazosin hydrochloride (TER) showed in Figure 1 is a α_1-adrenoceptor blocker with a long lasting action. α_1-adrenoceptor antagonists are clinically useful for the improvement of urinary obstruction due to benign prostatic hyperplasia (BPH), and their pharmacologic effect is mediated through the blockade of prostatic α_1-adrenoceptor.[1-3] It is used in the management of hypertension and in benign prostate hyperplasia to relieve symptoms of urinary obstruction. TER is rapidly and almost completely absorbed from the gastrointestinal tract after oral administration and is extensively metabolized in the liver to yield piprazine and three other inactive metabolites. Absorption is not affected by the presence of food. The major route of elimination is via the biliary tract and the drug is excreted in faeces (60%) and urine (40%). 10% is excreted as the parent drug and the remainder as its metabolites. Renal impairment shows no significant effect on pharmacokinetics.[4]
TER could be determined by using several analytical techniques, potentiometry,[5] voltammetry,[6,7] spectrophotometry,[8,9] fluorimetry,[10,11] and HPLC.[12-14] Thermal analysis including TGA, DTG, DTA and DSC are useful techniques that have been successfully applied in the pharmaceutical industry to reveal important information regarding the physicochemical properties of drug and excipients such as

polymorphism, stability and purity.[15-21] DSC can be used as an analytical tool of great importance for the identification and purity testing of active drugs, yielding results rapidly and efficiently. DSC has been applied for the quality control of raw materials used in pharmaceutical products.[22]

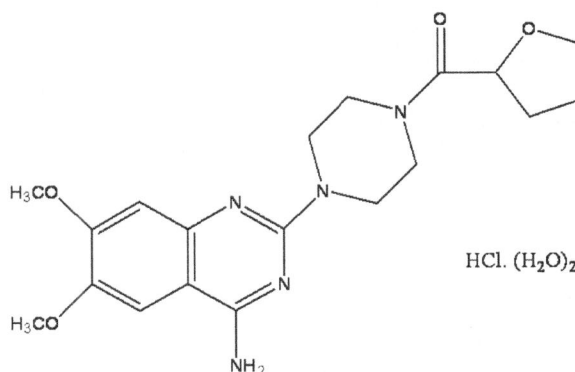

Figure 1. The molecular structure of TER

The present work represents the study of the thermal behavior of TER, in comparison with the methods employed for purity testing in the pharmaceutical industry in relation to the application of thermal techniques in the quality control of medications.

*Corresponding author: Ali Kamal Attia, National Organization for Drug Control and Research, P.O. Box 29, Cairo.
Email: alikamal1978@hotmail.com

Materials and Methods

Materials

Terazosin hydrochloride was provided from the reference standard department of NODCAR, which manufactured by Pharaonia Amriya for Pharmaceutical Company, Alexandria, Egypt. The purity of terazosin hydrochloride was found to be 99.85% and the impurities content was found to be 0.15% according to the potentiometric and liquid chromatographic methods which reported in the British pharmacopoeia, BP 2011.

Methods

The thermal analysis of TER was performed using Shimadzu thermogravimetric analyzer TGA-60H in a dynamic nitrogen atmosphere. Highly sintered α-Al_2O_3 was used as a reference. The mass losses of samples and heat response of the change of the sample were measured from room temperature up to 750 °C. The heating rate was 10 °C/min.

Thermodynamic parameters such as activation energy (E*), enthalpy (ΔH^*), entropy (ΔS^*) and Gibbs free energy change of the decomposition (ΔG^*) were obtained by using the Horowitz-Metzger and Coats-Redfern relations which applied for the first order kinetic process.[23,24]

Horowitz and Metzger Method [23]

The Horowitz-Metzger equation can be represented as follows:

$$\log.[\log \frac{W_f}{W_f - W}] = \frac{\theta.E^*}{2.303 RT_s^2} - \log 2.303$$

Where W_f was the mass loss at the completion of the decomposition reaction, W was the mass loss up to temperature T, R was the gas constant, T_s was the DTG peak temperature and $\theta = T - T_s$. A plot of log [log W_f / (W_f - W)] against θ would give a straight line and E^* could be calculated from the slope.

Coats-Redfern Method [24]

The Coats-Redfern method equation can be represented as follows:

$$\log\left(\frac{\log\left[\frac{W_f}{W_f - W}\right]}{T^2}\right) = \log\left[\frac{AR}{\phi E^*}\left(1 - \frac{2RT}{E^*}\right)\right] - \frac{E^*}{2.303 RT}$$

Where ϕ was the heating rate. Since 1- 2RT / $E^* \cong 1$, the plot of the left-hand side of equation against 1/T would give a straight line. E^* was then calculated from the slope and the Arrhenius constant (A) was obtained from the intercept.

The entropy ΔS^*, enthalpy ΔH^*, and free energy ΔG^* of activation were calculated using the following equations:

$$\Delta S^* = 2.303 \, [\log (Ah / kT)] \, R$$
$$\Delta H^* = E^* - RT$$
$$\Delta G^* = H^* - T_s \Delta S^*$$

Where k and h were the Boltzman and Planck constants, respectively. So the calculated values of E^*, ΔS^*, ΔH^*, and ΔG^* could be obtained.

DSC curves were measured on Shimadzu DSC-50 cell. Approximately 2 mg of samples was weighed and placed in a sealed aluminum pan. An empty aluminum pan was used as a reference. The purity determination was performed using a heating rate of 10 °C/min in the temperature range from 25 to 320 °C in nitrogen atmosphere with flow rate of 30 ml/min. DSC equipment was calibrated with indium.

Results and Discussion

Thermal Analysis of TER

Thermal analysis data containing thermogravimetric analysis (TGA), Derivative thermal analysis (DTG) and Differential thermal analysis (DTA) curves of the drug are shown in Figure 2. Thermal degradation pattern of TER was shown in Figure 3. The weights losses, physical and chemical changes during thermal degradation of the drug are presented in Table 1.

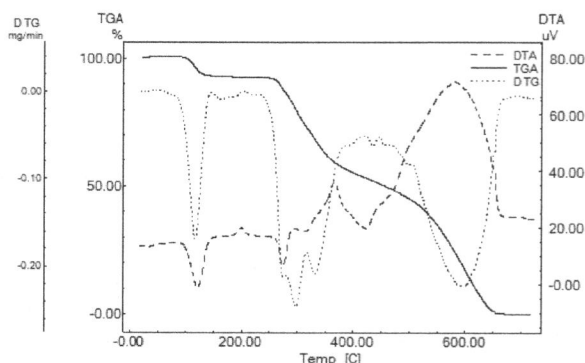

Figure 2. TGA, DTG and DTA curves of TER.

The TGA curve shows that TER is thermally decomposed in four steps. The first step occurs at 25-150 °C as a result of 7.59% estimated weight loss which may be due to the loss of two crystal water molecules. The second step occurs at 150-280 °C with about 7.71% weight loss which may be due to the loss of HCl molecule. The third step occurs in two stages at 280-320 °C with an estimated weight loss of 14.98% which may be attributed to the loss of C_4H_7O molecule and at 320-341 °C with an estimated weight loss of 6.18% which may be attributed to the loss of CO molecule. The fourth step occurs in two stages at 341-490 °C with an estimated weight loss of 18.56% which may be attributed to the loss of $C_4H_8N_2$ molecule and at 490-700 °C with an estimated weight loss of 45.31% which may be attributed to the loss of $C_{10}H_{10}N_3O_2$ molecule. The weight losses appeared in DTA as endothermic and exothermic peaks which refer to several chemical processes occur as a result of thermal degradation of the used drug at the temperature ranges were given in Table 1. These results indicate the compatibility between mass fragmentation and thermal degradation of the used drug.[4]

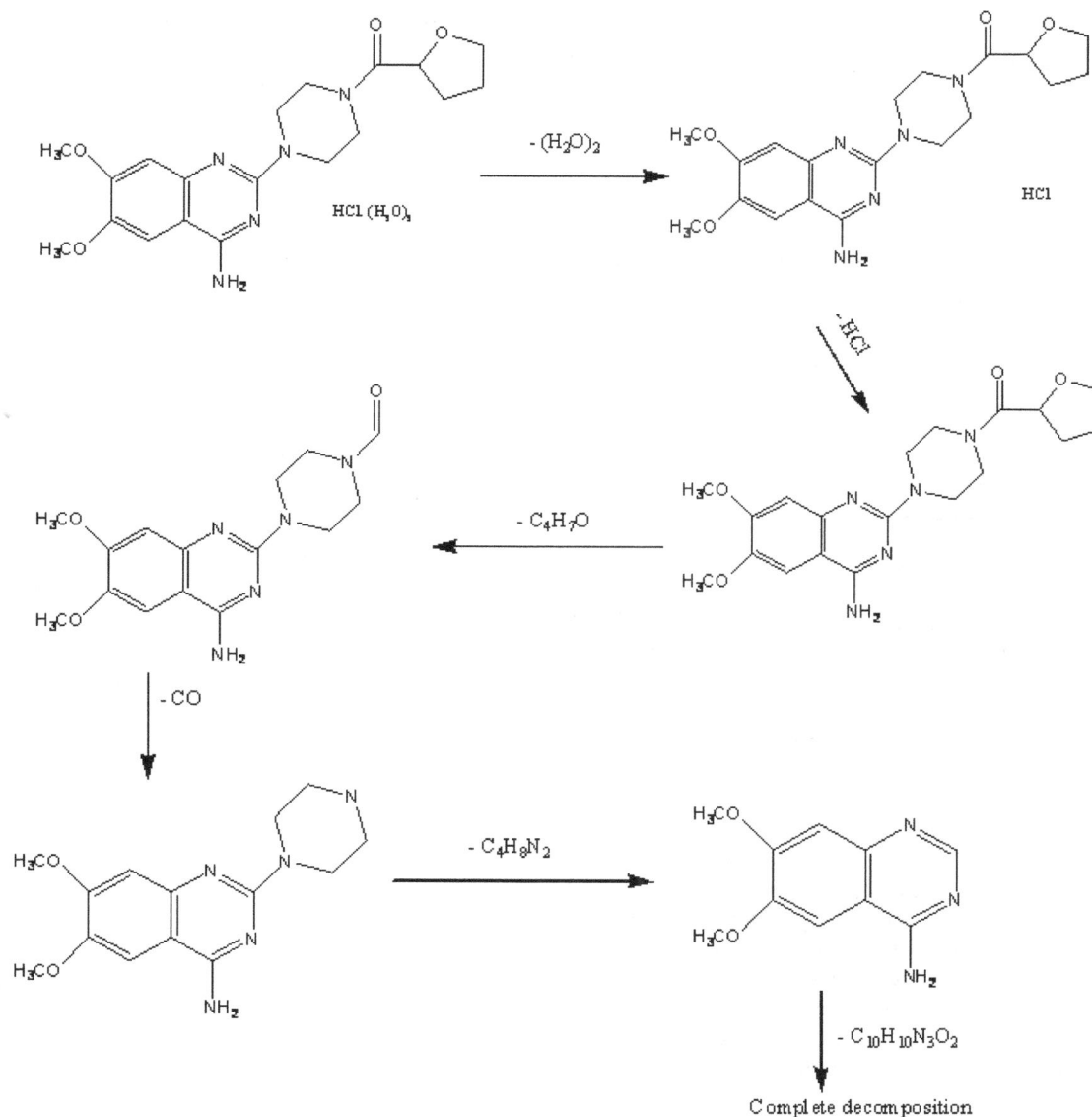

Figure 3. Thermal degradation pattern of TER.

Table 1. Thermogravimetric data (TGA, DTG and DTA) of TER.

Temperature range (°C)	DTG_{max} (°C)	Mass loss (%)	Assignment	DTA[#] (°C)
25-150	117	7.59	Loss of water molecules	119 (+)
150-280	275	7.71	Loss of HCl molecule and melting	199 (-), 273 (+)
280-320	296	14.98	Loss of C_4H_7O molecule	--------
320-341	332	6.18	Loss of CO molecule	--------
341-490	433	18.56	Loss of $C_4H_8N_2$ molecule	367 (-)
490-700	595	45.31	Loss of $C_{10}H_{10}N_3O_2$ molecule	578 (-)
# (+) = endothermic, (-) = exothermic				

Both Horowitz-Metzger (HM) and Coats-Redfern (CR) methods were applied for calculating the different thermodynamic parameters of the thermal decomposition steps of TER. The results were listed in Table 2.

Table 2. Thermodynamic parameters of the thermal decomposition of TER

Temperature range (°C)	E* (kJ/mol) HM (CR)	A (S⁻¹) HM (CR)	ΔS* (kJ/mol. K) HM (CR)	ΔH* (kJ/mol) HM (CR)	ΔG* (kJ/mol) HM (CR)
25-150	152.10 (131.47)	2.84×10^{17} (9.50×10^{16})	144.44 (77.88)	148.87 (128.23)	92.53 (97.85)
150-280	51.81 (53.42)	6.47×10^{-2} (2.41×10^{-3})	-272.78 (-300.15)	625.39 (782.71)	150.11 (165.26)
280-320	112.95 (104.70)	9.82×10^{9} (8.55×10^{8})	-59.01 (-79.31)	108.21 (99.96)	141.80 (145.09)
320-341	132.31 (121.38)	1.16×10^{11} (1.30×10^{10})	-39.02 (-57.20)	127.29 (116.34)	150.89 (150.95)
341-490	32.35 (18.80)	1.93×10 (1.14)	-227.49 (-251.05)	26.48 (12.93)	187.10 (190.17)
490-700	121.18 (99.67)	3.79×10^{6} (7.61×10^{4})	-127.87 (-160.37)	113.96 (92.45)	224.95 (231.65)

Determination of Purity of TER

DSC can be successfully used as a complementary or an alternative technique to verify purity of a compound provided that the material is at least 98% pure. Main advantages of purity analysis by DSC are minimal sample requirement and shorter analysis time as compared to chromatographic analysis.[25] Van't Hoff equation [$T_f = T_0 - [(R\ T_0^2\ X/\Delta H_f).\ 1/F]$] was used to determine the purity value, where T_f is the melting temperature of the sample, T_0 is the melting point of pure substance in Kelvin (K), R is the gas constant, ΔH_f is the heat of fusion, F is the fraction melted and X is the mole fraction of impurities. The determination of purity is based on the assumption that impurities lower the melting point of a pure substance. The melting transition of a pure, 100% crystalline substance should be infinitely sharp, but impurities or defects in the crystal structure will broaden the melting range and lower the melting point.[26]

DSC thermogram of TER is shown in Figure 4. An endothermic reaction with a broad peak at 141 °C, a weak exothermic peak at 199 °C and an endothermic sharp peak at 274 °C correspond to the loss of water molecules, the loss of HCl molecule and the drug melting, respectively. These results are in close agreement with that obtained from the DTA profile. Applying DSC method and Van't Hoff equation indicated that the sample is very pure (99.97%). This value was in close agreement with the results obtained by using the official method (99.85%) confirming low impurity content (Table 3).[27]

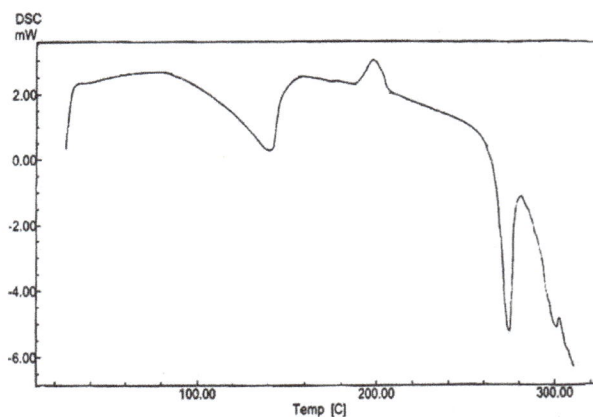

Figure 4. The DSC curve of TER.

Table 3. Melting point and degree of purity of TER.

Melting point (°C)				Degree of purity (%)	
DTA method	Melting point apparatus	DSC Method	Literature[4]	DSC Method	Official Method[27]
273	272	274	271-274	99.97%	99.85%

Thermal Analysis Application of TER

Different quality parameters such as water content and ash content were determined by using thermal analysis method. No significant difference was observed between the obtained results when compared with reported official method as shown in Table 4.[27]

Table 4. Quality control parameters obtained from the thermal analysis of TER compared with reported method

Water content (%)		Ash content (%)	
Thermal analysis method	Reported method[27]	Thermal analysis method	Reported method[27]
7.49	8.0 (7.0-8.6)	zero	0.02 (Max. 0.1%)

Conclusion

The comparison between mass fragmentation and thermal degradation of TER could show the agreement or the disagreement between the two techniques used in studying the drug fragmentation pathways. The obtained results indicate the compatibility between mass fragmentation and thermal degradation of TER. Therefore fragmentation pathway of TER was correctly determined. Thermal analysis methods are widely used in all fields of pharmaceutical sciences. These techniques are unique for the characterization of compounds and mixtures. Differential scanning calorimetry provides a satisfactory result for purity determination of the drug when compared with the official methods. Thermal analysis method might be a very useful tool to determine some quality control parameters such as water content and ash content comparing with results obtained by using the official methods.

Conflict of Interest

There is no conflict of interest in this study.

References

1. Yamada S, Suzuki M, Kato Y, Kimura R, Mori R, Matsumoto K, et al. Binding characteristics of naftopidil and alpha 1-adrenoceptor antagonists to prostatic alpha-adrenoceptors in benign prostatic hypertrophy. *Life sci* 1992;50(2):127-35.
2. Kazvabe K, Moriyama N, Yamada S, Taniguchi N. Rationale for the use of a-blockers in the treatment of benign prostatic hyperplasia (BPH). *Int J Urol* 1994;1(3): 203-11.
3. Rossi C, Kortmann BB, Sonke GS, Floratos DL, Kiemeney LA, Wijkstra H, et al. Alpha-blockade improves symptoms suggestive of bladder outlet obstruction but fails to relieve it. *J Urol* 2001;165(1):38-41.
4. Anthony CM, Osselton MD, Widdop B. Clark's Analysis of Drugs and Poisons. 3rd ed. London: Pharmaceutical Press;2004.
5. Lamie NT, Badawey AM, Abd El-Aleem AB. Membrane sensors for the selective determination of terazosin hydrochloride dihydrate in presence of its degradation product. *Int J Comprehen Pharm* 2011;2(7):1-5.
6. Atta NF, Darwish SA, Khalil SE, Galal A. Effect of surfactants on the voltammetric response and determination of an antihypertensive drug. *Talanta* 2007;72(4):1438-45.
7. Ghoneim MM, El Ries MA, Hammam E, Beltagi AM. A validated stripping voltammetric procedure for quantification of the anti-hypertensive and benign prostatic hyperplasia drug terazosin in tablets and human serum. *Talanta* 2004;64(3):703-10.
8. Sarsambi PS, Raju SA. Spectrophotometric determination of terazosin hydrochloride. *Asian J Chem* 2001;13(2):760-2.
9. Abdine HH, El-Yazbi FA, Blaih SM, Shaalan RA. Spectrophotometric and spectrofluorimetric methods for the determination of terazosin in dosage forms. *Spectrosc Lett* 1998;31(5):969-80.
10. Prasad CVN, Gautham A, Bharadwaj V, Praimoo P. Quantitative determination of terazosin HCl in tablet preparation by fluorimetry. *Indian J Pharm Sci* 1998;60(3):167-9.
11. Wang CC, Luconi MO, Masi AN, Fernandez L. Determination of terazosin by cloud point extraction-fluorimetric combined methodology. *Talanta* 2007;72(5):1779-85.
12. Srinivas JS, Avadhanulu AB, Anjaneyulu Y. HPLC determination of terazosin hydrochloride in its pharmaceutical dosage forms. *Indian Drugs* 1998;35(5):269-73.
13. Cheah PY, Yuen KH, Liong ML. Improved high-performance liquid chromatographic analysis of terazosin in human plasma. *J Chromatogr B Biomed Sci Appl* 2000;745(2):439-43.
14. Bakshi M, Ojha T, Singh S. Validated specific hplc methods for determination of prazosin, terazosin and doxazosin in the presence of degradation products formed under ich-recommended stress conditions. *J Pharm Biomed Anal* 2004;34(1):19-26.
15. Macedo RO, Nascimento TG, Veras JWE. Compatibility and stability studies of propranolol hydrochloride binary mixtures and tablets for TG and DSC photovisual. *J Therm Anal Calorim* 2002;67(2):483-9.
16. Oliveira GGG, Ferraz HG, Matos JSR. Thermoanalytical study of glibenclamide and excipients. *J Therm Anal Calorim* 2005;79(2):267-70.
17. El-Ries MA, Ahmed IS, Salem WM. The thermal analysis study of the tenoxicam. *J Drug Res* 2010;31(1):89-92.
18. Freitas MN, Alves R, Matos JR, Marchetti JM. Thermal analysis applied in the osmotic tablets pre-formulation studies. *J Therm Anal Calorim* 2007;87:905-11.
19. Yoshida MI, Gomes EC, Soares CD, Cunha AF, Oliveira MA. Thermal analysis applied to verapamil hydrochloride characterization in pharmaceutical formulations. *Molecules* 2010;15(4):2439-52.
20. Attia AK, Hassan NY, El-bayoumi A, Abdel-hamid SG. Thermoanalytical study of alfuzosin HCl. *Int J Curr Pharm Res* 2012;4(3):101-5.
21. Attia AK, Abdel-Moety MM, Abdel-hamid SG. Thermal analysis study of antihypertensive drug doxazosin mesilate. *Arab J Chem* 2012; in press.
22. Giron D. Applications of thermal analysis in the pharmaceutical industry. *J Pharm Biomed Anal* 1986;4:755-70.
23. Horowitz HH, Metzger G. A new analysis of thermogravimetric traces. *Anal Chem* 1963;35:1464-8.
24. Coats AW, Redfern JP. Kinetic parameters from thermogravimetric data. *Nature* 1964;201:68-9.

9

Extractive Spectrophotometric Determination of Ambrisentan

Namasani Santhosh Kumar[1], Avula Prameela Rani[1], Telu Visalakshi[1], Chandra Bala Sekaran[2]*

[1] University College of Pharmaceutical Sciences, Acharya Nagarjuna University, Nagarjuna nagar, India-522 510.

[2] Department of Biotechnology, Jagarlamudi Kuppuswamy Choudary College, Guntur, India - 522 006.

ARTICLE INFO

Keywords:
Ambrisentan
Methylene blue
Safranine O
Ion-Pair complex

ABSTRACT

Purpose: Ambrisentan (ABS) is an antihypertensive drug used in the treatment of pulmonary atrial hypertension. The survey of literature for ABS revealed only two spectrophotometric methods for its quantification. The reported methods lack the sensitivity. This study is aimed at developing two sensitive extractive spectrophotometric methods for the determination of ABS in bulk and in tablets. *Methods*: The proposed methods are based on the formation of colored chloroform extractable ion-pair complexes of ABS with methylene blue (MB method) and safranine O (SO method) in buffered solution at pH 9.8. The extracted complexes showed maximum absorbance at 525 and 515 nm for methylene blue and safranine O, respectively. *Results*: In both the methods, the calibration curve was linear from 1–15 μg mL^{-1} of drug. Apparent molar absorpitivities were 1.7911×10^5, 2.3272×10^5 L mol^{-1} cm^{-1}; Sandell's sensitivities were 0.0215, 0.0162 μg cm^{-2}; LOD were 0.182, 0.175 μg mL^{-1}; LOQ were 0.551, 0.531 μg mL^{-1} for methods MB and SO, respectively. The relative standard deviation and percent recovery ranged from 0.206–1.310% and 99.0–101.5%, respectively. *Conclusion*: The results demonstrate that the proposed methods are sensitive, precise, accurate and inexpensive. These methods can easily be used for the assay of ABS in quality control laboratories.

Introduction

Ambrisentan (ABS), a non-peptide, is a highly selective endothelin-1 type A receptor antagonist.[1-5] ABS belongs to antihypertensive class of drugs and used in the treatment of pulmonary atrial hypertension in patients with WHO Class II or III symptoms. Endothelin is a peptide that constricts blood vessels and elevates blood pressure. ABS blocks the effects of endothelin-1 and thus decreases blood pressure in lungs. The thickening of blood vessels in the lungs and heart is also inhibited by ABS. ABS is chemically known as (2S)-2-(4,6-dimethylpyrimidin-2-yloxy)-3-methoxy-.3,3- diphenylpropionic acid (Figure 1).

To the best of our knowledge, the assay of ABS is not official in pharmacopoeias. Due to the vital significance of the ABS, the development of a sensitive, simple and fast method for its quantification is of significant need. The detailed survey of literature revealed that very few methods have been reported for the estimation of ABS. Douša and Gibala developed and validated highperformance liquid chromatography (HPLC) method for the determination of ABS enantiomers. Enantioseparation was achieved on Chiralcel OZ-3R (cellulose 3-chloro-4-methylphenylcarbamate) using mixture of 20 mM sodium formate (pH 3.0) with acetonitrile (55:45; *v/v*).[6] Ramakrishna et al. reported a HPLC–positive ion electrospray tandem mass spectrometry method for the quantification of ABS in plasma using armodafinil as

internal standard.[7] This method was applied to quantify ABS concentration in a rodent pharmacokinetic study.

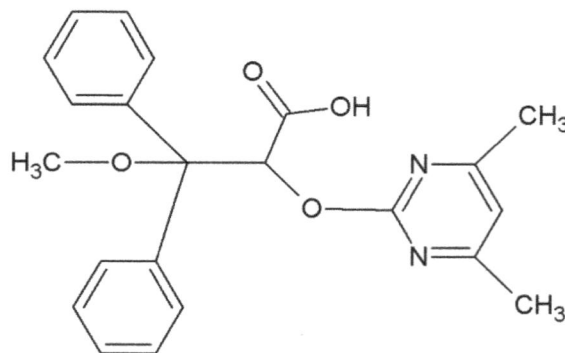

Figure 1. Structure of ambrisentan.

Spectrophotometric method of analysis is extensively used in the analysis of drugs in pharmaceutical formulations owing to its good sensitivity, selectivity and cost effectiveness. Ambrisentan can be estimated by using UV spectroscopy in tablets. But the selectivity of the method is less because the interference from the tablet excipients increases in UV region. Two visible spectrophotometric methods have been reported for the assay of ABS by Vinaya Kumar et al.[8] The first method is based on the reaction between ABS and 1,2-naphthoquinone-4-sulphonate.[8] The second method is

*Corresponding author: Chandra Bala Sekaran, Department of Biotechnology, Jagarlamudi Kuppuswamy, Choudary College, Guntur, Andhra Pradesh-522006. Email: balumphil@gmail.com

based on the oxidation of ABS by ammonium metavanadate in presence of H_2SO_4.[8] Beer's law is obeyed in the concentration ranges between 10-60 and 10-50 µg/mL ABS for 1,2-naphthoquinone-4-sulphonate (first method) and ammonium metavanadate (second method), respectively. The reported visible spectrophotometric methods are associated with lack of sensitivity.

Methylene blue[9-12] (MB) and safranin O[12-15] (SO) have been used as ion-pair complexing dyes in the development of extractive spectrophotometric method for the determination of many pharmaceutical compounds. The present study is aimed to investigate the ion-pair complexation of ABS with MB (MB method) and SO (SO method) at pH 9.8, and employment of this reaction in the development of two new simple and sensitive extractive spectrophotometric methods for the determination of ABS in bulk and in its pharmaceutical dosage forms.

Materials and Methods
Instrumentation
A systronics (Ahemadabad, India) digital double beam UV-Visible spectrophotometer, model Visiscan-167 with 1 cm matched quartz cell is used for the spectral and absorbance measurements. A Shimazdu (Tokyo, Japan) electronic weighing balance, model BL 220 H is used for weighing the samples.

Chemicals and Reagents
Standard Sample and Tablets
ABS Standard was kindly donated by MSN laboratories, Hyderabad, India. Letairis tablets (Gilead Sciences, Inc., CA, US) labeled to contain 10 mg ABS per tablet were employed in the present study.

Stock and Working Standard Solutions
The ABS stock solution (1 mg/mL) was prepared by dissolving 100 mg of the ABS in 20 mL of 0.1 N NaOH (Fisher Scientific, Mumbai, India) and then diluted to 100 mL with distilled water. The ABS stock solution was diluted with distilled water to get working concentration of 100 µg/mL ABS for MB and SO methods.

Dye Solutions (0.1% MB and 0.05% SO)
Aqueous solutions of 0.1% MB (Fisher Scientific, Mumbai, India) and 0.05% SO (Sdfine-Chem limited, Mumbai, India) were prepared for methods MB and SO, respectively.

Buffer
Ammonia-ammonium chloride buffer solution (pH 9.8) was prepared by mixing 7 g of ammonium chloride (Sdfine-Chem limited, Mumbai, India) with 56.8 mL of 25% liquor ammonia (Merck, Mumbai, India) and diluted to 100 mL with distilled water and pH was adjusted to 9.8.

General Procedure
To a set of 125 mL separating funnels, aliquot volumes (0.1-1.5 mL) containing the ABS in the working concentration range of 1-15 µg/mL were transferred. The volume in each funnel was adjusted to 1.5 mL with 0.1 N NaOH. To each funnel 2 mL of buffer (pH 9.8) followed by 1 mL dye solution [0.1% MB in MB method or 0.05 % SO in SO method] were added and mixed well. The funnels were shaken vigorously with 5 mL of chloroform (Merck, Mumbai, India) for 2 min. The funnels were allowed to stand at room temperature for the clear separation of the two phases. The separated colored organic phase was transferred into a 10 mL volumetric flask, made up to the mark with chloroform and mixed well. The absorbance of the colored organic phase was measured at 525 and 515 nm against the corresponding reagent blank for methods MB and SO, respectively. In both the methods, the calibration graphs were constructed by plotting the absorbance versus the final concentration of the ABS (µg/mL). On the other hand, the corresponding regression equation was derived.

Procedure for Letairis Tablets
The content of twenty tablets of Letairis was weighed. An exactly weighted portion equivalent to 100 mg ABS was transferred into a beaker and then 25 mL of methanol (Merck, Mumbai, India) was added. The solution was shaken for 20 minutes. The solution was filtered using Whatman No. 1 filter paper. The filtrate was evaporated to dryness on a water bath. Then, the residue was transferred into a 100 mL calibrated flask containing 20 ml of 0.1 N NaOH and mixed well. The beaker was washed with few ml of 0.1 N NaOH to make use of the residue completely without any wastage. The washings were transferred to the flask and the volume was made up to the mark with distilled water. Suitable aliquots of the ABS solution (100 µg/mL) were used for analysis and treated as described in the above methods MB and SO. The recovery of ABS was calculated from either the corresponding linear regression equation or the calibration curve.

Validation of the Proposed Methods
According to ICH guidelines,[16] the proposed methods were validated for linearity, sensitivity, precision, accuracy and robustness.

For assessment of linearity, determination of ABS was done at six concentration levels (1, 3, 6, 9, 12, and 15 µg/mL) by the proposed methods. Least square regression analysis was carried out for calculating the slope, intercept and regression coefficient values.

The sensitivity parameters such as molar absorptivity, Sandell's sensitivity, limit of detection (LOD) and limit of quantification (LOQ) for ABS in each proposed method were calculated.

The precision and accuracy of the proposed methods were evaluated by performing five replicate analysis of pure ABS solution at three different concentrations (2,

8 and 14 µg/mL) on the same day and in three consecutive days for intra- and inter-day studies, respectively. The precision is expressed as standard deviation and relative standard deviation while accuracy is expressed as percent recovery and percent error. The accuracy and validity of the proposed methods were further assessed by recovery studies. Recovery studies were performed using the standard addition method. The recovery studies were carried out by measuring percent recovery using powdered tablets spiked with ABS at three different concentration levels (50, 100 and 150% of the labeled claim).

The robustness of the proposed methods was established by the constancy of the absorbance with the deliberated minor changes in the experimental parameters such as change in pH (9.8± 0.1), change in the volume of buffer (2 ± 0.2 mL) and change in the volume of 0.1% MB (1 ± 0.1 mL) for MB method. For SO method these changes include; change in pH (9.8 ± 0.1), change in the volume of the buffer (2 ± 0.2 mL) and change in the volume of 0.05 % SO (1 = 0.1 mL).

Results and Discussion

An ion-pair complex consists of a positive ion and a negative ion bonded together by the electrostatic force of attraction between them at suitable pH. The ion pair complex is extractable into organic solvents from aqueous phase. In the recent years, ion pair complex extraction has been applied to the estimation of numerous compounds using extractive spectrophotometric method.[17-21] A major advantage of the extractive spectrophotometric method is that they

can be applied to the assay of individual substances in a complex mixture with high sensitivity.

Basic dyes such as MB and SO have been used as ion-pair complexing dyes in the development of extractive spectrophotometric method for determination of many pharmaceutical compounds with carboxylic group.[9-15] Since ABS contains a carboxylic group in its structure, it reacts with MB (MB method) and SO (SO method) in ammonia-ammonium chloride buffer (pH 9.8) to give colored chloroform soluble ion-pair complexes [ABS-MB (MB method) and ABS-SO (SO method)], which exhibit absorption maxima at 525 and 515 nm for MB and SO, respectively (Figure 2).

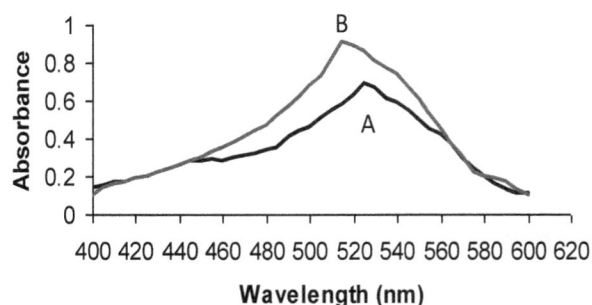

Figure 2. Absorption spectrum: A) ABS-MB ion-pair complex (λ_{max} – 525 nm), B) ABS-SO ion pair complex (λ_{max} – 515 nm).

Under the experimental conditions, the colorless blanks have virtually negligible absorbance. ABS-MB and ABS-SO ion-pair complexes were found to be stable at the room temperature approximately for 1 and 2 hr, respectively. The possible reaction mechanism was based on the reported methods is given in Figures 3 and 4.[9-15]

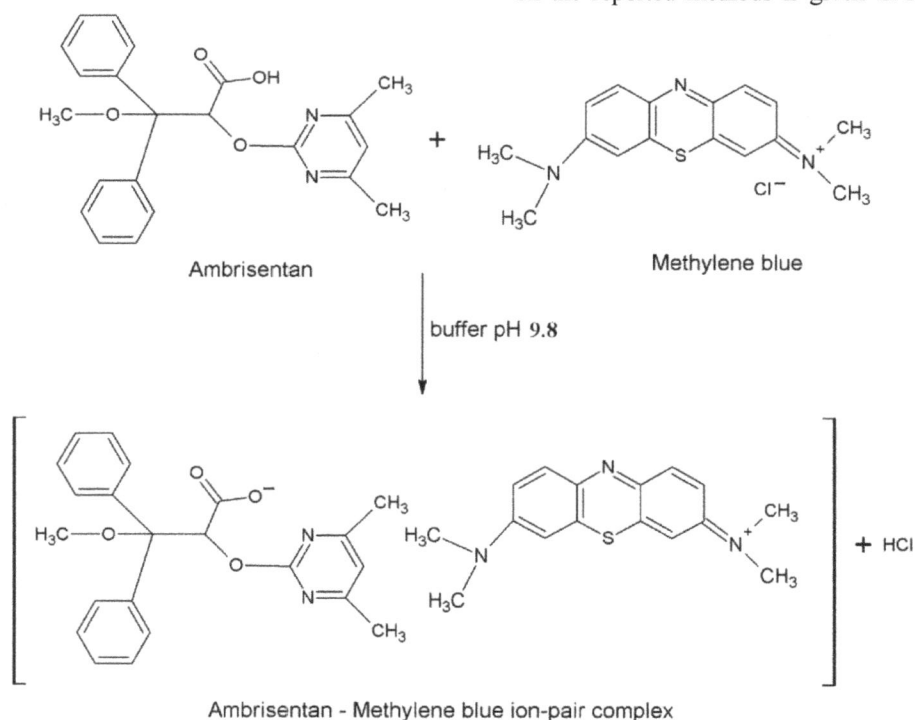

Ambrisentan - Methylene blue ion-pair complex

Figure 3. Ion pair complexation of ambrisentan with methylene blue.

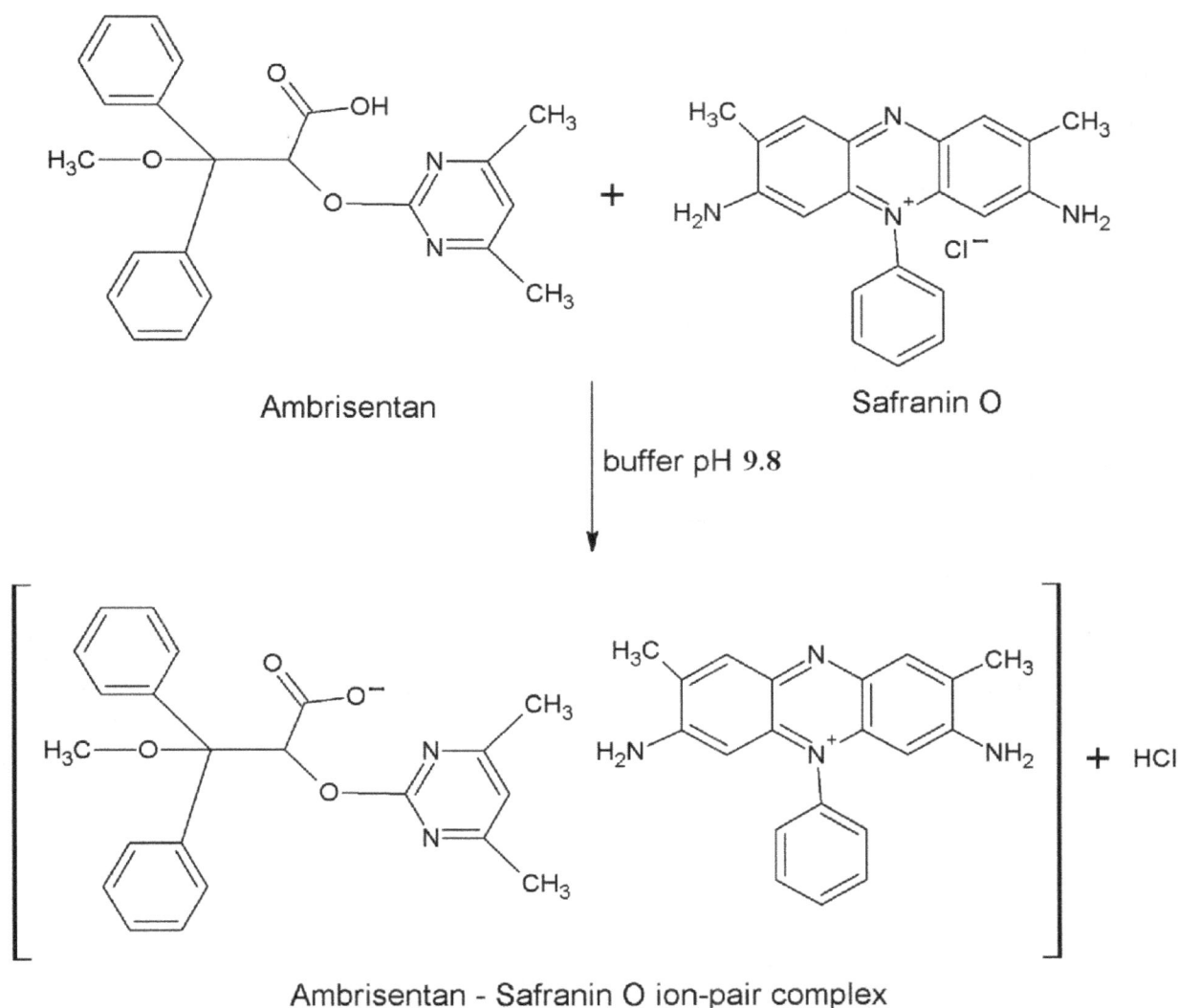

Ambrisentan   +   Safranin O

buffer pH 9.8

Ambrisentan - Safranin O ion-pair complex

Figure 4. Ion pair complexation of ambrisentan with safranin O.

Optimization of the Methods

In order to optimize the developed MB and SO methods, the effect of experimental parameters such as, dye concentration, pH of the buffer, volume of buffer and extraction solvent, on the formation of ABS-MB and ABS-SO ion-pair complexes has been tested.

Effect of Concentration of Methylene Blue (MB Method) and Safranine O (SO Method)

The influence of the concentration of MB (MB method) or SO (SO method) was studied by treating 10 μg/mL ABS with 2 mL of buffer and varying volumes (0.2–2.0 mL) of 0.1% MB or 0.05% SO. The absorbance of the ABS-MB and ABS-SO ion-pair complexes was increased with increasing volume of 0.2% MB and 0.05% SO, respectively and became constant at 1.0 mL; above this volume, the absorbance remained unchanged (Figure 5). Therefore, 1 mL of 0.2% MB (MB method) and 0.05% SO (SO method) dye solution was chosen as the optimal volume for the quantification process.

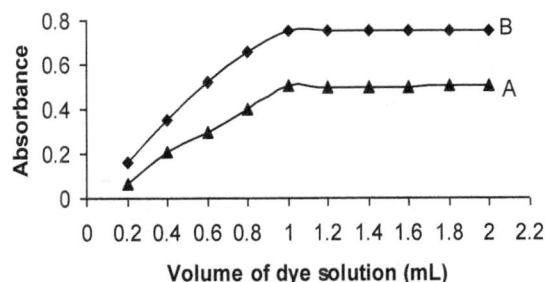

Figure 5. Effect of volume of dye solution: A) 0.1% Mb solution (λ_{max} – 525 nm), B) 0.05% SO solution (λ_{max} – 515 nm).

Effect of PH

At a fixed concentration of ABS (10 μg/mL), the formation of ABS-MB (MB method) and ABS-SO (SO method) ion-pair complexes were investigated over the pH range of 8.0-11.0 using ammonia-ammonium chloride buffer. The absorbance of the ion-pair complexes in both the methods varies only slightly between pH 8-9.8. However the absorbance at pH 9.8 is slightly higher than the absorbance at other pH values.

After pH 9.8, the absorbance decreases (Figure 6). Therefore, pH 9.8 was selected as the optimum pH for the reaction.

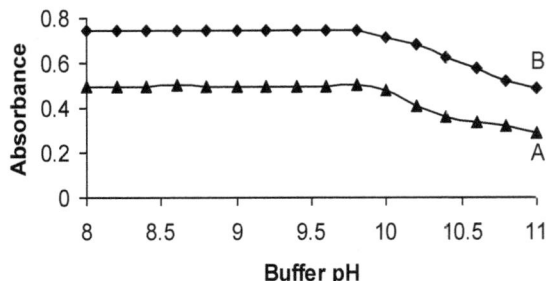

Figure 6. Effect of buffer pH: A) ABS-MB ion-pair complex (λ_{max} – 525 nm), B) ABS-SO ion pair complex (λ_{max} – 515 nm).

Effect of Volume of Buffer

The influence of the volume of ammonia-ammonium chloride buffer (pH 9.8) on the absorbance value of the ion-pair complexes was studied by treating 10 µg/mL ABS with varying volumes (0.5–4.0 mL) of buffer and 1 mL of 0.1% MB (MB method) or 0.05% SO (SO method). As shown in Figure 7, 2 mL of ammonia-ammonium chloride buffer (pH 9.8) was sufficient to get the optimum pH value (pH 9.8). Therefore, 2 mL was chosen as the optimum buffer volume.

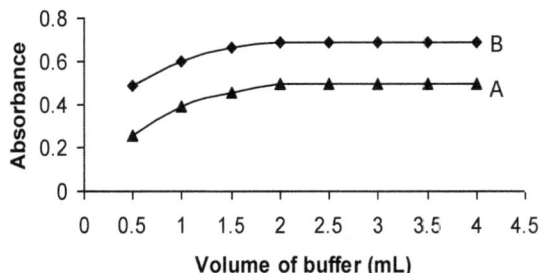

Figure 7. Effect of buffer volume: A) ABS-MB ion-pair complex (λ_{max} – 525 nm), B) ABS-SO ion pair complex (λ_{max} – 515 nm).

Effect of Extraction Solvent

The effect of extraction solvent was tested using different solvents such as chloroform, benzene, dichloromethane and butanol. Using chloroform as extraction solvent, the ion-pair complexes showed the highest absorbance value and reproducibility. Therefore, chloroform was chosen as the best extraction solvent for extraction of ABS-MB and ABS-SO ion-pair complexes.

Method Validation

Calibration curve was constructed by plotting the absorbance *vs* concentration of ABS. Linearity was found to be 1-15 µg/mL ABS for MB and SO methods. The linear regression equations for MB and SO methods were:

MB method: y = 0.0458x + 0.0095 ($R^2 = 0.9991$)
SO method: y = 0.0602x + 0.0140 ($R^2 = 0.9999$)
Where y is absorbance and x is the concentration of ABS (µg/mL)

Sensitivity of the proposed methods was evaluated by molar absorptivity, Sandell's sensitivity, LOD and LOQ. The results, presented in Table 1, indicated the high sensitivity of the proposed methods.

Table 1. Sensitivity parameters of the propose methods.

Parameters	Method	
	MB	SO
Molar Absorbtivity(L mole^{-1} cm^{-1})	1.7911×10^5	2.3272×10^5
Sandell's sensitivity(µg cm^{-2}/0.001 Absorbance unit)	0.0215	0.0162
LOD (µg mL^{-1})	0.182	0.175
LOQ (µg mL^{-1})	0.551	0.531

The intra day and inter day assays were performed by conducting five replicate analyses of ABS at the 2, 8 and 14 µg/mL concentration levels using the proposed methods on one day and on three consecutive days. The results are summarized in Table 2. The standard deviation, relative standard deviation, percent recovery and percent error values can be considered to be very reasonable. Thus the proposed methods are precise and accurate.

Table 2. Precision and accuracy of the proposed methods.

Method	Assay type	Concentration of ABS (µg mL^{-1})		RSD (%)	Recovery (%)	Error (%)
		Taken	Found ± SD[a]			
MB	Intra-day	2	1.98 ± 0.013	0.656	99.00	1.00
		8	7.94 ± 0.041	0.516	99.25	0.75
		14	13.93 ± 0.044	0.315	99.50	0.50
	Inter-day	2	1.98 ± 0.017	0.858	99.00	1.00
		8	7.95 ± 0.053	0.666	99.37	0.63
		14	13.92 ± 0.092	0.660	99.42	0.58
SO	Intra-day	2	2.03 ± 0.027	1.310	101.50	1.50
		8	7.97 ± 0.054	0.654	99.62	0.38
		14	14.03 ± 0.029	0.206	101.21	1.21
	Inter-day	2	1.98 ± 0.021	1.076	99.00	1.00
		8	8.04 ± 0.048	0.592	100.50	0.50
		14	13.94 ± 0.098	0.703	99.57	0.43
a-Average of five determinations						

The accuracy and validity of the proposed methods were further assessed by performing recovery studies using standard addition technique. The results are presented in the Table 3. The recovery of pure ABS added indicates that common excipients did not interfere in the assay procedures. The results obtained were reproducible with low relative standard deviation.

Table 3. Recovery results of ABS by the proposed methods.

| Method | Concentration of ABS (mg) | | | RSD (%) | Recovery (%) |
	Tablet	Pure drug added	Total found ± SD[a]		
MB	10	5	15.08 ± 0.121	0.802	100.53
	10	10	19.86 ± 0.175	0.881	99.30
	10	15	25.15 ± 0.260	1.033	100.60
SO	10	5	14.96 ± 0.118	0.788	99.73
	10	10	20.10 ± 0.096	0.477	100.50
	10	15	24.97 ± 0.184	0.736	99.88
a-Average of three determinations					

The robustness of the proposed methods was investigated by making small intentional changes in the experimental parameters at two different concentration levels (2 and 14 µg/mL). The results (Table 4) revealed that the slight changes expected to take place did not adversely influence the absorbance intensity.

Table 4. Robustness of the proposed methods.

| Method | Experimental Parameter | | ABS Taken (2 µg mL^{-1}) | | ABS Taken (14 µg mL^{-1}) | |
			Absorbance	RSD (%)	Absorbance	RSD (%)
MB	0.1% MB (mL)	0.9	0.101		0.634	
		1.0	0.104	1.666	0.638	0.470
		1.1	0.103		0.640	
	Buffer pH	9.7	0.100		0.628	
		9.8	0.104	1.960	0.631	0.270
		9.9	0.102		0.630	
	Buffer volume (mL)	1.8	0.099		0.632	
		2.0	0.101	1.700	0.635	0.315
		2.2	0.102		0.636	
SO	0.05% SO (mL)	0.9	0.132		0.838	
		1.0	0.134	1.278	0.842	0.238
		1.1	0.135		0.841	
	Buffer pH	9.7	0.134		0.836	
		9.8	0.137	1.111	0.840	0.309
		9.9	0.135		0.841	
	Buffer volume (mL)	1.8	0.128		0.842	
		2.0	0.129	0.781	0.848	0.355
		2.2	0.129		0.846	

Application to Letairis Tablets

Applicability of the proposed methods was evaluated by determination of ABS in its dosage form, Letairis tablets. The results are presented in Table 5. Excellent recoveries with low SD and RSD values were obtained. Common excipients present in the tablet dosage form did not interfere with the assay in the two applied methods.

Conclusion

Two simple, rapid, accurate, precise and robust extractive spectrophotometric methods were developed for the estimation of ABS, using MB and SO as ion-pair complexing dyes, in bulk drug and in tablet. The reagents used in the proposed methods are cheaper and readily available. The developed methods have the advantages over the reported spectrophotometric methods in being more sensitive, stable colored complex, robust, precise and accurate. Furthermore, the developed methods are inexpensive and do not require sophisticated instrumentation & elaborate treatments allied with chromatographic methods. Therefore, the proposed methods can be used for the routine analysis of ABS in quality control laboratories.

Table 5. Analysis of tablet dosage form by the proposed methods.

Formulation	Labelled claim (mg)	Method	Found ± SD[a]	RSD (%)	Recovery (%)
Letairis	10	MB	9.96 ± 0.098	0.968	99.60
		SO	10.04 ± 0.071	0.707	100.40
a: Average of five determinations					

Acknowledgements

The authors, Namasani Santhosh Kumar and Telu Visalakshi, express their gratitude to the principal, University College of Pharmaceutical Sciences, Acharya Nagarjuna University, Nagarjuna nagar, Andhra Pradesh for providing research facilities.

Conflict of Interest

The authors report no conflicts of interest in this work.

References

1. Frampton JE. Ambrisentan. *Am J Cardiovasc Drugs* 2011;11(4): 215-26.
2. Galie N, Olschewski H, Oudiz RJ, Torres F, Frost A, Ghofrani HA, et al. Ambrisentan for the treatment of pulmonary arterial hypertension: results of the ambrisentan in pulmonary arterial hypertension, randomized, double-blind, placebo-controlled, multicenter, efficacy (ARIES) study 1 and 2. *Circulation* 2008;117(23):3010-9.
3. Oudiz RJ, Galie N, Olschewski H, Torres F, Frost A, Ghofrani HA, et al. Long-term ambrisentan therapy for the treatment of pulmonary arterial hypertension. *J Am Coll Cardiol* 2009;54(21):1971-81.
4. Vatter H, Seifert V. Ambrisentan, a non-peptide endothelin receptor antagonist. *Cardiovasc Drug Rev* 2006;24(1):63-76.
5. Klinger JR, Oudiz RJ, Spence R, Despain D, Dufton C. Long-term pulmonary hemodynamic effects of ambrisentan in pulmonary arterial hypertension. *Am J Cardiol* 2011;108(2):302-7.
6. Dousa M, Gibala P. Rapid determination of ambrisentan enantiomers by enantioselective liquid chromatography using cellulose-based chiral stationary phase in reverse phase mode. *J Sep Sci* 2012;35(7):798-803.
7. Nirogi R, Kandikere V, Komarneni P, Aleti R, Padala N, Kalaikadhiban I. LC-ESI-MS/MS method for quantification of ambrisentan in plasma and application to rat pharmacokinetic study. *Biomed Chromatogr* 2012;26(10):1150-6.
8. Vinaya Kumar Y, Murali D, Rambabu C. New visible spectrophotometric methods for determination of ambrisentan. *Bull Pharm Res* 2010;1(S): 194.
9. Duan YL, Du LM, Chen CP. Study on extractive spectrophotometry for determination of amoxicillin with ionic associate. *Guang pu xue yu guang pu fen xi* 2005;25(11):1865-7.
10. Koh T, Okazaki T, Ichikawa M. Spectrophotometric of determination of gold(III) by formation of dicyanoaurate(I) and its solvent extraction with methylene blue. *Anal Sci* 1986;2:249-53.
11. Kishore M, Jayaprakash M, Vijayabhaskara Reddy T. Spectrophotometric determination of azelaic acid in pharmaceutical formulations. *J Pharm Res* 2010;3(12):3090-2.
12. Krishna MV, Sankar DG. Spectrophotometric determination of gemifloxacin mesylate in pharmaceutical formulations through ion-pair complex formation. *E J Chem* 2008;5(3):515-20.
13. Madhavi L, Shireesha M, Tuljarani G. Spectrophotometric estimation of valsartan and benazepril hydrochloride in pure and pharmaceutical formulations. *Int J ChemTech Res* 2011;3(4):1830-4.
14. Sharma S, Sharma MC. Extractive spectrophotometric methods for the determination of emtricitabine in dosage form using safranin O. *Am-Euras J Toxicol Sci* 2011;3(3):138-42.
15. Prajapati PB, Bodiwala KB, Marolia BP, Rathod IS, Shah SA. Development and Validation of Extractive spectrophotometric method for determination of Rosuvastatin calcium in pharmaceutical dosage forms. *J Pharm Res* 2010;3(8):2036-8.
16. International Conference on Harmonization of Technical Requirements for Registration of Pharmaceuticals for Human Use, ICH Harmonised Tripartite Guidelines, Validation of Analytical Procedures: Text and Methodology Q2 (R1), Current Step 4 version, Nov. 1996, Geneva, Nov. 2005.
17. Li XM, Chen ZP, Wang SP, Tang J, Liu CY, Zou MF. Extractive spectrophotometric determination of trodat-1 hydrochloride in lyophilized kit. *Pharmazie* 2008;63(9):638-40.
18. Chaple DR, Bhusari KP. Spectrophotometric estimation of fluroquinolones as ion-pairs with bromocresol green in bulk and pharmaceutical dosage form. *Asian J Chem* 2010;22(4):2593-8.
19. Ulu ST, Aydogmus Z. A new spectrophotometric method for the determination of tianeptine in tablets using ion-pair reagents. *Chem Pharm Bull (Tokyo)* 2008;56(12):1635-8.
20. Basavaiah K, Zenita O. Spectrophotometric determination of famotidine using sulphonphthalein dyes. *Quim Nova* 2011;34(5):735-44.
21. Sridevi N, Jahnavi G, Sekaran CB. Spectrophotometric analysis of perindopril erbumine in bulk and tablets using bromophenol blue. *Der Pharmacia Lettre* 2012;4(1):159-69.

10

Toxicity Effect of *Nigella Sativa* on the Liver Function of Rats

Mohammad Aziz Dollah[1], Saadat Parhizkar[2]*, Latiffah Abdul Latiff[3], Mohamad Hafanizam Bin Hassan[1]

[1] *Biomedical Department, Faculty of Medicine and Health Sciences, University Putra Malaysia, Selangor, Malaysia.*

[2] *Medicinal Plants Research Centre, Yasuj University of Medical Sciences (YUMS), Yasuj, Iran.*

[3] *Community Health Department, Faculty of Medicine and Health Sciences, University Putra Malaysia, Selangor, Malaysia.*

ARTICLE INFO

Keywords:
Enzyme
Liver
Function
Nigella sativa
Toxicity
Rat

ABSTRACT

Purpose: The aim of this study was to determine the toxic effect of Nigella sativa powder on the liver function which was evaluated by measuring liver enzymes and through histopathological examination of liver tissue. *Methods:* Twenty four male Sprague Dawley rats were allotted randomly to four groups including: control (taking normal diet); low dose (supplemented with 0.01 g/kg/day Nigella sativa); normal dose (supplemented with 0.1 g/kg/day Nigella sativa) and high dose (supplemented with 1 g/kg/day Nigella sativa). All of supplements administered in powder form mixed with rats' pellet for 28 days. To assess liver toxicity, liver enzymes measurement and histological study were done at the end of supplementation. *Results:* The finding revealed that there was no significant change in serum alanine aminotransferase (ALT) and aspartate aminotransferase (AST) between treatment groups. Histopathological study showed very minimal and mild changes in fatty degeneration in normal and high doses of Nigella sativa treated group. Inflammation and necrosis were absent. *Conclusion:* The study showed that supplementation of Nigella sativa up to the dose of 1 g/kg supplemented for a period of 28 days resulted no changes in liver enzymes level and did not cause any toxicity effect on the liver function.

Introduction

Herbal medicines have been used by human for thousands years to treat medical illness or to improve physical performance. Plants have been always a major source of nutrition and health care for both humans and animals.[1] In recent years, there has been growing interest in alternative therapies and the therapeutic use of natural products, especially those derived from plants.[2] Despite the move toward synthetic medicine and use of sophisticated drugs, traditional plant-based remedies still play an important role in the world's medicine.[3] Extremely, 80% of the world's population use plant-based remedies as their primary form of healthcare and the world market of herbal medicines based on traditional knowledge are estimated at USD 60 thousand million.[4] *Nigella sativa* (Black seed) is an annual plant belongs to the botanical family of Ranunculaceae[5] (Figure 1 A,B) and commonly grows in Europe, Middle East and Western Asia. *Nigella sativa* (NS) is usually used as a traditional medicine in Arabian countries,[6] Indian sub-continent and Europe,[7] for a wide range of therapeutic purpose including immunomodulative,[8] antibacterial,[9] anti-tumor,[10] diuretic and hypotensive,[11] genoprotective,[12] hepato-protective and antidiabetic[11] as well as bronchodilator activity[8] and estrogenic activity.[13] Since 1970 to 2001,

about 530 studies have been conducted on the *Nigella sativa* and only 3.4% concern about its toxicity.[14] Another study showed *Nigella sativa* fixed oil has a low toxicity with the evidence of high value of LD50 and no morphological changes on the histopathological examination on heart, liver, kidney, and pancreas tissue of treated rats.[15] There are a wide range of studies which proved hepato-protective effect of *Nigella sativa*[16,17] as well as its mild hepatotoxicity in animals.[18] Even though it is now commercially found in supplement, but the consumption in raw form is still popular. People usually consume it at a low dose because of unknown effect at high dose. This study aimed to determine the toxic effect of *Nigella sativa* seed consumption at different doses on the liver function of rat. Liver contains enzymes which help the body detoxifying poisonous substances.[19] Therefore, high dose of *Nigella sativa* might cause damage to the liver tissue and this can be evaluate by measuring several liver enzymes levels and microscopic examination of liver tissue after receiving *Nigella sativa* supplementation for 28 days. Therefore current study aimed to determine the toxic effect of *Nigella sativa* powder on the rats' liver function which was evaluated by Alanine aminotransferase (ALT) and

*Corresponding author: Saadat Parhizkar, Medicinal Plants Research Centre, Yasuj University of Medical ciences (YUMS), Iran.
Email: parhizkarsa@gmail.com

aspartate aminotransferase (AST) and through histopathological examination of liver tissue.

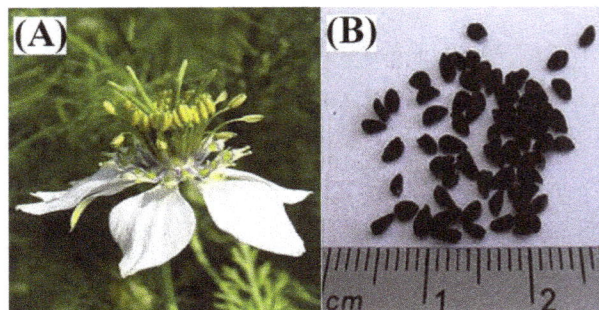

Figure 1. (A) *Nigella sativa* flower   (B) *Nigella sativa* seeds

Materials and Methods
Plant Materials
Nigella sativa seeds (imported from India) were purchased from a local herb store in Serdang, Malaysia. Voucher specimens of seeds were kept at the Cancer Research Laboratory of Institute of Biosciences and the seed was identified and authenticated by Professor Dr. Nordin Hj Lajis, Head of the Laboratory of Natural Products, Institute of Bioscience, University Putra Malaysia. After cleaning the seeds under running tap water for 10 min, they were rinsed twice with distilled water and air dried in an oven at 40 °C overnight until a constant weight was attained. The seeds were grounded to a powder shape using an electric grinder (National, Model MX-915, Kadoma, Osaka, Japan) for 6 minutes and were mixed with rat chow pellet powder and water into different doses including 0.01 (low dose), 0.1 (Normal dose) and 1 (High dose) g/kg body weight. Afterward, dough was baked in an oven at 40 °C until it received instant weight.

Animals
The protocol of the study was approved by Animal Care and Use Committee (ACUC), Faculty of Medicine and Health Sciences, University Putra Malaysia (UPM) with UPM/FPSK/PADS/BR/UUH/F01-00220 reference number for notice of approval. Twenty four male Sprague Dawley rats with 300-350 g body weight were supplied by Faculty of Medicine and Health Sciences, University Putra Malaysia and placed in the Animal House of the Faculty. They were housed individually in cages under standard laboratory conditions with a period of 12 h light/dark at 29 to 32°C and 70 to 80% relative humidity in the Animal House, Faculty of Medicine and Health Sciences, University Putra Malaysia. The animals were allowed to acclimatize for at least 10 days before the start of the experiments. The rats were fed with a standard rat chow pellet and allowed to drink water *ad libitum*. All animal received human care according to the criteria outlined in the "Guide for care and use of laboratory animals" prepared by the ACUC of Faculty of Medicine and Health Sciences, University Putra Malaysia and animal handling were conducted between 08.00 and 10.00 am

to minimize the effects of environmental changes. The treatments were given to the rats for 4 weeks. The body weight was measured once a week.

Experimental Design
Animals were assigned into four treatment groups which are considered as control, low, normal, and high. Control groups were given normal pellet without *Nigella sativa* while the other treatment groups are given pellet containing different doses of *Nigella sativa* respectively. The dosages were chosen based on human *Nigella sativa* consumption which is equal to 2 g/day and considering conversion rate to rats, 0.1 g/kg was selected as normal dose. The low dose was ten times (10 X) less than the normal dose while the high dose was ten times (10 X) higher than the normal dose. The treatments were given to the rats for 4 weeks.

Blood Collection
The blood samples were collected at the end of study. The rats were fasted for 12 h before blood collection. Prior to blood sampling, the rats were anesthetized with diethyl ether to ease handling. The blood samples were collected by cardiac puncture using 25 G, 1" needle. Approximately 5 ml of blood volume were taken and dispensed into labelled plain tubes. The blood samples were then centrifuged at 3000 rpm for 10 min to separate the serum. The serum was stored at -40°C until enzyme assays were carried out.

Biochemical Analysis
Stocks and working solutions were maintained at 0°C in a refrigerator. Serum was obtained by high speed centrifugation. The hepatic enzymes were measured by an automatic analyzer (Hitachi 902) using Roche Liver Enzyme Kits based on the manufacturer's instructions.

Histological Examination
All rats were sacrificed by cervical dislocation under and then midline laparotomy was performed. Resected liver specimens of each rat in all groups were fixed in 10% buffered formaldehyde for 24 hours and embedded into paraffin after 16 h of alcohol process. Five μm thick sections were obtained from the paraffin blocks and stained with hematoxylin and eosin. Each slide was examined under a light microscope by the same pathologist, who was blinded to the study group allocations. Central venous congestion, congestion and dilation of the hepatic sinusoids and inflammation of the portal tracts were noted and graded from 0 to 3, with "0" indicating no change, "1" slight change, "2" moderate change and "3" severe change. A sum of all grades was regarded as total score, which ranged between 0-9.

Statistical Analysis
Data were expressed as means ± standard deviation. The data were analyzed using SPSS windows program version 15 (SPSS Institute, Inc., Chicago, IL, USA).

The One-way Analysis of Variance (ANOVA) and General linear Model (GLM) followed by Duncan Multiple Range Test (DMRT) were used for analysis of data. A p-value less than 0.05 ($P<0.05$) was considered to be significant.

Results
Body Weight
The means of rats' body weight supplemented with *Nigella sativa* powder at various doses for 4 weeks period illustrated graphically in Figure 2. Measurement of the body weight was used to evaluate the health status of the rats during the treatment period. There was a slight weight reduction in treated rat groups compared to control, which was not statistically significant. This is indicating the healthy status of rats following *Nigella sativa* supplementation.

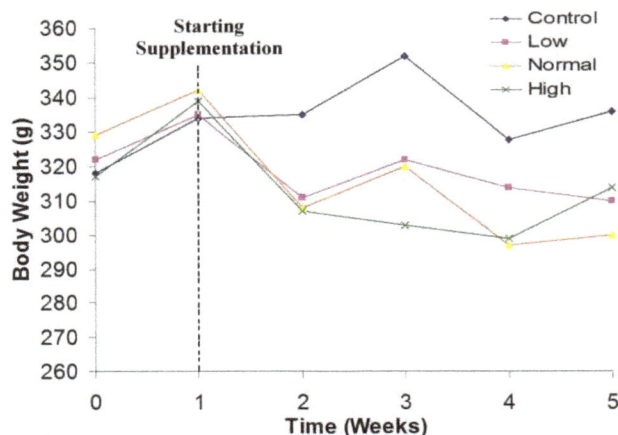

Figure 2. Changes in body weight of rats supplemented with various doses of *Nigella sativa* for 4 weeks.

Alanine Aminotransferase (ALT)
The results obtained in Figure 3 showed no significant decrease in serum ALT following supplementation with *Nigella sativa*. This small reduction of ALT was dose dependent. It means that consumption of high dose NS resulted in higher reduction of serum ALT level compared to other groups.

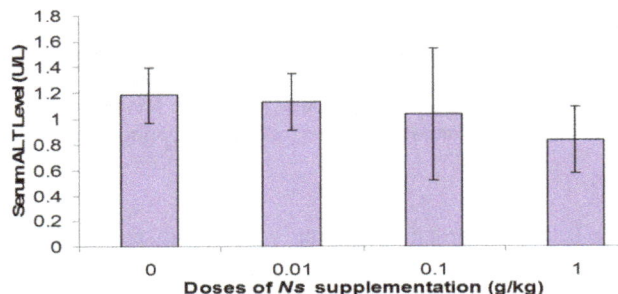

Figure 3. Changes in serum ALT level of rats supplemented with various doses of *Nigella sativa* for 4 weeks

Aspartate Aminotransferase (AST)
The results of liver function tests in this study revealed reduction in serum AST concentration in all NS group in comparison with control group, while the serum AST level was decreased in High dose NS administrated group more than other treatment group (Figure 4). It was indicated that AST level has not been affected by supplementation.

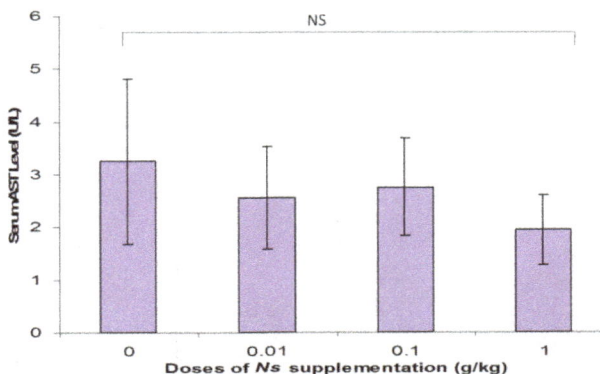

Figure 4. Changes in serum AST level of rats supplemented with various doses of *Nigella sativa* for 4 weeks

Histopatological Finding
The results of liver histopathologic examination are shown in Table 1. The results of histopathologic examination of the liver showed no hepatic vacuolization, degeneration, inflammation and necrosis. Among treatment group, there were very minimal and mild fatty degeneration in the portal tracts of normal and high doses (0.1 g/kg and 1.0 g/kg body weight) *Nigella sativa* treated rats as shown in Figure 5 (A, B, C, D).

Table 1. Histopathology scoring of liver tissue for rats supplemented with different doses of *Nigella sativa* supplementation for 28 days.

Doses (g/kg) of Nigella sativa	0.0					0.01					0.1					1				
Score	0	1	2	3	4	0	1	2	3	4	0	1	2	3	4	0	1	2	3	4
Hepatic vacuolization	6	0	0	0	0	6	0	0	0	0	6	0	0	0	0	6	0	0	0	0
Hepatic degeneration	6	0	0	0	0	6	0	0	0	0	6	0	0	0	0	6	0	0	0	0
Hepatic inflammation	6	0	0	0	0	6	0	0	0	0	6	0	0	0	0	6	0	0	0	0
Necrosis	6	0	0	0	0	6	0	0	0	0	6	0	0	0	0	6	0	0	0	0
Fatty degeneration	0	0	0	0	0	0	5	1	0	0	0	5	1	0	0	0	2	4	0	0

Discussion
The present study was designed to investigate the toxicity effect of *Nigella sativa* on liver function evaluating Alanine aminotransferase (ALT), Aspartate aminotransferase (AST) and histopathological changes of liver. ALT is an enzyme normally present in liver and heart cells. When the liver or heart is damaged, ALT in blood will increased, and thus indicates liver or

heart injury. During hepatocellular injury, enzymes which are normally located in the cytosol are released into the blood flow. Their qualification in plasma is useful biomarkers of the extent and type of hepatocellular damage.[20] ALT and AST are used to assess the hepatocellular integrity of liver tissue. ALT is more predominantly found in liver while AST is normally found in equal amounts in the liver, heart, muscle, kidney and brain. Therefore, ALT is more liver-specific than AST. Normal range both for ALT and AST in human is 25 U/L to 50 U/L.[21] From the biochemical study, it showed that the treatment doses (low dose 0.01 g/kg body weight, normal dose 0.1 g/kg body weight and high dose 1.0 g/kg body weight) of *Nigella sativa* supplementation reduced the liver enzymes (ALT and AST) level in treated rats compared to control group of rats. However, there was no significant different between dosage. The slowdown of body weight in *Nigella sativa* treated rats might be related to the liver enzyme (ALT and AST) level decrease, possibly effect of *Nigella sativa* treatment in rats with different doses for 28 days period.

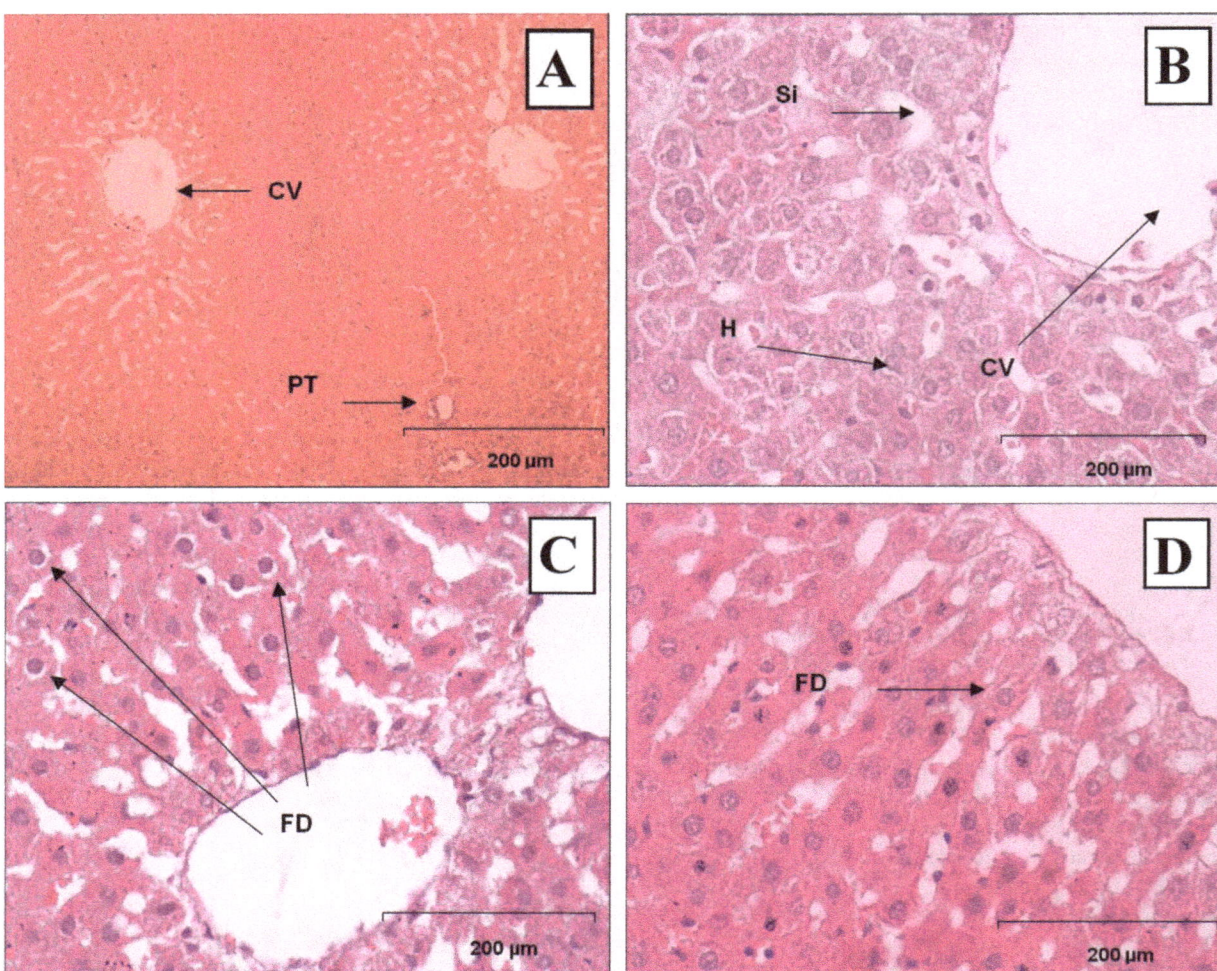

Figure 5. Histopathological section in the liver tissue of **A)** control group(0 g/kg NS), displaying central vein (CV) and portal triad (PT) **B)** Supplemented with Low dose NS(0.01 g/kg NS), displaying central vein (CV), sinusoid (Si), and hepatocyte (H), **C)** Supplemented with Normal Dose NS(0. 1 g/kg NS), displaying very minimal change, fatty degeneration (FD) was observed in normal doses treatment. Normal central vein (CV) and portal tract (PT) infiltrated with lymphocytes. **D)** Supplemented with High Dose NS (1 g/kg NS) displaying very minimal change, fatty degeneration (FD) was observed in high doses treatment. Normal central vein (CV) and portal tract (PT) infiltrated with lymphocytes. (H&E, X200).

The results of present study showed that the supplementation of *Nigella sativa* to the diets of rats for 28 days did not change the biochemical parameters of liver function as well as histopathological examinations which illustrated normal architecture of liver. It's proved by no significant changes of serum ALT and AST level in treatment group compare to the control group. Absent of pathological condition of liver tissue in histological evaluation confirmed the result. This study also found that body weights of the rats in all groups are maintained during the experiment which indicating healthy status of animals.

In accordance, the oral administration of aqueous extract of *Nigella sativa* seeds showed no significant changes in liver function evaluating hepatic enzymes level as well as histopathological changes of liver tissue.[22] Al Ammen and his colleagues[16] reported no toxic effects of *Nigella sativa* on hepatic enzymes among asthmatic patients. Another studies also failed to show any toxicity for *Nigella sativa* fixed oil in mice.[9,16]

Our study showed that oral administration of *Nigella sativa* has no toxicity in the doses used. These results agree with previous data reporting that *Nigella sativa* has a wide margin of safety.[23,24] Current study showed that *Nigella sativa* did not give any toxicity effect on liver to the parameters used, alanine aminotransferase (ALT) and aspartate aminotransferase (AST). The supplementations of *Nigella sativa* reduce the ALT level and AST level treated rats compared to the control doses of rats. This indicated that *Nigella sativa* dose up to 1.0 g/kg body weight showed no hepatocllular damage or hepatobiliary obstructive diseased and did not cause toxicity to the liver. Serum ALT and AST should increase as Itraconazole will induce liver damage.[25] Histopathology examination showed very minimal and mild fatty degeneration change in the portal tracts in normal (0.1 g/kg) and high doses (1.0 g/kg body weight) *Nigella sativa* supplementation for 28 days. There are no hepatic vacuolization, degeneration, inflammation and necrosis in liver tissues. Therefore, histopathological changes can be due to environmental factors such as malnutrition or loss body weight. Almost of studies suggested a hypoprotective effects of *Nigella sativa* due to some components such as either thymoquinone and monoterpenes[26] or tocopherols, phytosterols, and phenols.[27] To the best of our knowledge two compounds of *Nigella sativa* probably exerted potent cytotoxic activity. These two compounds were found to be terpenoids, one of which showed presence of carbonyl functionality whereas the other showed the presence of both carbonyl and hydroxyl functionalities.

Conclusion

With the evidence of normal ALT and AST level in blood and normal liver tissue in histology examination for all treatment groups, it is suggested that there are no toxic effect on liver function of *Nigella sativa* at different doses for 4 weeks period. As a conclusion, popular consumption of *Nigella sativa* powder by human did not cause any toxicity effect on the liver function and safe to be consumed for many purposes.

Acknowledgments

The authors would like to thank the authorities of Faculty of Medicine and Health Sciences, University Putra Malaysia, for providing analytical facilities.

Conflict of Interest

There is no conflict of interest in this study.

References

1. The World Medicine Situation 2011. 3rd ed. Geneva: World Health Organization; 2011.
2. Schwartsmann G, Ratain MJ, Cragg GM, Wong JE, Saijo N, Parkinson DR, et al. Anticancer drug discovery and development throughout the world. *J Clin Oncol* 2002;20(18 Suppl):47S-59S.
3. Newman DJ, Cragg GM. Natural products as sources of new drugs over the last 25 years. *J Nat Prod* 2007;70(3):461-77.
4. WHO traditional medicine strategy 2002-2005. Geneva: World Health Organization; 2002.
5. Saad SI. Classification of flowering plants. 2nd ed. Alexandria: The general Egyptian Book Co; 1975. p.412–3.
6. Sayed MD. Traditional medicine in health care. *J Ethnopharmacol* 1980;2(1): 19–22.
7. Nadkarni AK. Indian Materia Medica. Bombay: Popular Parkishan; 1976. p.854.
8. Boskabady MH, Keyhanmanesh R, Khameneh S, Doostdar Y, Khakzad MR. Potential immunomodulation effect of the extract of nigella sativa on ovalbumin sensitized guinea pigs. *J Zhejiang Univ Sci B* 2011;12(3):201-9.
9. Zaoui A, Cherrah Y, Lacaille-Dubois MA, Settaf A, Amarouch H, Hassar M. Diuretic and hypotensive effects of nigella sativa in the spontaneously hypertensive rat. *Therapie* 2000;55(3):379-82.
10. Turkdogan MK, Agaoglu Z, Yener Z, Sekeroglu R, Akkan HA, Avci ME. The role of antioxidant vitamins (c and e), selenium and nigella sativa in the prevention of liver fibrosis and cirrhosis in rabbits: New hopes. *Dtsch Tierarztl Wochenschr* 2001;108(2):71-3.
11. Kanter M, Meral I, Yener Z, Ozbek H, Demir H. Partial regeneration/proliferation of the beta-cells in the islets of langerhans by nigella sativa l. In streptozotocin-induced diabetic rats. *Tohoku J Exp Med* 2003;201(4):213-9.
12. Babazadeh B, Sadeghnia HR, Safarpour Kapurchal E, Parsaee H, Nasri S, Tayarani-Najaran Z. Protective effect of *Nigella sativa* and thymoquinone on serum/glucose deprivation-induced DNA damage in PC12 cells. *Avicenna Journal of Phytomedicine* 2012:2(3):125-132.
13. Parhizkar S, Latiff L, Rahman S, Dollah MA. Assessing estrogenic activity of *Nigella sativa* in ovariectomized rats using vaginal cornification assay. *Afr J Pharm Pharmacol* 2011;5(2): 137-142.
14. Anwar MA. *Nigella sativa*: A bibliometric study of the literature on Habbatul-Barakah. *Malays J Libr & Inf Sci* 2005;10(1):1-18.
15. Al Mofleh IA, Alhaider AA, Mossa JS, Al-Sohaibani MO, Al-Yahya MA, Rafatullah S, et al. Gastroprotective effect of an aqueous suspension of black cumin nigella sativa on necrotizing agents-induced gastric injury in experimental animals. *Saudi journal of gastroenterology : official journal of the Saudi J Gastroenterol* 2008;14(3):128-34.

16. Al-Ghamdi MS. Protective effect of nigella sativa seeds against carbon tetrachloride-induced liver damage. *Am J Chin Med* 2003;31(5):721-8.

17. Ilhan N, Seçkin D. Protective effect of nigella sativa seeds on ccl4-induced hepatotoxicity. *FÜ Sağlık Bil Dergisi* 2005;19(3):175-9.

18. Ezzat S, Daly EL. The effect of *Nigella sativa* seeds on certain aspects of carbohydrates and key hepatic enzymes in serum of rat. *J Islamic Acad Sci* 1994;7(2):93-9.

19. Marieb EN. The digestive system. In *Human anatomy and physiology*, 6th ed. San Francisco: Pearson Education; 2004. P.912-5.

20. Pari L, Murugan P. Protective role of tetrahydrocurcumin against erythromycin estolate-induced hepatotoxicity. *Pharmacol Res* 2004;49(5):481-6.

21. Anderson SC, Cockayne S. Liver function. In: Clinical Chemistry: Concepts and Applications, New York: McGrow-Hill; 2003. P. 286-96.

22. Mohammed AK. Ameliorative effect of black seed (*Nigella sativa L*) on the toxicity of aluminum in rabbits. *Iraqi J Vet Med* 2010;34(2): 110-6.

23. EL-Kholy WM, Hassan HA, Nour SE, Abe Elmageed ZE, Matrougui K. Hepatoprotective effects of *Nigella sativa* and bees' honey on hepatotoxicity induced by administration of sodium nitrite and sunset yellow. *FASEB J* 2009;23: 733.

24. Al Ameen NM, Altubaigy F, Jahangir T, Mahday IA, Mohammed EA, Musa OAA. Effect of *Nigella sativa* and bee honey on pulmonary, hepatic and renal function in Sudanese in Khartoum state. *J Med Plants Res* 2011;5(31):6857-63.

25. Somchit N, Norshahida AR, Hasiah AH, Zuraini A, Sulaiman MR, Noordin MM. Hepatotoxicity induced by antifungal drugs itraconazole and fluconazole in rats: A comparative in vivo study. *Hum Exp Toxicol* 2004;23(11):519-25.

26. El Tahir KE, Ashour MM, Al-Harbi MM. The respiratory effects of the volatile oil of the black seed (nigella sativa) in guinea-pigs: Elucidation of the mechanism(s) of action. *Gen Pharmacol* 1993;24(5):1115-22.

27. Ramadan MF, Kroh LW, Morsel JT. Radical scavenging activity of black cumin (nigella sativa l.), coriander (coriandrum sativum l.), and niger (guizotia abyssinica cass.) crude seed oils and oil fractions. *J Agric Food Chem* 2003;51(24):6961-9.

Analgesic Activity of Some 1,2,4-Triazole Heterocycles Clubbed with Pyrazole, Tetrazole, Isoxazole and Pyrimidine

Shantaram Gajanan Khanage[1]*, **Appala Raju**[2], **Popat Baban Mohite**[3], **Ramdas Bhanudas Pandhare**[4]

[1] *Research scholar, Department of Pharmacy, Vinayaka Missions University, Salem, Sankari main road, NH-47, Tamilnadu, India-636308.*

[2] *Department of Pharmaceutical chemistry, H.K.E.'S College of Pharmacy, Sedam road, Gulbarga, Karnataka, India-585105.*

[3] *Department of Pharmaceutical chemistry, M.E.S. College of Pharmacy, Sonai, Tq-Newasa, Dist.-Ahmednagar, Maharashtra, India-414105.*

[4] *Department of Pharmacology, M.E.S. College of Pharmacy, Sonai, Tq-Newasa, Dist.-Ahmednagar, Maharashtra, India-414105.*

ARTICLE INFO

Keywords:
Triazole
Analgesic Activity
Pyrazole
Tetrazole
Isoxazole
Pyrimidine

ABSTRACT

Purpose: In the present study *in vivo* analgesic activity of some previously synthesized 1,2,4-triazole derivatives containing pyrazole, tetrazole, isoxazole and pyrimidine ring have been evaluated. *Methods*: Acetic acid induced writhing method and Hot plate method has been described to study analgesic activity of some 1,2,4-triazole derivatives containing pyrazole, tetrazole, isoxazole and pyrimidine as a pharmacological active lead. *Results*: Thirty six different derivatives containing 1,2,4-triazole ring were subjected to study their *in vivo* analgesic activity. Chloro, nitro and methoxy, hydroxy and bromo substituted derivatives showed excellent analgesic activity and dimethylamino, furan and phenyl substituted derivatives showed moderate analgesic activity in both of the methods. Compounds IIIa, IIId, IIIf, IIIi, IIIj, IVa, IVb, IVd, IVf, IVh, IVj IV3a and IIj were found to be superior analgesic agents after screening by Acetic acid induced writhing method. Compounds IIIb, IIId, IIIf, IIIh, IIIj, IVa, IVb, IVd, IVf, IVh, IVi, IV3c, IV3e and IIj were showed analgesic potential after screening of Hot plate method. *Conclusion*: All tested compounds containing 1,2,4-triazole were found to be promising analgesic agents, for this activity pyrazole, tetrazole, isoxazole and pyrimidine leads might be supported.

Introduction

Analgesic and anti-inflammatory drugs are one of the most valuable medicaments that used in many of disease for relief of pain and inflammation. Most analgesic and anti-inflammatory drugs available in the market, still present a wide range of many problems such as efficacy and undesired effects including GIT disorders and other unwanted effects,[1] that limit their clinical usefulness and remain to be solved and leaving an open door for new and better compounds.[2] This situation highlights the need for advent of safe, novel and effective analgesic and anti-inflammatory compounds.[3] 1,2,4-triazole received sheer attention of medicinal chemists because of their many therapeutic applications like anticancer,[4,5] antimicrobial,[6-9] anticonvulsant,[10] anti-inflammatory, analgesic,[11] antidepressant,[12] antitubercular,[13] antimalarial[14] and hypoglycemic[15] activities.
We have reported that 5-methyl-2-[(5-substituted aryl-4*H*-1,2,4-triazol-3-yl)methyl]-2,4-dihydro-3*H*-pyrazol-3-one and 5-phenyl-1-[(5-substituted aryl-4*H*-1,2,4-triazol-3-yl)methyl]-1*H*-tetrazole had significant

anticancer activity specially on renal cancer cell lines (UO-31) as well *in vitro* antibacterial activity against gram positive bacterial *S. aureus* NCIM 2079, *B. subtillis* NCIM 2063 and gram negative bacterial *E. coli* NCIM 2065, *P. aeruginosa* NCIM 2863 strains.[16] More recently we have reported antimicrobial, antitubercular and anticancer activity of 1-[5-(substituted aryl)-1,2-oxazol-3-yl]-3,5-diphenyl-1*H*-1,2,4-triazole (4a-g).[17] In continuation of our previous work[18-20] in this article the attempts have been made to explore the analgesic potential of some formerly synthesized 1,2,4-triazoles clubbed with pyrazole, tetrazole, isoxazole and pyrimidine heterocycles.

Materials and Methods

The standard analgesic drugs Ibuprofen and Pentazocine, solvents used for the experimental work were commercially procured from E. Merck India and Qualigens India. Swiss strain albino mice for study were procured from National Toxicology Center, Pune.

---

*Corresponding author: Shantaram Gajanan Khanage, College of Pharmacy, Sonai. At post-Sonai, Tq-Newasa, Dist.-Ahmednagar, Maharashtra-414105, India. Email: shantaram1982@gmail.com

Evaluation of analgesic activity
Study protocol was approved by the Institutional Animal Ethics Committee for the purpose of control and supervision of experiments on animals (IAEC, Approval No.1211/ac/08/CPCSEA) before experiment. Swiss strain albino mice of either sex weighing 25–30 g were used for this study. The test compounds were administered intraperitoneally in 10% v/v Tween 80 suspension.

Acute toxicity study
The acute toxicity for the test compounds was determined by the Miller and Tainter method administering the compounds intraperitoneally. LD_{50} of the test compounds calculated by Miller and Tainter (1944) method,[21] initially least tolerated (smallest) dose (100% mortality) and most tolerated (highest) dose (0% mortality) were determined by hit and trial method. After determination of two doses we have selected five doses in between the least tolerated and most tolerated doses were given intraperitoneally to 5 groups of mice, 10 animals in each group. The animals were observed for first 2 hours and then at 6th and 24th hour for any toxic symptoms. After 24 hours, the number of deceased animals was counted in each group and percentage of mortality calculated. From the obtained data determined the LD_{50} of the test compounds by using probit value transformations.

Acetic acid induced writhing method (Abdominal Constriction Test)
The animals were divided into 38 groups of six mice each. The control group of animals was administered with 10% v/v Tween 80 (0.5 ml) suspension. The animals of another group were injected intraperitoneally with standard drug Ibuprofen (10 mg/kg). After 20 min of the administration the test compounds, all the groups of mice were given with the writhing agent 3% v/v aqueous acetic acid in a dose of 2 ml/kg intraperitoneally. The writhing produced in these animals was counted visually for 15 min and the numbers of writhings produced in treated groups were compared with control group. The results of analgesic activity are recorded in Table 1. Analgesic activity in percent was calculated by using following formula.
Protection = 100-[{(No. of writhes in treated mice)/(No. of writhes in untreated mice)}×100]

Hot plate method
The method of Eddy and Leimbach was adopted for the study. The temperature of a metal surface in the hot plate test was set at 55±1.0°C. The time taken by the animals to lick the fore or hind paw or jump out of the place was taken as the reaction time. Latency to the licking paws or jumping from plate was determined before and after treatment. The latency was recorded at the time of 0 (just before any treatment) and 15, 30 and 60 min after intraperitoneal administration of test compounds. A latency period of 15 sec was defined as complete analgesia as cut off time to prevent damage to mice. The reference compound Pentazocine was administered in a dose of 5 mg/kg. The time course of hot plate latency was expressed as the percentage of the maximum possible effect (%MPE) according to the following formula:

$$\%MPE = \frac{(\text{post drug latency}) - (\text{pre} - \text{drug latency})}{(\text{cut} - \text{off time}) - (\text{pre} - \text{drug latency})} \times 100$$

After the treatment of test and reference compounds, the pain thresholds of the animals were observed and presented in Table 2.

Statistical analysis
Data were presented as arithmetic mean±SEM. Statistical analysis was performed by one way variance (ANOVA) followed by Dunnett's test. "p" value of less than 0.05 was considered as statistically significant.

Results and Discussion
Acetic acid induced writhing method
Abdominal construction responses induced by acetic acid is a sensitive procedure to establish efficacy of peripherally acting analgesics, it may causes increase in the level of PGE_2 and PGF2a by intraperitoneally administration of acetic acid. The analgesic activity was expressed as percentage of protection. All tested compounds exhibited activity in a dose range of 25-100 mg/kg. Writhing episodes and percent protection of tested compounds for analgesic activity are summarized in Table 1. Compound IIIa, IIId, IIIf, IIIi, IIIj, IVa, IVb, IVd, IVf, IVh, IVj IV3a and IIj (Figure 1 and 2) were found to be superior analgesic agents with 55, 60, 57, 57, 57, 57, 55, 60, 60, 56, 63, 60 and 60% analgesic activity respectively as compared to other tested compounds. Chloro, nitro, methoxy, hydroxy and bromo substituted derivatives exhibited excellent analgesic activity where as dimethylamino, furan and phenyl substituted derivatives showed moderate analgesic activity. Substituted phenyl ring present on isoxazole, pyrimidine and 1,2,4-triazole nucleus might have attributed crucial role to show analgesic activity. Compounds with substitution of chloro, methoxy, bromo on 4th position of phenyl ring present on isoxazole, pyrimidine and triazole nucleus showed maximum analgesic activity. Compounds IIId, IVd, IVf, IVj, IV3a and IIj were exhibited comparative analgesic property (up to 60% protection) with standard drug Ibuprofen (66%) as illustrated in Table 1. because of 4-methoxy, 4-chloro, 2-chloro, 2,4-dimethoxy groups present on phenyl ring of pharmacologically active isoxazole, pyrimidine, and triazole chalcone heterocycles.

Hot plate method
All compounds tested by Eddy's hot plate method exhibited activity in a dose range of 25-100 mg/kg. The analgesic activity measured by central analgesia.

Pentazocine 5 mg/kg significantly increased the hot plate latency producing a highest %MPE at 69.02. Compounds IIIb, IIIj, IVa, IVd, IVf, IVh, IVi, and IIj significantly increased the hot plate latency when compared to the control group. The highest antinociception induced by compounds IIIj, IVd and IVf at dose of 50 mg/kg were observed with 64.82, 66.98 and 67.21 %MPE respectively. The analgesic activity of compounds IIIb, IIId, IIIf, IIIh, IIIj, IVa, IVb, IVd, IVf, IVh, IVi, IV3c, IV3e and IIj were comparable to Pentazocine after 15, 30 and 60 min. 2-chloro, 3-nitro, 4-chloro, 4-methoxy, 4-bromo, 4-hydroxy and 2,4-dimethoxy substituted analogs exhibited dynamic analgesic activity. 4-dimethyl amino and 2-furyl substituted compound of tested series of 1-(3,5-diphenyl-1H-1,2,4-triazol-1-yl)-3-(substituted aryl) prop-2-en-1-one (Chalcones) were also acquired higher hot plate latency with 10.76 and 10.74 sec respectively after 60 min. Compounds from series of 1-[5-(substituted aryl)-1,2-oxazol-3-yl]- 3,5-diphenyl-1H-1,2,4-triazoles and 6-(substituted aryl)-4-(3,5-diphenyl-1H-1,2,4-triazol-1-yl)-1,6-dihydropyrimidine-2-thiol obtained excellent analgesic potential.

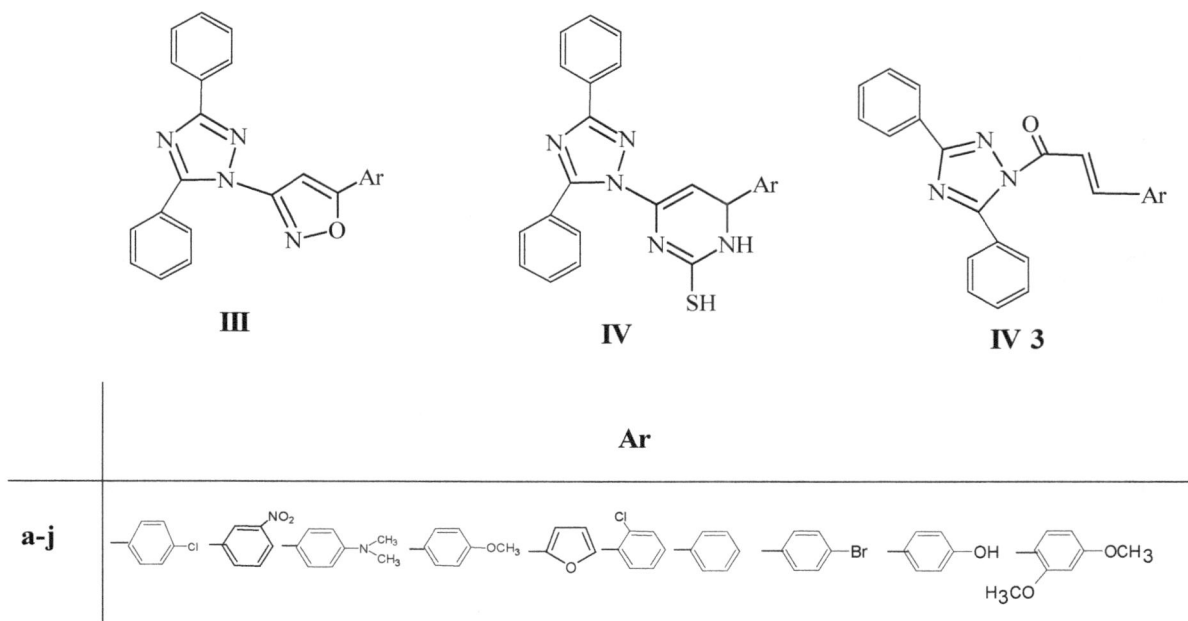

Figure 1. Structures of compounds of scheme III, IV and IV3.

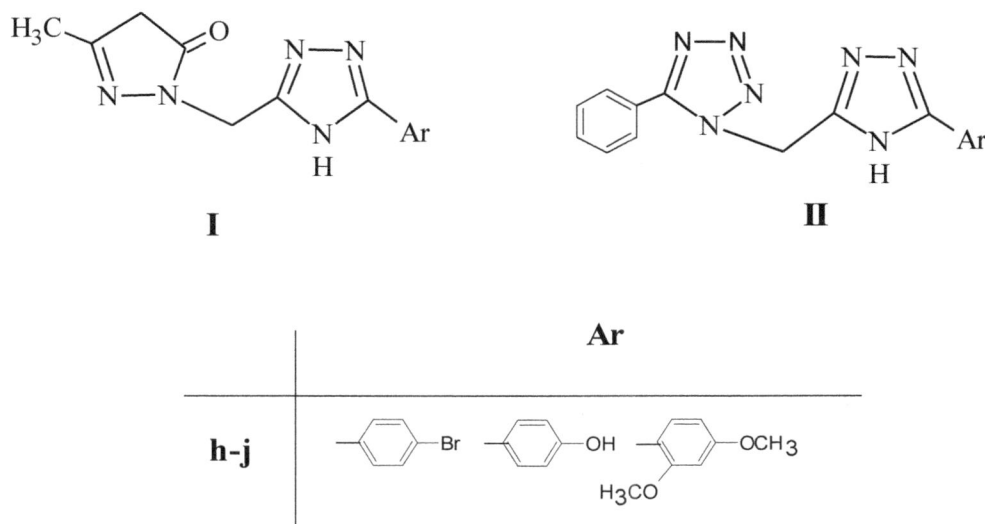

Figure 2. Structures of compounds of scheme I and II.

Table 1. Evaluation of analgesic activity by acetic acid induced writhing method.

Sr. No.	Treatment	Dose mg/kg	Writhing episodes in 15 min (Mean ± S.E.M.)	Percent protection
1	Control	--	38.70±0.5547	-
2	Ibuprofen	10	13.19±0.6921**	66
3	IIIa	50	17.28±0.6647**	55
4	IIIb	50	18.24±0.6425**	53
5	IIIc	50	24.89±0.5354**	36
6	IIId	50	15.65±0.7845**	60
7	IIIe	50	26.45±0.8121**	32
8	IIIf	50	16.46±0.5744**	57
9	IIIg	50	27.65±0.5478**	29
10	IIIh	50	18.57±0.4545**	52
11	IIIi	50	16.49±0.6545**	57
12	IIIj	50	16.47±0.2254**	57
13	IVa	50	16.45±0.5456**	57
14	IVb	50	17.49±0.5641**	55
15	IVc	50	21.73±0.5974**	44
16	IVd	50	15.44±0.6133**	60
17	IVe	50	22.45±0.5525**	42
18	IVf	50	15.36±0.6455**	60
19	IVg	50	19.65±0.7322**	49
20	IVh	50	17.22±0.4855**	56
21	IVi	50	19.47±0.6513**	50
22	IVj	50	14.24±0.4745**	63
23	IV3a	100	15.44±0.4454**	60
24	IV3b	100	22.65±0.5546**	42
25	IV3c	100	19.47±0.5941**	50
26	IV3d	100	21.77±0.4423**	44
27	IV3e	100	25.49±0.4473**	34
28	IV3f	100	19.42±0.6651**	50
29	IV3g	100	26.56±0.4329**	31
30	IV3h	100	28.56±0.7325**	26
31	IV3i	100	23.58±0.6423**	39
32	IV3j	100	19.26±0.4523**	50
33	Ih	25	20.54±0.6425**	47
34	Ii	25	22.89±0.5214**	41
35	Ij	25	18.34±0.4527**	53
36	IIh	25	20.57±0.8592**	47
37	IIi	25	22.44±0.6854**	42
38	IIj	25	15.47±0.8957**	60

** $P < 0.01$ represent significant difference when compared with control groups.

Table 2. Evaluation of analgesic activity by Hot plate method.

Treatment	Average Reaction Time in seconds before treatment (Mean ± S.E.M.)	Reaction time in seconds after treatment (Mean ± S.E.M.)			%MPE
		15 min	30 min	60min	
Control	4.75±0.1547	4.75±0.1583	4.75±0.2563	4.75±0.4941	-
Pentazocine	4.70±0.4012**	7.70±0.5211**	9.67±0.4302**	11.81±0.3254**	69.02
IIIa	4.56±0.5221**	7.23±0.6326**	9.23±0.5745**	10.76±0.4369**	59.38
IIIb	4.63±0.4785**	7.49±0.2234**	9.87±0.3865**	11.15±0.5356**	62.87
IIIc	4.67±0.4523**	6.52±0.6542**	9.34±0.5413**	9.53±0.4356**	47.04
IIId	4.63±0.6374**	7.46±0.7585**	9.52±0.2658**	10.47±0.7541**	56.31
IIIe	4.69±0.4474**	6.45±0.5428**	8.36±0.6756**	9.27 ±0.5854**	44.42
IIIf	4.65±0.4469**	7.42±0.3769**	9.49±0.5369**	10.71±0.5775**	58.55
IIIg	4.56±0.5854**	6.70±0.4459**	8.49±0.7474**	9.27±0.6525**	45.11
IIIh	4.43±0.3544**	7.50±0.7585**	9.57±0.6456**	10.52 ±0.6785**	57.61
IIIi	4.71±0.4675**	6.39±0.3646**	9.03±0.5236**	9.46±0.5359**	46.16
IIIj	4.68±0.7548**	7.56±0.5636**	9.52±0.6552**	11.37±0.6426**	64.82
IVa	4.72±0.5957**	7.68±0.4523**	9.56±0.3356**	11.09±0.5517**	61.96
IVb	4.67±0.4358**	7.45±0.6984**	9.16±0.3548**	10.59±0.5478**	57.30
IVc	4.55±0.4785**	6.59±0.4578**	9.44±0.5349**	9.69±0.8689**	49.18
IVd	4.58±0.5878**	7.66±0.6689**	9.50±0.4245**	11.56±0.6741**	66.98
IVe	4.39±0.4589**	6.89±0.7481**	8.59±0.6478**	9.75 ±0.4589**	50.51
IVf	4.66±0.5958**	7.53±0.3549**	9.80±0.3358**	11.61±0.6358**	67.21
IVg	4.45±0.5869**	7.72±0.5269**	9.58±0.5895**	10.46±0.5692**	56.96
IVh	4.41±0.5321**	7.80±0.4781**	9.57±0.5696**	10.82 ±0.3324**	60.52
IVi	4.64±0.2966**	7.56±0.3826**	9.45±0.7851**	10.89±0.5369**	60.32
IVj	4.52±0.2853**	7.70±0.5239**	9.43±0.4665**	10.44±0.6745 **	56.48
IV3a	4.64±0.4789**	7.34±0.3545**	9.12±0.3456**	10.12±0.2985**	52.89
IV3b	4.56±0.5884**	7.11±0.5789**	8.36±0.6398**	9.47±0.6489**	47.03
IV3c	4.67±0.3956**	7.49±0.5212**	9.27±0.3369**	10.76±0.6245**	58.95
IV3d	4.73±0.4525**	7.13±0.2845**	9.10±0.3235**	9.46±0.5469**	46.05
IV3e	4.59±0.5823**	6.93±0.5861**	9.14±0.6478**	10.74 ±0.4369**	59.07
IV3f	4.54±0.4969**	7.23±0.5326**	9.50±0.3756**	10.32±0.6542**	55.25
IV3g	4.49±0.5478**	7.02±0.4689**	8.48±0.5225**	8.93±0.5692**	42.24
IV3h	4.61±0.4526**	6.80±0.4369**	8.55±0.5236**	9.51 ±0.5236**	47.16
IV3i	4.67±0.6325**	6.56±0.3989**	8.47±0.5364**	9.37±0.6346**	45.49
IV3j	4.71±0.5963**	7.31±0.2845**	9.46±0.3623**	10.20±0.4126 **	53.35
Ih	4.46±0.6522**	7.25±0.4545**	8.55±0.2625**	9.88±0.4121**	51.18
Ii	4.29±0.3532**	7.45±0.4666**	9.12±0.3644**	9.83±0.5481**	51.72
Ij	4.34±0.5418**	7.75±0.6641**	9.85±0.4236**	10.24±0.3678**	55.34
IIh	4.54±0.6645**	6.96±0.4425**	8.86±0.3356**	9.87±0.4356**	50.95
IIi	4.59±0.5414**	6.45±0.3784**	8.22±0.3541**	9.45±0.4678**	46.68
IIj	4.74±0.4775**	7.35±0.4125**	9.45±0.5925**	10.96±0.6486**	60.62

Dose: 25 mg/kg for compounds Ih-Ij, 50mg/kg for IIIa-j and IVa-j, 100mg/kg for IV3a-j and 5mg/Kg for Pentazocine.
** p<0.01 represent the significant difference when compared control group.

Conclusion

The results of the present investigation reveals that the increase in analgesic activity is attributed to the presence of 2-chloro, 3-nitro, 4-chloro, 4-methoxy, 4-bromo, 4-hydroxy and 2,4-dimethoxy groups on phenyl ring of isoxazole, pyrimidine, pyrazole, tetrazole and triazole. All tested heterocycles posses central and peripheral analgesic property. Perceptibly the comparative evaluation of active compounds will required in the further studies, the data reported in this article may be helpful guide for the medicinal chemist who is working in this area.

Acknowledgments

Authors are highly thankful to National Toxicology Center, Pune, for providing animals to caring out analgesic activity and acute toxicity study. We are also grateful of Principal M.E.S. College Pharmacy, Sonai and Prashant Patil Gadakh, Secreatary, Mula Education Society for providing excellent research facilities for this work.

Conflict of interest

All the authors report no conflicts of interest.

References

1. Girard P, Verniers D, Coppe MC, Pansart Y, Gillardin JM. Nefopam and ketoprofen synergy in rodent models of antinociception. *Eur J Pharmacol* 2008; 584: 263-71.
2. Tao YM, Li QL, Zhang CF, Xu XJ, Chen J, Ju YW, et al. LPK-26, a novel κ- opioid receptor agonist with potent antinociceptive effects and low dependence potential. *Eur J Pharmacol* 2008; 584: 306-11.
3. Kolesnikov Y, Soritsa D. Analgesic synergy between topical opioids and topical non-steroidal anti-inflammatory drugs in the mouse model of thermal pain. *Eur J Pharmacol* 2008; 579: 126-33.
4. Bhat KS, Poojary B, Prasad DJ, Naik P, Holla BS. Synthesis and antitumor activity studies of some new fused 1,2,4-triazole derivatives carrying 2,4-dichloro-5-fluorophenyl moiety. *Eur J Med Chem* 2009; 44:5066-70.
5. Al-Soud YA, Al-Masoudi NA, Ferwanah AE. Synthesis and properties of new substituted 1,2,4-triazoles: Potential antitumor agents. *Bioorg Med Chem* 2003; 11:1701-8.
6. Lingappa B, Girisha KS, Kalluraya BN, Rai S, Kumari NS. Regioselective reaction: Novel Mannich bases derived from 3-(4,6-disubstituted-2-thiomethyl)3-amino-5-mercapto-1,2,4-triazoles and their antimicrobial properties. *Ind J Chem* 2008; 47B:1858-64.
7. Rao G, Rajasekran S, Attimarad M. Synthesis and Antimicrobial activity of Some 5-phenyl-4-substituted amino-3-mercapto (4*H*) 1,2,4-triazoles. *Ind J Pharm Sci* 2000; 6:475-7.
8. Jalilian AR, Sattari S, Bineshmarvasti M, Shafiee A, Daneshtalab M. Synthesis and in vitro antifungal and cytotoxicity evaluation of thiazolo-*4H*-1,2,4-triazoles and 1,2-thiadiazolo-4H-1,2,4-triazoles-thiazoles-1,2,3-thiadiazoles. *Arch Der Pharm* 2000; 333:347-54.
9. Lazarevic M, Dimova V, Molnar GD, Kakurinov V, Colanceska RK. Synthesis of some N1-aryl/heteroarylaminomethyl/ethyl-1,2,4-triazoles and their antibacterial and antifungal activities. *Hetero Comm* 2001; 7:577-82.
10. Chimirri A, Bevacqua F, Gitto R, Quartarone S, Zappala MD, Sarro A, et al. Synthesis and anticonvulsant activity of new 1-*H*-triazolo[4,5-c][2,3]benzodiaze-pines. *Med Chem Res* 1999; 9:203-12.
11. Hunashal RD, Ronad PM, Maddi VS, Satyanarayana D, Kamadod MA. Synthesis, anti-inflammatory and analgesic activity of 2-[4-(substituted benzylideneamino)-5-(substitutedphenoxymethyl)-4*H*-1,2,4-triazol-3-yl-thio] acetic acid derivatives. *Arab J Chem* 2011; 1-9.
12. Kane MJ, Dudley MW, Sorensen MS, Miller FP. Synthesis of 1,2,4-Dihydro-3*H*-1,2,4-triazole-3-thiones as potential antidepressant agents. *J Med Chem* 1988; 31:1253-8.
13. Husain MI, Amir M, Singh E. Synthesis and antitubercular activities of [5-(2furyl)-1,2,4-triazoles-3yl thio] acehydrazide derivatives. *Ind J Chem* 1987; 26B:2512-54.
14. Xiao Z, Waters NC, Woodard CL, Li PK. Design and synthesis of pfmrk inhibitors as potential antimalarial agents. *Bioorg Med Chem Lett* 2001; 11:2875-8.
15. Deliwala CV, Mhasalkar MY, Shah MH, Pilankar PD, Nikam ST, Anantanarayan KG. Synthesis and hypoglycaemic activity of 3-aryl(or pyridyl)-5-alkyl amino-1,3,4, Thiadiazole and some sulfonyl ureas derivatives of 4*H*-1,2,4 triazoles. *J Med Chem* 1971; 14:1000-3.
16. Khanage SG, Mohite PB, Raju SA. Synthesis, Anticancer and Antibacterial Activity of Some Novel 1,2,4-Triazole Derivatives Containing Pyrazole and Tetrazole Rings. *Asian J Res Chem* 2011; 4(4):567-73.
17. Khanage SG, Mohite PB, Pandhare RB, Raju SA. Synthesis and pharmacological evaluation of isoxazole derivatives containing 1,2,4-triazole Moiety. *Mar Pharm J* 2012; 16(2):134-40.
18. Khanage SG, Mohite PB, Pandhare RB, Raju SA. Investigation of pyrazole and tetrazole derivatives containing 3,5 disubstituted-4*H* 1,2,4-triazole as a potential antitubercular and antifungal agent. *Bioint Res App Chem* 2012; 2(2):277-83.
19. Khanage SG, Mohite PB, Pandhare RB, Raju SA. Study of analgesic activity of novel 1,2,4-triazole derivatives bearing pyrazole and tetrazole moiety. *J Pharm Res* 2011; 4(10):3609-11.
20. Khanage SG, Raju SA, Mohite PB, Pandhare RB. Synthesis and Pharmacological Evaluation of Some New Pyrimidine Derivatives containing 1, 2, 4-triazole. *Adv Pharm Bull* 2012; 2(2): 213-22.
21. Miller LC, Tainter ML. Estimation of LD$_{50}$ and its error by means of log-probit graph paper. *Proc Soc Exp Bio Med* 1944; 57: 261.

12

Formulation, Characterization and Physicochemical Evaluation of Ranitidine Effervescent Tablets

Abolfazl Aslani*, Hajar Jahangiri

Department of Pharmaceutics, School of Pharmacy and Novel Drug Delivery Systems Research Center, Isfahan University of Medical Sciences, Isfahan, Iran.

ARTICLE INFO	ABSTRACT
Keywords: Effervescent tablet Ranitidine HCl Fusion method Direct compression method	*Purpose:* The aim of this study was to design, formulate and physicochemically evaluate effervescent ranitidine hydrochloride (HCl) tablets since they are easily administered while the elderly and children sometimes have difficulties in swallowing oral dosage forms. *Methods:* Effervescent ranitidine HCl tablets were prepared in a dosage of 300 mg by fusion and direct compression methods. The powder blend and granule mixture were evaluated for various pre-compression characteristics, such as angle of repose, compressibility index, mean particle size and Hausner's ratio. The tablets were evaluated for post-compression features including weight variation, hardness, friability, drug content, dissolution time, carbon dioxide content, effervescence time, pH, content uniformity and water content. Effervescent systems with appropriate pre and post-compression qualities dissolved rapidly in water were selected as the best formulations. *Results:* The results showed that the flowability of fusion method is more than that of direct compression and the F_5 and F_6 formulations of 300 mg tablets were selected as the best formulations because of their physicochemical characteristics. *Conclusion:* In this study, citric acid, sodium bicarbonate and sweeteners (including mannitol, sucrose and aspartame) were selected. Aspartame, mint and orange flavors were more effective for masking the bitter taste of ranitidine. The fusion method is the best alternative in terms of physicochemical and physical properties.

Introduction

Oral dosage forms of drugs are the main popular routes in spite of some disadvantages such as slow absorption and delayed onset of action. On the other hand, liquid forms of drugs are not stable enough and slow release dosage forms have longer routes for changing throughout the gastrointestinal tract. These two forms are thus limited in applications. Hence, effervescent tablets seem to be an appropriate alternative for oral dosage forms.[1]

Effervescent tablets are designed to be dissolved or dispersed in water before administration.[2] The tablet is promptly broken apart by internal release of CO_2 in water and the CO_2 reaction is created by an interaction of tartaric acid and citric acid with alkali metal carbonates or bicarbonates in the presence of the water. Effervescent tablets are uncoated tablets that usually consist of acids and bicarbonates or carbonates.[3,4] Some products are useful for pharmaceuticals that damage the stomach or those which are susceptible to stomach pH. In addition, the drugs prescribed commonly in high doses may be used in the form of effervescent tablets.[3,5]

Moreover, since effervescent tablets are administrated in liquid form, they are easily swallowed so they are preferred over tablets or capsules with a difficult

consumption for some patients. On the other hand, one dose of effervescent tablet is often dissolved in 3-4 ounces of water. Being previously dissolved in a buffer solution, effervescent products do not get in direct contact with the gastrointestinal tract. They can thus be tolerated in stomach and intestine well due to reduced gastrointestinal irritation.

Another advantage relating to effervescent tablet is that when they are taken by the patient, exactly the taken amount enters the stomach. In fact, the CO_2 produced in an effervescence reaction increases the penetration of active substances into the paracellular pathway and consequently their absorption.[6,7]

These products contain active ingredients, mixtures of acids/acid salts (citric, tartaric and malic acids or any other suitable acid or acid anhydride), and bicarbonate or carbonate salts (sodium, potassium or any other carbonate or bicarbonate relating to alkali metals) and they all release CO_2 when mixed with water.[3] Effervescent tablets also contain other materials such as fillers, binders, sweeteners, flavors and lubricants. Water soluble lubricants are used to prevent the adhesion of the tablet to the device and formation of insoluble scum on water

---

*Corresponding author: Abolfazl Aslani, Department of Pharmaceutics, School of Pharmacy and Pharmaceutical Sciences, Isfahan University of Medical Sciences, Isfahan, Iran. E-mail: aslani@pharm.mui.ac.ir

surface. Sweeteners are also essential in these formulations. Since sucrose is hygroscopic and it leads to an increase tablet bulk, therefore other sweeteners such as aspartame, maltitol and sucralose are frequently used.[1,8]

Various methods including wet granulation, fusion method, fluid-bed granulation and direct compression are employed in producing the effervescent tablets. Controlled environmental conditions are very important in producing the effervescent tablets. Since these products are sensitive to moisture and temperature, a relative humidity (RH) of 25% or less and moderate temperatures (25 °C) are essential in manufacturing areas to prevent granulation or adhesion of tablets to the machinery as a result of absorbed moisture.[2,5] Currently, the most commonly used effervescent tablet is aspirin tablet.[3]

Ranitidine is a potent histamine H_2 receptor antagonist extensively used in the treatment of conditions like duodenal and gastric ulceration, reflux esophagitis and Zollinger-Ellison syndrome. It is also used in postoperative prophylaxis and in the treatment of allergic and inflammatory conditions related to histamine receptors.[9] Ranitidine is more effective than omeprazole in treating gastric ulcer among the children who develop this condition two weaks after taking non-steroidal anti-inflammatory drugs (NSAIDs).[10] Ranitidine has both oral (tablets, capsules and syrups) and injectable dosage forms. The aim of this study was to design, prepare and physicochemically evaluate effervescent tablets of ranitidine HCl. Ranitidine effervescent tablets are of a faster action onset and a more effective treatment for gastrointestinal diseases. Ranitidine of 300 mg effervescent tablets aren't available. The advantages of formulations prepared in this study are their equal properties with other effervescent tablets i.e suitable flavor and weight. Since the weight of effervescent tablets in this study are about half that of other effervescent tablets, so they are economical for pharmaceutical industries.

Effervescent tablets are more suitable for the children due to their better flavor and acceptability. Patients' compliance to the drug can be increased due to the appearance of this product during effervescence, convenience of usage and use of attracting colors and flavors in these products.

Materials and Methods
Chemicals
The pharmaceuticals including ranitidine HCl was purchased from Saraca (India). Citric acid, tartaric acid, sodium bicarbonate, mannitol, sorbitol, sucrose, povidone k-30 (PVP), polyethylene glycol 6000 (PEG 6000), sodium benzoate, and aspartame were obtained from Merck (Germany). Flavoring agents were gifted by Farabi Pharmaceutical Company (Isfahan, Iran).

Spectrophotometeric Analysis
Different aliquots (1.0-7.0 ml) of a standard 100 µg/ml drug solution were transferred into a series of 10 ml volumetric flasks. Adequate purified water was then added to fill the flasks. The amount of ranitidine HCl was determined by measuring the drug absorbance at 315.3 nm using a Shimadzu UV-1240 model UVmini-visible spectrophotometer.

Determination of Effervescent Components
The effervescent components and the ratios between them were determined according to the neutralization of acids and alkali and the allowed amount of each component. All components were then mixed with ranitidine HCl. Afterwards, the effects of citric acid and tartaric acid on solubility, effervescence time and pH were investigated using changing the acid amounts as follows: 0.5, 0.75□ 1, 1.5 and 2 times. The same experiment was repeated for sodium bicarbonate (Table 1).

Table 1. Determination of effervescent components based on ratio of effervescent materials (Mean ± SD).

Code	Citric Acid (mg)	Tartaric Acid(mg)	Sodium bicarbonate(mg)	Effervescent time (s)	*Solubility	pH
P_1	85.9	171.8	292.2	55± 2.08	2	5.35± 0.01
P_2	85.9	85.9	292.2	50± 3.21	3	6.30± 0.1
P_3	85.9	128.8	292.2	67± 1.53	2	6.11± 0.07
P_4	85.9	257.7	292.2	73± 3.51	1	3.51± 0.05
P_5	85.9	343.6	292.2	75± 1.83	1	2.72± 0.04
P_6	171.8	171.8	292.2	67± 2.87	2	3.45± 0.06
P_7	42.9	85.9	292.2	53± 1.52	3	6.74± 0.04
P_8	64.4	85.9	292.2	60± 2.31	3	6.47± 0.03
P_9	128.8	85.9	292.2	67± 1	3	6.13± 0.02
P_{10}	171.8	85.9	292.2	80± 2.08	3	5.37± 0.08
P_{11}	-	85.9	292.2	68± 2.52	2	6.48± 0.1
P_{12}	85.9	-	292.2	75± 1.15	5	6.57± 0.05
P_{13}	171.8	-	292.2	77± 2	5	6.10± 0.02
P_{14}	128.8	-	292.2	58± 1.53	5	6.42± 0.05
P_{15}	128.8	-	146.1	60± 2.50	5	5.59± 0.07
P_{16}	128.8	-	219.2	67± 1.53	5	6.23± 0.09
P_{17}	128.8	-	438.3	65± 2.31	3	6.73± 0.04
P_{18}	128.8	-	584.4	65± 3.64	3	6.75± 0.06

*Solubility of formulations using a standard table [15] (1=insoluble; 2=slightly soluble; 3=sparingly soluble; 4=soluble; 5=freely soluble)

Since ranitidine HCl has a bitter taste and a sulfur-like smell, using sweeteners and flavoring agents is necessary. We used different sweeteners at different levels in F_1 formulation. After adding the sweeteners and flavors, formulations were surveyed by the Latin square design.[11] The formulation with the highest mean score was selected as the best formulation (Table 2).

Table 2. Panel test for sweeteners and flavors by Latin Square method (on 40 volunteers).

Ingredients(mg)	Formulations													
	S1	S2	S3	S_4	S5	S6	S_7	S_8	S_9	S_{10}	S_{11}	S_{12}	S_{13}	S_{14}
Ranitidine	336	336	336	336	336	336	336	336	336	336	336	336	336	336
Citric acid	171.8	171.8	171.8	171.8	171.8	171.8	171.8	171.8	171.8	171.8	171.8	171.8	171.8	171.8
Na bicarbonate	292.2	292.2	292.2	292.2	292.2	292.2	292.2	292.2	292.2	292.2	292.2	292.2	292.2	292.2
Mannitol	80	–	100	100	–	100	100	150	150	150	150	150	200	150
Sorbitol	–	50	50	80	–	–	80	80	100	100	100	100	100	100
Aspartame	–	–	–	–	20	30	40	60	70	–	80	–	80	80
Sucrose	20	–	–	–	–	–	–	–	–	20	–	20	20	20
Acesulfame k	–	–	–	–	35	–	–	–	–	–	–	50	–	–
Mint	5	15	20	25	20	–	–	–	–	–	–	–	–	–
Cherry	–	–	–	–	–	–	20	30	–	–	–	–	–	–
Tutti-frutti	–	–	–	–	–	–	–	–	20	30	–	–	–	–
Raspberry	–	–	–	–	–	20	20	–	–	–	25	–	–	–
Orange	–	–	–	–	–	–	–	–	–	–	–	20	25	40

Evaluating the Mixture of Powders and Granules
The main flowability properties of granules and powders (before compression) were characterized by the angle of repose, compressibility index (Carr's index), and Hausner's ratio.

Angle of Repose (θ)
The frictional forces in a loose powder or granules may be measured by repose angle. It is defined as the maximum possible angle between the surface of a powder pile or granules and the horizontal plane. The granules were allowed to flow through a funnel fixed to a stand at a definite height. The angle of repose (θ) was then calculated by measuring the height (h) and radius (r) of the formed granules heap and putting the values into the formula :
Tan θ = (h/r).[12]

Compressibility Index
The flowability of powder may be evaluated by comparing the bulk density (ρ_b) and tapped density (ρ_t) of powder and the rate at which it packs down. The percentage of compressibility index was calculated as
$\frac{\rho\ tapped - \rho\ bulk}{\rho\ tapped} \times 100$.[13]

Hausner's Ratio
Hausner's ratio is an important character to determine the flow property of powder and granules. This can be calculation by the following formula: ρ_t/ρ_b.[14]

Particle Size Distribution
In order to evaluate particle size distribution, powders and granules are sieved. Powders or granules were then disposed on a series of sieves sized 20, 25, 30, 35, 40, 70, and 100 and placed on the device. The remaining powders or granules on each sieve were weighed and the mean particle size (d) was calculated as d= $\frac{\sum xidi}{100}$ where x_i was the average size of both upper and lower sieves and d_i was the percent of value i in the range of that bulk (Figure 1).[15]

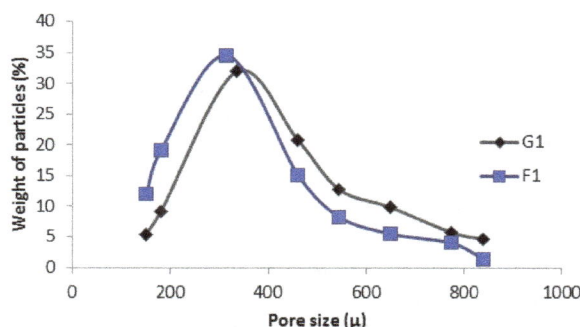

Figure 1. Particle size distribution of F_1 and G_1 300 mg tablets formulations

Preparation of Effervescent Tablets by Direct Compression Method
After mixing the powder with appropriate characteristics, the tablets were made. Ranitidine was first triturated with sweeteners and then mixed with the effervescent base. The powder was subsequently pressed in a single punch machine (Kilian & Co, Germany) with a rod number 14. The prepared tablets were dried in an oven at 60°C for 1 hour. They were finally packaged.

Preparation of Effervescent Tablets by Fusion Method

The selected acid and alkali were placed on a heater at 54°C to release the crystallization water of citric acid. The formed granules were then dried in an oven at 60°C. Afterwards, the mixture of ranitidine and the sweeteners was added. The powders were pressed in a single punch machine (Kilian & Co, Germany) with a rod number 14. The tablets were again dried in an oven at 60°C for 1 hour and finally packaged.

Physicochemical Evaluation of the Effervescent Tablets

The following physicochemical tests were conducted to evaluate the tablets.

Weight Variation

Twenty tablets were randomly selected and weighed individually and the weights of tablets were compared with the calculated mean weight. In this method, not more than two tablets should have a deviation greater than pharmacopoeia limits ± 5% of the weight.[16]

Friability Test

Friability of the tablets was determined using friabilator (Erweka, TAP, Germany). It subjected the tablets to the combined abrasion and shock in a plastic chamber revolving at 25 rpm for 4 minutes and dropping a tablet at height of 6 inches in each revolution. The tablets were reweighed. Tablets were de-dusted using a soft muslin cloth and reweighed. The percentage of the tablets friability was calculated as $\frac{initial\ weight\ of\ tablets - final\ weight\ of\ tablets}{initial\ weight\ of\ tablets} \times 100$. The desirable friability was determined as lower than 1%.[16]

Thickness

A vernier caliper (For-Bro Engineers, India) was used to determine the thickness of randomly 10 selected tablets.[17]

Hardness Test

The force required to break down a tablet in a compression is defined as the hardness or crushing strength of a tablet. In this study, ten tablets were randomly selected and individually placed in a hardness tester (Erweka, 24-TB, Germany) and then the hardness of tablets reported in N.[18]

CO_2 Content

Three tablets were placed in 100 ml of sulphuric acid solution 1N in 3 separate beakers. In order to determine the amount of released CO_2 (mg), the difference in weight before and after dissolving the tablets was calculated.[19]

Evaluating the Solution pH

Using a pH meter (Metrohm, 632, Switzerland), the pH of the solution was measured by dissolving 3 tablets in 3 beakers containing 200 ml of water.[20]

Effervescence Time

Three tablets were put in 3 beakers of water and the effervescence time was measured using a stopwatch. Effervescence time was defined as the moment when a clear solution was obtained.[18]

Assay

Twenty tablets were weighed and grounded into a fine powder. An amount of powder equivalent to 200 mg of ranitidine HCl was weighed accurately and mixed with 70 ml of pure water in a 100 ml volumetric flask. The mixture was shaken for about 20 minutes. Purified water was then added to fill the flask. After mixing well, the solution was filtered using a Whatman No. 42 filter paper. The first 10 ml of the filtrate was discarded. A suitable aliquot was subsequently subjected to analysis by titrimetry. The filtrate (equivalent to 2 mg/ml) was diluted appropriately to obtain a 100 µg/ml solution which is then analyzed by spectrophotometry.[21]

Content Uniformity

After selecting 10 tablets randomly, the content of each tablet was determined separately.[15]

Water Content

Ten tablets were dried for 4 hours in a desiccator containing silica gel. The percentage of water content was calculated as $\frac{tablet\ weight\ before\ drying - tablet\ weight\ after\ drying}{tablet\ weight\ before\ drying} \times 100$.[18]

Equilibrium Moisture Content

Three tablets were placed in 3 desiccators containing saturated salt solutions of sodium nitrite (RH, 60%), sodium chloride (RH, 71%), and potassium nitrate (RH, 90%). The percentage of equilibrium moisture content was determined on the first and seventh days by the following method. First, about 50 ml of methanol was poured in Autotitrator (Mettler, TOLEDO-DL53, Switzerland) while a dry magnet was present with methanol. It was titrated by the endpoint with Karl Fischer reagent. In a dry mortar, the pellets were grounded to fine powder of which 100 mg was accurately weighed and transferred to the titration vessel quickly. It was stirred by the end point.[20] The equilibrium moisture content was then calculated as $V \times F \times 100$ in which F was a factor of Karl Fischer reagent and V, the volume of Karl Fischer reagent consumed for sample titration in ml.

Results

Examining the standard curves of ranitidine HCl in purified water led to the curve equation, y=0.044x+0.086 and the regression $R^2 = 0.998$.

Finally, some of the formulations were obtained by measuring effervescent components and eighteen formulations listed in Table 1. The formulations were selected with the best solubility, effervescence time and pH. The formulation with an effervescence time of over

180 seconds or a sediment formation were deleted. The P_1-P_5 formulations were fixed in amount of citric acid and sodium bicarbonate but variable in amount of tartaric acid. The P_7-P_{11} formulations varied in the amount of citric acid and according to the previous results, tartaric acid was 85.9 mg but sodium bicarbonate was fixed. Thus, citric acid was not less than its original value because of its pH rises. The P_{14}-P_{18} formulations varied in the amount of sodium bicarbonate but citric acid was fixed. Therefore, the amount of sodium bicarbonate should be 146.1- 292.2 mg. After altering the ratio of effervescent components, the materials had a lot of effect on solubility and pH. The P_{12}-P_{16} formulation were selected as the appropriate base formulations in tableting process.

To improve the unpleasant taste of ranitidine HCl, various sweeteners were used and then the sweeteners added to the formulation of F_6 (according to Table 3) and the mixture of sweeteners utilized (S_{14} formulation). Different flavors were then added to the formulations and surveyed by Latin square method. Mint and orange flavors were finally selected as the best flavors (Table 2).

Based on the previous stages, 6 formulations for 300 mg tablets were selected as the best (Table 3).

Table 3. Compositions of 300 mg ranitidine HCl effervescent tablets.

Ingredients (mg)	Formulations					
	F_1	F_2	F_3	F_4	F_5	F_6
Ranitidine	336	336	336	336	336	336
Citric acid	128.8	171.8	128.8	171.8	128.8	171.8
Na bicarbonate	146.1	146.1	219.2	219.2	292.2	292.2
Mannitol	150	150	150	150	150	150
Sorbitol	100	100	100	100	100	100
Aspartame	80	80	80	80	80	80
Sucrose	20	20	20	20	20	20
PVP	8	8	8	8	8	8
PEG 6000	15	15	15	15	15	15
Mint	20	20	20	20	20	20

Evaluation of Powders Blend and Granules

The results for evaluation of powder blend and granular formulations are provided in Table 4, and their results were compared with standard tables.[15]

Table 4. Evaluation of physical characteristics of powders and granules blend in 300 mg tablets.

Physical characteristics	Formulations											
	F_1	G_1	F_2	G_2	F_3	G_3	F_4	G_4	F_5	G_5	F_6	G_6
Angle of repose (θ)	27.7	26.3	29.7	27.3	29.3	25.5	30.1	25.3	28.2	27.6	27.3	26.1
Compressibility index	7.35	3.72	5.26	5.21	3.74	1.74	3.2	2.41	8.79	4.92	5.40	4.32
Hausner's ratio	1.08	1.04	1.06	1.06	1.04	1.02	1.03	1.02	1.1	1.05	1.06	1.04
Mean particle size	302.9	385.3	304.6	385.4	303.6	375.9	304.5	380.7	318.6	383.9	308.5	371.6

Physicochemical Evaluation

Tablets were prepared by direct compression and fusion methods. They was exposed to all of the physicochemical tests. The weight of formulated effervescent tablets met the pharmacopoeia criteria. Physicochemical tests were conducted on complete tablets including assay, hardness, friability, thickness, weight variation, CO_2 content, water content and equilibrium moisture content (Tables 5, 6). All tablets had similar conditions in the weight variation test in pharmacopoeia limits i.e $\pm$ 5% .[21] The drug content of the whole formulations were put down in the range of 85-115%.[1]

Table 5. Physicochemical evaluation of 300 mg effervescent ranitidine HCl tablets by direct compression method (Mean ± SD).

Physicochemical evaluation	Formulations					
	F1	F_2	F_3	F_4	F_5	F_6
Weight variation (%)	1.95±0.04	2.32±0.04	1.76±0.05	1.12±0.08	1.08±0.05	1.30±0.04
Friability test (%)	0.78±0.10	0.89±0.18	0.78±0.18	0.84±0.22	0.57±0.13	0.43±0.13
Thickness (mm)	5.08±0.03	5.73±0.04	5.18±0.05	5.23±0.08	5.50±0.01	5.75±0.06
Hardness (N)	58±8.50	42±6.46	59±4.12	47.5±3.30	65±4.28	66±6.43
pH	5.36±0.03	5.02±0.02	5.85±0.02	5.38±0.01	6.1±0.04	5.94±0.02
Effervescence time (sec)	98±1.53	82±3	82±2.50	67±3.61	90±4.04	83±3.79
CO_2 content (mg)	239±1	240±0.58	244±1.53	247±1.16	248±0.58	250±1.15
Assay (mg)	340±0.02	330.3±0.05	341.4±0.04	336.7±0.02	336±0.01	335±0.04
Content uniformity (%)	99.4±3.55	99.2±4.15	100±4.92	100.1±2.96	100.1±3.94	99.5±5.02
Water content (%w/w)	0.14±0.006	0.18±0.012	0.17±0.007	0.14±0.007	0.20±0.003	0.16±0.009

Friability of the all formulations was found to be lower than 1%. The hardness of the tablets was determined using a hardness tester. The values were within the range of 40-80 (N). The thickness of the tablets varied between 3 and 6 mm. The tablets produced by the fusion method were thicker. The effervescence test was carried out in 200 ml of water. Effervescence times of all formulations were 67-98 seconds. The G_1 and F_1 formulations of 300 mg tablets had the longest effervescence time (91 and 98 seconds, respectively). Effervescent compounds basically absorb a lot of moisture. Water content of all formulations was lower than 0.5%.

Table 6. Physicochemical evaluation of 300 mg effervescent ranitidine HCl tablets by fusion method (Mean ± SD).

Physicochemical evaluation	Formulations					
	G_1	G_2	G_3	G_4	G_5	G_6
Weight variation (%)	1.89±0.003	1.53±0.018	1.09±0.004	1.11±0.012	1.03±0.004	1.05±0.004
Friability test (%)	0.55±0.11	0.63±0.34	0.49±0.12	0.59±0.23	0.39±0.12	0.33±0.19
Thickness (mm)	5.12±0.02	5.15±0.03	5.25±0.03	5.34±0.05	5.40±0.02	5.45±0.05
Hardness (N)	64±5.34	54±4.35	65±6.57	63±6.73	68±5.27	73±3.15
pH	5.31±0.03	4.93±0.02	5.75±0.02	5.32±0.006	6.12±0.04	5.95±0.01
Effervescence time (sec)	91±3.05	72±1.53	70±2.52	69±2.51	86±2.52	72±2.64
CO_2 content (mg)	236±1.16	238±0.58	241±1	244±1	245±1.16	249±0.58
Assay (mg)	336±0.03	340.6±0.06	337.5±0.03	336.7±0.02	336.5±0.06	338.9±0.04
Content uniformity (%)	99.6±4.30	99.6±3.63	99.7±4.41	99.9±3.87	99.6±4	99.9±4.40
Water content (%w/w)	0.020±0.003	0.04±0.001	0.05±0.002	0.04±0.001	0.05±0.001	0.04±0.002

Among 300 mg tablets, the F_6 and G_6 formulations had the lowest friability. In both methods, the F_6 and F_2 formulations had the highest and lowest hardness, respectively.

The pH of formulations should be within the range of 5.5 and 6.2, otherwise they may not be acceptable due to lack of stability and sediment production.
The results of equilibrium moisture content (%) of effervescent powders and granules formulations (F_5 and F_6) are provided in Table 7.

Table 7. Equilibrium moisture content (%) in effervescent powder and granular mixing of the F_4 and F_5 in temperature 18 °C.

Formulations	Microclimates	Powder effervescent mixing		Variation (%w/w)	Effervescent granule		Variation (%w/w)
		1st Day	7th Day		1st Day	7th Day	
F_5	RH 90%	11.54(0.02)*	15.63(0.03)	26	13.32(0.01)	19.39(0.01)	31
	RH 71%	4.98 (0.02)	6.25(0.01)	20	5.12 (0.02)	7.18(0.01)	28
	RH 60%	2.22 (0.02)	2.73(0.03)	18	3.11(0.01)	3.65 (0.03)	14
F_6	RH 90%	12.93(0.01)	18.67(0.01)	44	14.77(0.02)	21.32(0.01)	44
	RH 71%	6.42 (0.02)	8.83(0.02)	38	7.18(0.02)	9.34 (0.01)	30
	RH 60%	3.85 (0.01)	5.29(0.02)	37	5.60(0.02)	6.78(0.02)	21

*Mean (standard deviation), n=3
The saturated salt solutions: sodium nitrite (RH, 60%), sodium chloride (RH, 71%), and potassium nitrate (RH, 90%).

Discussion

Most of the oral pharmaceutical dosage forms such as conventional tablets and capsules are formulated to be swallowed or chewed. Old people and children frequently have difficulties in swallowing these dosage forms. Such problems are more serious for those confined to bed patients. Despite the attractiveness of effervescent pharmaceutical forms, 300 mg ranitidine HCl is not available in this form. Since it is better tolerated by patients and results in a faster recovery, as the previous studies show,[22] we decided to formulate and research the 300 mg effervescent ranitidine HCl tablets.
The standard curve of ranitidine HCl in purified water was plotted using the UV spectrophotometer with λ_{max} of 315.3 nm. This was in agreement with the results obtained from the other studies.[23]
Since the effervescent reaction in effervescent products requires acid and alkali resources, so they were used in all formulations. Then, pH of the solution, the solubility and the effervescence time were tested.[24] Formulations containing tartaric acid (P_1-P_{12}) were eliminated due to the formation of clearly observed sediment and a lower pH. The P_{17} and P_{18} formulations with a higher amount of sodium bicarbonate were eliminated due to the observed sediment and the highest pH. Ratios of effervescent components in the formulations of P_{12}-P_{16} led to a better solubility, a pH less than 6 and an appropriate effervescent reaction.

As mentioned earlier, the very bitter taste and the sulphur-like smell of ranitidine HCl are major problems for the patients. Hence, the next step was to add flavor and sweeteners to improve the taste of final product and to increase patient acceptance. A previous study also reported similar findings.[25]

Consequently, several sweeteners were used in this stage and none of them could not mask the unpleasant taste, so a mixture of sweeteners was used. Different flavors were used and 40 volunteers chose the best formulation in 3 stages and the formulation with a score about 4 was selected as the best (Table 2). The S_{14} formulations were the best.

Each of the physical properties listed in Table 4 were compared with USP tables. In both methods, most of the formulations had a suitable flowability. As the results showed, angle of repose was reduced in fusion method. For example, angles of repose of F_6, G_6 (the same formulations, but different manufacturing methods) were reported as 27.3, 26.1, respectively. Hausner's ratio and compressibility index are reduced in fusion method. Fusion method increases flowability and decreases angle of repose due to increasing the particle size and its spherical shape.[26] Compressibility of the granules was higher due to internal porosity of granules.

The mean diameter of particles in the fusion method is larger than the average diameter of the particles in the direct compression due to the adhesion of smaller particles and formation of larger particles. The particle size of all formulations was in the range of 150-800 microns. Effervescent granules had the particle size larger than of the effervescent powders blend.

The majority of formulations had the weight variation and friability of pharmacopoeia limits.[26] The F_5, F_6, G_3, G_5, and G_6 formulations were suitable friability. The F_1, F_3, F_5, F_6, G_1-G_6 formulations had the desired hardness. Due to a lower hardness of direct compression method, the friability of tablets was increased compared to the fusion method. Another study found similar results.[27]

CO_2 content of fusion method is lower than that of the direct compression method. These differences are found in manufacturing process of the granules. In the studied formulations, CO_2 contents of G_5 and G_6 were 245 and 249 mg, respectively. Other study reported that in each grams of formulas containing citric acid and sodium bicarbonate CO_2 content, was 292 mg which is comparable with these results.[20] In formulation G_1, lower level of CO_2 was obtained.

The pH of formulations should be within the range of 5.7 and 6.2. Therefore, the F_3, F_5 and F_6 formulations of 300 mg tablets were selected.

The effervescence times of the all formulations were less than 3 minutes and all were in the range mentioned in BP.[7] All of the formulations showed effervescence within 67 to 98 seconds.

Finally, a drug content was established in a range of 330.25-338.89 mg for 300 mg tablets which was within

the normal range. Drug content of all formulations was in the range mentioned in USP.[15]

Water content was lower in formulations of fusion method, since they had lost some water during granulation process.

Measurements of relative humidity in some formulations revealed more moisture absorption in the fusion method, compared with direct compression method. Moreover, formulations with higher amounts of sodium bicarbonate absorbed more moisture. Therefore, the F_5 and F_6 formulations absorbed the highest amount of moisture.

Conclusion

Effervescent ranitidine HCl tablets were prepared by fusion and direct compression methods to replace the conventional tablets of ranitidine HCl in treatment of gastric and duodenal ulcers. The results obtained at each stage of formulation were utilized and the best formulations selected.

After performing the required studies, citric acid, sodium bicarbonate and sweeteners (including mannitol, sucrose and aspartame) were selected. Pre and post-compression tests were conducted on the prepared tablets. Aspartame, mint and orange flavors were more effective in masking the bitter taste of ranitidine.

Finally, the F_5 and F_6 formulations of 300 mg tablets were selected as the best formulation because of their physicochemical characteristics. It is significant that fusion method resulted in better tablets compared to direct compression method.

Acknowledgments

This study was supported by Isfahan University of Medical Sciences as a thesis research project numbered 390181.

Conflict of Interests

Authors have no conflict of interests.

References

1. Rajalakshmi G, Vamsi CH, Balachandar R, Damodharan N. Formulation and evaluation of diclofenac potassium effervescent tablets. *Int J Pharm Biomed Res* 2011;2(4):237-43.
2. Prabhakar C, Krishna KB. A review on effervesent tablets. *Int J Pharm Technol* 2011;3:704-12.
3. Palanisamy P, Abhishekh R, Yoganand Kumar D. Formulation and evaluation of effervescent tablets of aceclofenac. *Int Res J Pharm* 2011;2(12):185-90.
4. Srinath KR, Chowdary CP, Palanisamy P, Krishna AV, Aparna S, et al. Formulation and evaluation of effervescent tablets of paracetamol. *Int J Pharm Res Dev* 2011;3(3):76-104.
5. Lee RE. Effervescent tablets. 2010; Available from: http://www.amerilabtech.com/wp-content/uploads/ EffervescentTabletsKeyFacts.pdf.

6. Wadhwani AR, Prabhu NB, Nadkarni MA, Amin PD. Consumer friendly mucolytic formulations. *Indian J Pharm Sci* 2004;7:506-7.

7. Bandeline FJ. Granulation. In: Liberman HA, Lachman L, Schwartz JB, editors. Pharmaceutical Dosage Forms: Tablets. New York: Marcel Dekker Inc; 1989. P. 287-92.

8. Bhusan SY, Sambhaji SP, Anant RP, Kakasaheb RM. New drug delivery system for elderly. *Indian Drug* 2000;37:312-8.

9. Brunton L, Lazo J, Parker K. Goodman and Gilman's the pharmacological basis of therapeutics. New York: McGraw-Hill; 2005.

10. Kitagami K, Yamao J. NSAID induced gastroduodenal lesions in patients with rheumatoid arthritis. *Jpn Gastroent.* 1990;87:2025-6.

11. Clarke-O'Neill S, Pettersson L, Fader M, Dean G, Brooks R, Cottenden A. A multicentre comparative evaluation: Washable pants with an integral pad for light incontinence. *J Clin Nurs* 2002;11(1):79-89.

12. Gunn C, Carter SJ. Cooper and Gunn's Tutorial Pharmacy. New Delhi: CBS Publishers; 1986.

13. Nagar P, Singh K, Chauhan I, Verma M, Yasir M. Orally disintegrating tablets: Formulation, preparation techniques and evaluation. *J Appl Pharm Sci* 2011;1(4):35-45.

14. Patil MG, Kakade SM, Pathade SG. Formulation and evaluation of orally disintegrating tablet containing tramadol HCL by mass extrusion technique. *J Appl Pharm Sci* 2011;1(6):178-81.

15. United States Pharmacopeia and National Formulary. 29th ed. Rockville, MD, USA: United States Pharmacopeial Convention; 2006.

16. Lachman L, Lieberman HA, Kanig JL. The Theory and Practice of Industrial Pharmacy. 3rd ed. Mumbai:Vargheese Publishing House;1991.

17. Tadros MI. Controlled-release effervescent floating matrix tablets of ciprofloxacin hydrochloride: development, optimization and in vitro-in vivo evaluation in healthy human volunteers. *Eur J Pharm Biopharm* 2010;74(2):332-9.

18. Masareddy R, Yellanki SK, Patil BR, Manvi V. Development and evaluation of floating matrix tablets of riboflavin. *Int J PharmTech Res* 2010;2(2):1439-45.

19. Prajapati ST, Patel LD, Patel DM. Gastric floating matrix tablets: design and optimization using combination of polymers. *Acta Pharm* 2008;58(2):221-9.

20. Yanze FM, Duru C, Jacob M. A process to produce effervescent tablets: fluidized bed dryer melt granulation. *Drug Dev Ind Pharm* 2000;26(11):1167-76.

21. Basavaiah K, Nagegowda P, Ramakrishna V. Determination of drug content of pharmaceuticals containing ranitidine by titrimetry and spectrophotometry in non-aqueous medium. *Sci Asia* 2005;31:207-14.

22. Gosai AR, Patil SB, Sawant KK. Formulation and evaluation of oro dispersible tablets of ondansetron hydrochloride by direct compression using superdisintegrants. *Int J Pharm Sci Nanotechnol* 2008;26(1):106-11.

23. Jaiswal D, Bahattacharya A, Yadav IK, Singh HP, Chandra D, Jain DA. Formulation and evaluation of oil entrapped floating alginate beads of ranitidine hydrochloride. *Int J Pharm Pharm Sci* 2009;1(3):128-40.

24. Moghimipour E, Akhgari A, Ghassemian Z. Formulation of glucosamine effervescent granules. *Sci Med J* 2010 ;9(1):21-34.

25. Sharma V, Chopra H. Formulation and evaluation of taste masked mouth dissolving tablets of levocetirizine hydrochloride. *Iran J Pharm Res* 2012;11(2):457-63.

26. Twitchell A. Mixing. In: Aulton ME, editor. Pharmaceutics: The Science of Dosage Form Design. 3rd ed. New York: Churchill Livingstone; 2007. P. 181-96.

27. Bhardwaj V, Bansal M, Sharma PK. Formulation and evaluation of fast dissolving tablets of amlodipine besylate using different super disintegrants and camphor as sublimating agent. *Am-Euras J Sci Res* 2010;5(4):264-9.

13

Mass-Production and Characterization of Anti-CD20 Monoclonal Antibody in Peritoneum of Balb/c Mice

Koushan Sineh Sepehr[1,2], Behzad Baradaran[1,2]*, Jafar Majidi[2], Jalal Abdolalizadeh[2], Leili Aghebati[2], Fatemeh Zare Shahneh[1,2]

[1] *Drug Applied Research Center, Tabriz University of Medical Sciences, Tabriz, Iran.*

[2] *Immunology Research Center, Tabriz University of Medical Sciences, Tabriz, Iran.*

ARTICLE INFO

Keywords:
Monoclonal antibody
Ascetic fluid
Affinity chromatography
Human CD20

ABSTRACT

Purpose: Monoclonal antibodies are important tools are used in basic research as well as, in diagnosis, imaging and treatment of immunodeficiency diseases, infections and cancers. The purpose of this study was to produce large scale of monoclonal antibody against CD20 in order to diagnostic application in leukemia and lymphomas disorders. *Methods:* Hybridoma cells that produce monoclonal antibody against human CD20 were administered into the peritoneum of the Balb/c mice which have previously been primed with 0.5 ml Pristane. After twelve days, approximately 7 ml ascetic fluid was harvested from the peritoneum of each mouse. Evaluation of mAb titration was assessed by ELISA method. In the present study, we describe a protocol for large scale production of MAbs. *Results:* We prepared monoclonal antibodies (mAbs) with high specificity and sensitivity against human CD20 by hybridoma method and characterized them by ELISA. The subclass of antibody was IgG2a and its light chain was kappa. Ascetic fluid was purified by Protein-A Sepharose affinity chromatography and the purified monoclonal antibody was conjugated with FITC and Immunofluorescence was done for confirming the specific binding. *Conclusion:* The conjugated monoclonal antibody could have application in diagnosis B-cell lymphomas, hairy cell leukemia, B-cell chronic lymphocytic leukemia, and melanoma cancer stem cells.

Introduction

The current era of monoclonal antibodies (MAb) was introduced with the hybridoma technology devised by Köhler and Milstein in 1975.[1] They fused a single antibody-producing cell from the spleen of an immunized mouse with a human myeloma cell to produce an immortal hybrid cell that secreted an antibody to a single antigenic epitope. The antibody-producing spleen cell provided the specificity and the myeloma cell provided the immortality.[2] The first monoclonal antibodies were primarily mouse monoclonal and used to identify antigens on cells, usually by immune-fluorescent techniques, particularly by automated flowcytometry. Currently, monoclonal antibodies play crucial roles in diagnosis applications, disease monitoring, identifying prognostic markers and therapy. Meanwhile each antibody is highly specific for a particular antigen; this characteristic feature of antibodies has led to their routine usage in diagnostic kits and in uncovering the function of such antigens in a number of physiological and pathological conditions.[3,4] By hybridoma technology, monoclonal antibodies have been prepared against an extensive range of antigens including growth factors, growth factor receptors, mutated antigens, viruses, bacterial products, hormones, drugs, enzymes, and differentiated antigens. Such antibodies are used commonly in the identification of the antigens in human tumor biopsies and sera, and in considering their role in tumor progression.[5]

CD20, a 33–36 KD non-glycosylated phosphoprotein that has stable expression and tightly bound to the membrane with little modulation during maturation, and it likely has an important role in B-cell activation and regulation of cell cycle. All these features make CD20 an ideal anti-B-cell target.[6-8] CD20 is expressed within key B-cell development stages that give rise to B-cell lymph-proliferative disorders. production of the first anti-CD20 monoclonal antibody could have application in diagnosis malignancies, disease monitoring, prognostication or therapy of B-cell lymphomas, hairy cell leukemia, B-cell chronic lymphocytic leukemia, and melanoma cancer stem cells.[9,10]

For mass-production of the monoclonal antibody, hybridoma cells should be reproduced in either of two methods: in vivo method; Injection of desired clone

---

Corresponding author: Behzad Baradaran, Assistant Professor of Immunology, Drug Applied Research Center, Tabriz University of Medical Sciences, Tabriz, Iran. Emails: behzad_im@yahoo.com, baradaranb@tbzmed.ac.ir

into the peritoneal cavity of the mouse or in vitro method; Culture of the cells in tissue culture flasks. In this regards, the required purity and concentration of mAb were obtained in mouse ascetic fluid and tissue-culture supernatant.[11]

When hybridoma cells are injected into the peritoneum of mouse, the cells grow and produce ascitic fluid.[12] The method of ascitic fluid production in peritoneum of mouse is economic, but reproduction of cells by in vitro method needs special skills, special medium.[13] Furthermore, the loss of antibody's original glycosylation by in vitro culture method affected mAb biologic functions like increased immunogenicity, reduced binding affinity, accelerated clearance in vivo and preferred pharmacokinetic characteristics. Furthermore, contaminated hybridoma cells producing mAb with infectious disease often be passed through mice. So, antibody production in ascitic fluid can be a suitable and economical method.[14] The diagnostic-industry scale of mAb production is usually small to medium and large. The therapeutic industry is significantly less concerned than the diagnostic commerce with cost and turn-around time, and its production scale is medium to large. In summary, by the in vivo method, hybridoma cells in high density allow abundant production of highly active and pure MAbs necessary for certain specific purposes.

Materials and Methods

Female BALB/c mice (4-6 weeks old) were obtained from Pasteur institute of Iran. 0.5 ml Pristane (2, 6, 10, 14 tetra methyl pentadecane, Sigma) was administered intra-peritoneally into each mouse. Twelve days after priming with Pristane, high cell densities of a desired mono clone (1×10^6 cells / 0.5 ml PBS) were injected intra-peritoneally into each mouse. The mice were assessed daily for production of ascetic fluid after the injection of hybridoma cells. Abdomen of the mice was completely enlarged and their skins were extended about ten days after the injection of cells. Their ascetic fluids were harvested by 19-gauge needle. After 4 days, ascitic fluid of the mice were harvested again and centrifuged and the related supernatants were collected for characterization.[15]

The titer of monoclonal antibody was assessed by ELISA method. In this assay, 100 µl BSA-conjugated peptide (10 µg/ml) was coated in 96 wells plate (Nunc) overnight at 4 °C. After twice washing with PBS-Tween 20 (0.05%), non-specific sites were blocked with 2% BSA and incubated at 37 °C for 45 minutes. The washing was repeated and then 100µl of the continuous dilution of ascitic fluid was added to each well and incubated for an hour at 37 °C. Then the plate was washed five times. 100 µl of Rabbit Anti-mouse Ig conjugated with HRP (100 µl, 1/4000 dilution) (Sigma-Aldrich Co. Louis, USA) was added to each well and incubated for 45 minutes at 37 °C. After five times of washing, 100 µl of Tetramethylbenzidine (TMB) substrate solution (Sigma) was added into each well

and incubated for 20 minutes in dark place at RT. After 20 min, the reaction was stopped by adding 100 µl stopping solution (0.16 M H2SO4) to each well and Optical Density (OD) was read by ELISA Reader at 450 nm. Therefore the titer of monoclonal antibody in ascitic fluid was determined.[16]

Isotyping

ELISA mouse mAb isotyping Kit (Thermo, USA) was used for determination the class and subclass of the mAbs. First, tris buffer saline (TBS) was used for 1/50000 dilution of the ascetic fluid and 50 µl of diluted antibody added to each well of the 8-well strip. At the next step 50 µl of the anti-mouse IgG + IgA+ IgM + HRP conjugated was added to each well of the 8-well strip and then the plate was incubated for an hour at room temperature. After 3 times washing, 75 µl of TMB substrate was added to each well and the plate was incubated at room temperature in a dark place. After 10 min, the reaction was stopped by adding 75 µl of stopping solution to each well. The subsequent color of the reactions was measured at 450 nm by an ELISA reader (Biotech, USA).[17]

Purification

The diluted ascetic fluid in PBS (1:2) was precipitated with saturated ammonium sulfate and dialyzed against PBS pH 7.4 and IgG2a class mAbs were purified by Protein-A-Sepharose column affinity chromatography. Briefly, ascetic fluids were filtered through 45 µm filter and pH was adjusted to pH 7.5. Antibodies were affinity purified using a column of Protein A Sepharose. The elution was performed using 0.1 mol/l glycine buffer, pH=2.7. Mouse IgG 2a elute with 0.1M citrate buffer in pH 4.5. The eluted antibodies were dialyzed overnight against PBS pH=7.5 and the reactivity of the antibodies were measured by ELISA as described above.

Confirmation of the MAb purity by SDS-PAGE

Confirmation of the MAb purity was monitored by SDS-PAGE in non-reducing condition. 10 µg of purified mAb was mixed with 10 µl of sample buffer, then boiled for 2-5 min and cooled on ice. Electrophoresis was done in a 12% SDS-PAGE gel with a mini- PROTEAN electrophoresis instrument (Bio- Rad Laboratories, Hercules, CA, USA) 100 mA for 1 hr. The gel was stained with Coomassie Brilliant Blue R-250 (Sigma).

Conjugation of Monoclonal Antibody with Fluorescein Isothiocyanate (Fitc)

For conjugation, 200 µl mAb (5mg/ml) was added in 800 µl Reaction Buffer (500 Mm Carbonate, pH = 9.2) and dialyzed against PBS buffer in 24 hours. The antibody concentration was measured after buffer equilibration in 280 nm. 10 mg of FITC was dissolved in 1 mL anhydrous DMSO immediately before use. FITC (SIGMA, Germany) was added to give a ratio of

80 µg per mg of antibody and mixed immediately. The tubes were wrapping in foil then incubate and rotate at room temperature for 1 hour. The unreacted FITC was removed and exchanged the antibody into Storage Buffer (10 mM Tris, 150 mM Nacl, 0.1% Nah3, pH=8.2) by dialysis during overnight.[5]

Direct Immunofluorescence Staining

This technique was used for confirming the result of conjugation method. Raji cell line as a positive control (CD20 +) and Molt-4 as a negative control (CD20 -) were cultured in microtiter plates and after reaching in 50% confluence, cell suspension were transferred to 15 mL conical tubes and washed with RPMI medium. 50 µL of the cell suspension (1×10^6 cells) was Added to each microtiter plate well and then 1/1000 dilution of fluorochrome-conjugated monoclonal antibody was added. The mixture was incubated for 45 minutes on ice and washed two times with 100 µL of cold PBS buffer. Cells were suspend in 200 µL of 3.7% formaldehyde solution for fixation of Raji cells in 10 min at Room temperature and after two times washing, stained cells were analyses by florescent microscope.[5]

Results

For priming the peritoneum of the mice, Pristane were administered. High cell densities of a desired mono clone (1×10^6 cells) were suspended in 0.5 ml of sterile PBS and injected to each mouse. About 5 ml ascetic fluid was harvested from each mouse after twelve day. About 2 ml ascetic fluid was harvested from their peritoneum for a second time, after 4 days. The titer of monoclonal antibody in ascetic fluid was assessed by ELISA method. The mean absorbance of non-immune mouse serum, Immune mouse serum, and ascetic fluid was compared in Table 1 at 450 nm.

Table 1. Comparison of the mean absorbance of ascetic fluid at 450 nm

NC (SP/0)	NC* (Non Immune mouse serum)	PC* (Immune mouse serum)	Ascetic fluid (1/16000 dilution)
0.07	0.1	1.2	1.08
* With 1/8000 dilution			

The results showed that its 1/16000 dilution has high absorbance with CD20 antigen (above 1). Determination of mAb class and subclasses in ascetic fluid was examined by mouse isotyping kit (Thermo, USA). The subclass of monoclonal antibody was IgG2a with "kappa" type light chain. The product was precipitated by saturated ammonium sulfate and dialyzed against PBS and assess by UV at 280 nm. 40 mg concentrated protein was harvested. Purification by Protein-A-Sepharose column affinity chromatography yielded about 5 mg of monoclonal antibody and only one 150 KD band was appeared in non-reducing SDS-PAGE Figure 1. The purified monoclonal antibody was conjugated with fluorescein isothiocyanate (FITC) and

then Direct Immunofluorescence Staining was used for confirming the result of conjugation method and mAb specification. Specific attachment of purified mAb with CD20 antigen was evaluated by immuno-floresance techniques in the completely.

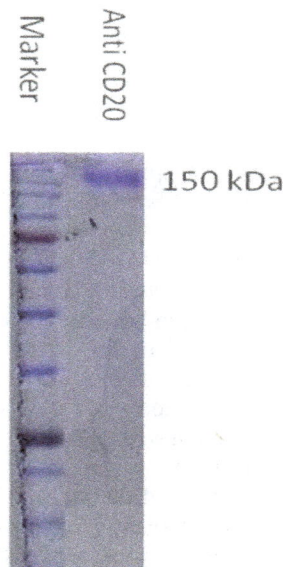

Figure 1. Non-reducing SDS-PAGE, one 150 KD band was appeared which could confirm purified antibody product.

Discussion

All branches of medical sciences have been touched with the hybridoma technology, in diagnosis malignancies, disease monitoring, prognostication or therapy.[18] Currently, monoclonal antibodies play crucial roles in diagnosis applications, disease monitoring, identifying prognostic markers and therapy. Since the introduction of the hybridoma technology by Kohler and Milstein in 1975, a variety of methodological technologies have been developed for large-scale production of mAbs.[1] To produce the desired mAb, the cells must be grown in either of two ways: by injection into the abdominal cavity of a suitably prepared mouse or by tissue culturing cells in plastic flasks. For efficient laboratory-scale production of monoclonal antibodies, hybridoma cells are injected into the peritoneum of mouse; the cells grow and produce ascetic fluid.[2] The production of monoclonal antibody in the ascetic fluid is commercially cost effective for large-scale production in comparison of expensive and time-consuming culture methods. In mouse method, two important factors for producing the required amount of cells are injected Pristane and the interval of priming with hybridoma cells. For example, for harvesting about 3-4 ml ascetic fluid from the peritoneum of each mouse, one million cells must be injected to the peritoneum of mouse.

In similar previous study, Baradaran et al produced large scale monoclonal antibody against EGFR in ascetic fluid efficiently and 10.4 mg antibody was purified with Ion exchange chromatography (IEC).[16]

In other study Galen et al used in vivo method for mass production of monoclonal antibodies against human rennin that ascites were produced after intra-peritoneal injection of cloned hybridoma cells into pristane-treated Balb/c mice. Then monoclonal antibodies were purified from ascites by affinity chromatography on protein A Sepharose.[19] Furthermore Mittal et al. used the same in production and characterization of murine monoclonal antibodies against *Haemophilus parasuis*.[20] In all these studies, In vivo methods were preferred for its cost effectiveness and high concentrations of mAbs produced.

Since analysis of mAb produced in tissue culture reveals that a desired antibody function is diminished or lost. In vitro methods are expensive and time-consuming and often fail to produce the required amount of antibody even with skilled manipulation.[8,9]

Considering to all issues, in this study injection into the abdominal cavity was preferred. Pristane were used for priming the peritoneum of the mice by high cell densities of a desired mono clone (1×10^{6} cells). Ascetic fluids were harvested from the mice and the titer of monoclonal antibody was assessed by ELISA method. The results showed that 1/16000 dilution has high absorbance with CD20 antigen (above 1).

For the class and subclass of mAbs determination, ELISA mouse mAb isotyping Kit was used and Monoclonal antibody class was IgG2a and its light chain was "kappa" type. Concentration of the dialyzed ascetic fluid product in assay with UV at 280 nm was about 40 mg and Protein-A Sepharose purification with affinity chromatography yielded about 5 mg of purified monoclonal antibody. Purity was monitored by SDS-PAGE in non-reducing condition, only one 150 KD band was appeared that demonstrate purified antibody. The purified monoclonal antibody was conjugated with fluorescein isothiocyanate (FITC). Direct Immunofluorescence Staining was used for confirming the result of conjugation method and mAb specification. Specific attachment of purified mAb with CD20 antigen was evaluated using immuno-floresance techniques in the surface of Raji cells (shown in Figure 2). CD20 is expressed within key B-cell development stages and generation of the first anti-CD20 monoclonal antibody could have application in diagnosis malignancies, disease monitoring, prognostication or therapy of B-cell lymphomas, hairy cell leukemia, B-cell chronic lymphocytic leukemia, and melanoma cancer stem cells.[18]

Conclusion

Taking all together, ascetic fluid production method seems to be a reasonable and economic approach for mAb production with suitable purity and concentration

Acknowledgements

We would like to thank for Drug Applied Research Center especially Animal House and Immunology Research Center (IRC) for kind assistance, respectively. This work was supported by a grant from Drug Applied Research Center.

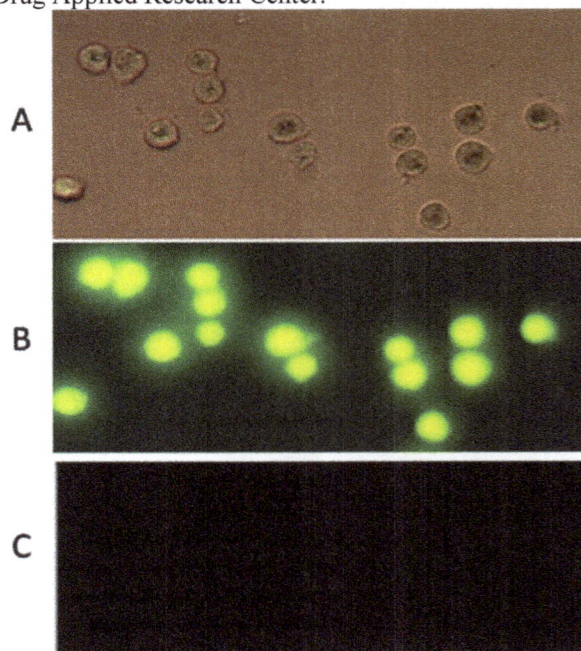

Figure 2. Direct Immunofluorescence Staining was used for confirming specific attachment of purified mAb with CD20 antigen in the surface of Raji cells. A. Raji cell before treatment, B. after treatment with purified mAb, C. Negative control.

Conflict of Interest

There is no conflict of interest in this study.

References

1. Kohler G, Milstein C. Continuous cultures of fused cells secreting antibody of predefined specificity. *Nature* 1975; 256(5517):495-7.
2. Modjtahedi H. Monoclonal Antibodies as Therapeutic Agents: Advances and Challenges. *Iran J Immunol* 2005; 2(1): 3-21.
3. Orfao A, Lopez A, Flores J, Almeida J. Diagnosis of hematological malignancies: new applications for flow cytometry. *Hematology* 2006; 2:6-13.
4. Richards S. Clinical application of flow cytometry: Immunophenotyping of leukemic cells: Approved guidelines. *National Committee on Clinical Laboratory Standards* 1998; 18(8): 1-73.
5. Yokoyama W. Production of Monoclonal Antibodies. *Curr Proto Immunol* 1995; 2: 2-17.
6. van Meerten T, Hagenbeek A. Cd20-targeted therapy: A breakthrough in the treatment of non-hodgkin's lymphoma. *Neth J Med* 2009;67(7):251-9.
7. Cheson BD, Leonard JP. Monoclonal antibody therapy for b-cell non-hodgkin's lymphoma. *N Engl J Med* 2008;359(6):613-26.
8. Tay K, Dunleavy K, Wilson WH. Novel agents for b-cell non-hodgkin lymphoma: Science and the promise. *Blood Rev* 2010;24(2):69-82.

9. Link BK, Friedberg JW. Monoclonal antibodies in lymphoma: The first decade. *Semin Hematol* 2008;45(2):71-4.

10. Renaudineau Y, Devauchelle-Pensec V, Hanrotel C, Pers JO, Saraux A, Youinou P. Monoclonal anti-cd20 antibodies: Mechanisms of action and monitoring of biological effects. *Joint Bone Spine* 2009;76(5):458-63.

11. Jackson LR, Trudel LJ, Fox JG, Lipman NS. Monoclonal antibody production in murine ascites. I. Clinical and pathologic features. *Lab Anim Sci* 1999;49(1):70-80.

12. Mc Ardle J. Alternatives to ascites production of monoclonal antibodies. *Ani Welf Inform Cent Newslett* 1998; 8: 3-4.

13. Lang AB, Schuerch U, Cryz SJ Jr. Optimization of growth and secretion of human monoclonal antibodies by hybridomas cultured in serum-free media. *Hybridoma* 1991;10(3):401-9.

14. Jackson LR, Trudel LJ, Fox JG, Lipman NS. Monoclonal antibody production in murine ascites. Ii. Production characteristics. *Lab Anim Sci* 1999;49(1):81-6.

15. Hadavi R, Zarnani AH, Ahmadvand N, Mahmoudi AR, Bayat AA, Mahmoudian J, et al. Production of Monoclonal Antibody against Human Nestin. *Avicenna J Med Biotech* 2010; 2(2): 69-76.

16. Baradaran B, Hosseini AZ, Majidi J, Farajnia S, Barar J, Saraf ZH, et al. Development and characterization of monoclonal antibodies against human epidermal growth factor receptor in balb/c mice. *Hum Antibodies* 2009;18(1-2):11-6.

17. Baradaran B, Majidi J, Hassan ZM, Abdolalizadeh J. Large scale production and characterization of anti-human IgG monoclonal antibody in peritoneum of Balb/c mice. *Am J Biochem Biotechnol* 2006; 1: 190-3.

18. Schrama D, Reisfeld RA, Becker JC. Antibody targeted drugs as cancer therapeutics. *Nat Rev Drug Discov* 2006;5(2):147-59.

19. Galen FX, Devaux C, Atlas S, Guyenne T, Menard J, Corvol P, et al. New monoclonal antibodies directed against human renin. Powerful tools for the investigation of the renin system. *J Clin Invest* 1984;74(3):723-35.

20. Tadjine M, Mittal KR, Bourdon S, Gottschalk M. Production and characterization of murine monoclonal antibodies against haemophilus parasuis and study of their protective role in mice. *Microbiol* 2004;150(Pt 12):3935-45.

14

Design and Characterization of Microemulsion Systems for Naproxen

Eskandar Moghimipour[1], Anayatollah Salimi[1]*, Soroosh Eftekhari[2]

[1] *Nanotechnology Research Center, Jundishapur University of Medical Sciences, Ahvaz, Iran.*

[2] *Department of Pharmaceutics, Faculty of Pharmacy, Jundishapur University of Medical Sciences, Ahvaz, Iran.*

ARTICLE INFO

Keywords:
Naproxen
Microemulsion
Phase Diagram
Characterization

ABSTRACT

Purpose: This research was aimed to formulate and characterize a microemolsion systems as a topical delivery system of naproxen for relief of symptoms of rheumatoid arthritis, osteoarthritis and treatment of dysmenorrheal. **Methods:** ME formulations prepared by mixing of appropriate amount of surfactant including Tween 80 and Span 80, co-surfactant such as propylene glycol (PG) and oil phase including Labrafac PG – transcutol P (10:1 ratio). The prepared microemolsions were evaluated regarding their particle size, zeta potential, conductivity, stability, viscosity, differential scanning calorimetry (DSC), scanning electron microscopy (SEM), refractory index (RI) and pH. **Results:** The mean droplets size of microemulsion formulation were in the range of 7.03 to 79.8 nm, and its refractory index (RI) and pH were 1.45 and 6.75, respectively. Viscosity range was 253.73- 802.63cps. Drug release profile showed that 26.15% of the drug released in the first 24 hours of experiment. Also, Hexagonal and bicontinuous structures were seen in the SEM photograph of the microemulsions. **Conclusion:** characterization, physicochemical properties and in vitro release were dependent upon the contents of S/C ratio, water and, oil phase percentage in formulations. Also, ME-6 may be preferable for topical naproxen formulation.

Introduction

Microemulsions are macroscopically isotropic mixtures of at least a hydrophilic, a hydrophobic and an amphiphilic component. Their thermodynamic stability and their nanostructure are two important characteristics that distinguish them from ordinary emulsions which are thermodynamically unstable. Microemulsions were first observed by Schulman[1] and Winsor[2] in the 1950s. Then, the term "microemulsions" has been used to describe multi-component systems comprising non-polar, aqueous, surfactant, and cosurfactant components. Conventional microemulsions can be classified oil-in-water, (o/w), water-in-oil (w/o) and bicontinuous phase microemulsions.[3] Some advantages offered by microemulsions include improvement in poorly drug solubility, enhancement of bioavailability, protection of the unstable drugs against environmental conditions and a long shelf life.

Naproxen (NAP, Figure 1) is a non-steroidal anti-inflammatory drug derived of propionic acid used widely as analgesic, antipyretic and for symptoms relief of dysmenorrheal pain.[1] The most widely reported side effect of NSAIDs includes, gastrointestinal ulcer, accompanied by anaemia due to the bleeding, which is also true for naproxen. In order to avoid the gastric irritation, minimize the systemic toxicity and achieve a better therapeutic effect, one promising method is to administer the drug via skin.[2] Transdermal drug delivery systems provide the most important route to achieve these goals.[3] The transdermal delivery system also enable controlled or sustained release of the active ingredients and an enhanced patient compliance.[4]

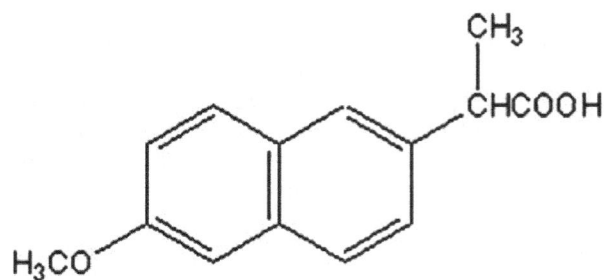

Figure 1. Chemical structure of naproxen.

Naproxen is poorly water solubility and it is possible to increase its solubility by utilizing microemulsion systems.[4] In this study, The main aim of our investigations was to design and evaluate a microemulsion based naproxen (1%, w/w) for topical delivery.

*Corresponding author: Anayatollah Salimi, Nanotechnology Research Center, Jundishapur University of Medical Sciences, Ahvaz, Iran.
E-mail: anayatsalimi2003@yahoo.com

Materials and Methods
Naproxen was purchased from Pars Darou company (Iran), Propylene glycol dicaprylocapraye (Labrafac^{TM} PG), Median chain triglycerides (Labrafac^{TM} Lipophile WL 1349), Diethylene glycol monoethyl ether (Transcutol P) was donated as gift by GATTEFOSSE Company (France). Span 80, Tween 80 and PG were obtained from Merck (Germany). All chemicals and solvents were of analytical grade. Freshly double distilled water was used in the experiments. Minitab15 software was used for experimental design and the evaluation of the effect of variables on responses. Sigma plot11 software was applied for providing tertiary phase diagrams.

Naproxen assay
The quantitative determination of naproxen was performed by UV spectrophotometry (BioWaveII,WPA) at λmax= 271 nm.

Solubility of naproxen
Solubility of naproxen was determined in different oil (Isopropyl myristate, Labrafac PG, Labrafac^{TM} Lipophile WL 1349, Labrafac PG+Transcutol P(10:1)), surfactants (Span 80, Tween 80) and co-surfactant (Propylen glycol) by dissolving an excess amount of naproxen in 3ml of oil, and other components using a stirrer at 37 °C±0.5 for 72 h. The equilibrated samples were then centrifuged at 10000 rpm for 30 min to remove undissolved drug, then the clear supernatant liquid was decanted.[5] The solubility of naproxen was measured by analyzing the filtrate spectrophotometrically using nanospecterophotometer (Biochrom WPA Bioware) at 271 nm.

Pseudo-ternary phase diagram construction
To investigate concentration range of components for the existing boundary of MEs, pseudo-ternary phase diagrams were constructed using the water titration method. Three phase diagrams were prepared with the 2:1, 4:1, and 6:1 weight ratios of (Span 80 /Tween 80) Propylen glycol respectively. Oil phase(Labrafac PG +Transcutol-P)(10:1) and the surfactant mixture were then mixed at the weight ratios of 1:9, 2:8, 3:7, 4:6, 5:5, 6:4, 7:3, 8:2, and 9:1.[6] These mixtures were diluted dropwise with double distilled water, under moderate agitation. The samples were classified as microemulsions when they appeared as clear liquids.[7]
Several parameters influence on final properties of microemulsions. Full factorial design was used concerning with 3 variables at 2 levels for formulations. Major variables take part in determination of microemulsion's properties includes surfactant/cosurfactant ratio (S/C), percentage of oil (% oil) and water percentage (%w). Eight different formulations with low and high values of oil (20% and 40%), water (5%, 10%), and S/Co mixing ratio (6:1, 4:1) were prepared for preparing of microemulsion formulation.

Preparation of naproxen Microemulsions
Various MEs were chosen from the pseudoternary phase diagram with 4:1, and 6:1 weight ratio of Span 80 /Tween 80/Propylen glycol. Naproxen (1%) was added to oil phase, then adding S/ CoS mixture and an appropriate amount of double distilled water was added to the mixture drop by drop and the MEs containing naproxen were obtained by stirring the mixtures at ambient temperature.[8,9]

Differential scanning calorimetry (DSC)
DSC measurements were carried out by means of a Metller Toldo DSC1 star^R system equipped with refrigerated cooling system (Hubert Tc45). Approximately 5-10mg of microemulsion samples were weighted into hermetic aluminium pans and quickly sealed to prevent water evaporation from microemulsion samples. Simultaneously an empty hermetically sealed pan was used as a reference. Microemulsion samples were exposed in a temperature ranging from +30 °C to - 50 °C (scan rate:10 °C/min). All measurements were preferred at least in triplicate.
 In order to ensure accuracy and repeatability of data, DSC instrument was calibrated and checked under the conditions of use by indium standard. Changes of Enthalpy quantities (ΔH) were calculated from endothermic and exothermic transitions of thermograms by Equation 1:[10]

$$\Delta H= \text{peak area/sample weight} \qquad \textbf{(Equation 1)}$$

Zeta potential determination
Zeta potential of samples were measured by Zetasizer (Malvern instrument ltd ZEN3600, UK). Samples were placed in clear disposable zeta cells and results were recorded.

Scanning electron microscopy (SEM)
Scanning electron microscopy (SEM) was used to characterize microstructure of micemulsions. SEM of samples were measured by LED 1455VP, Germany.

Particle size measurements
The average droplet size of samples was measured at 25 °C by SCATTER SCOPE 1 QUIDIX (South Korea) and their refractory indices (RI) were also calculated.

Viscosity measurements
Viscosity of samples was measured at 25 °C with a Brookfield viscometer (DV-II+Pro Brookfield., USA) using spindle no. 34. With shear rate 50 rpm. Each measurement was performed in triplicate.[11-13]

Conductivity measurements
Electrical conductivity of MEs was measured with a conductivity meter (Metrohm Model 712) using conductivity cells with a cell constant of 1.0 and consisting of two platinum plates separated by desired distance and having liquid between the platinum plate acting as a conductor.

Surface tension measurement

The surface tension of microemulsion was measured at 25 °C with a Torsion balance (WHITE ELEC Model NO. 83944E).

Determination of pH

The pH values for microemolsion was determined at 25 °C by pH meter (Mettler Toledo seven easy, Switzerland). All measurements were carried out in triplicate.[12]

Physical stability study

The physical stability of microemulsions was studied regarding the temperature stability and centrifugation. Microemulsions were kept in various temperatures (4 °C, 25 °C and 37 °C) and observed for phase separation, flocculation or precipitation. Also, Microemulsions were centrifuged by HIGH SPEED BRUSHLESS CENTERIFUGE (Vs-35sMTi, vision) 10000 rpm for 30 minute at 25 °C and inspected for any change in their homogeneity.[14]

Release study

Franz diffusion cells (area 3.4618 cm^2) with a cellulose membrane were used to determine the release rate of naproxen from different microemulsion formulations. The cellulose membrane was first hydrated in distilled water at 25 °C for 24 hours. The membrane was then clamped between the donor and receptor compartments of the cells. Each Diffusion cell was filled with 25 ml of phosphate buffer (pH =7.4). The receptor fluid was constantly stirred by externally driven magnetic bars at 300 rpm throughout the experiment. Naproxen microemulsion (5g) was accurately weighted and placed in donor compartment. At 0.5, 1, 2, 3, 4, 5, 6, 7, 8 and 24h time intervals, 2ml sample was removed from receptor for spectrophotometric determination and replaced immediately with an equal volume of fresh receptor medium. Samples were analyzed by UV visible spectrophotometer (BioWaveII,WPA) at 271nm. The results were plotted as cumulative released drug percentage versus time.[15]

Statistical methods

All the experiments were repeated three times and data were expressed as the mean value±SD. Statistical data were analyzed by one-way analysis of variance (ANOVA) and P<0.05 was considered to be significant with 95% confidence intervals.

Results and discussion

The results of solubility of naproxen are tabulated in Table 1. The maximum solubility of naproxen was found in Labrafac PG:Transcotol P (10:1) (14.067±0.023) as compared to other oils. In addition, the highest drug solubility of naproxen in surfactants were found in Span 80 (15.033±0.208), and Tween 80 (0.576±0.012). Based on the solubility studies of naproxen in oil, surfactant and co-surfactant and the

preformulation studies it was found that Labrafac PG-Transcutol P, span 80, Tween 80 and propylene glycol could be the most appropriate combination for preparation of microemulsion.

Table 1. Solubility of Naproxen in different oils, surfactants and co-surfactants (mean±SD, n=3)

Phase type	Excipient	Solubility (mg/ml)
oil	Labrafac PG	13.697 ± 0.536
	Isopropyl Myristat	12.820 ± 0.044
	Labrafac^{TM} Lipophile WL 1349	10.930 ± 0.100
	Labrafac PG+Transcutol P(10:1)	14.067 ± 0.023
surfactant	Tween 80	0.576 ± 0.012
	Span 80	15.033 ± 0.208
Co-surfactant	Propylene glycol	14.120 ± 0.368

Pseudo-ternary phase diagrams of the investigated quaternary system water/ Labrafac PG, Transcotol P (10:1)/ Span 80-Tween 80/ PG are showed in figure 2. Microemulsions were formed at ambient temperature. The phase diagrams clearly indicated that microemulsion existence region increased with increase in the weight ratio of surfactant/cosurfactant (Km=2-6). The mean particle size of formulations was from 7 to 79 nm (Table 2). Particle size of free drug MEs and drug loaded MEs were determined and there was no significant difference observed in average particle size after loading the drug. The ME 1 formulation had the lowest average particle size 7.03 ± 0.2nm with polydispersity index (PI) of 0.362±0.032 (Table 2). PI is a measure of particle homogeneity and it varies from 0.0 to 1.0. The closer to zero the PI value the more homogenous are the particles.

The PI indicated that ME formulations had narrow size distribution. Analysis of variance showed that correlation between mean particle size, PI and independent variables are not significant (p>0.05).

The refractive index (RI) of the ME formulation was found 1.45 that is near to oil phase which indicates ME formulations have water-in-oil structures. Analysis of variance is showed significant correlation between RI and independent variables (%w) and (% oil) (p<0.05). Equation 2 showed the effect of independent variables on RI.

$$RI=1.46+0.0000s/c-0.000257(\%oil)-0.000800(\%water)$$
(Equation 2)

There was a strong correlation between the specific structure of the microemulsion systems and their electrical conductive behavior.[16] The phase systems (o/w or w/o) of the microemulsions were determined by measuring the conductivity of the microemulsions.[17] The ME formulations had the average conductivity in the range of 0.046-0.136ms/cm that is showed w/o structure of MEs. Also, w/o structure of MEs is confirmed with colour tests.

The ME formulations had appropriate observed pH value (6.750±0.09) that is best for topical application. Incorporation of naproxen did not significantly affect the observed pH value of the ME formulations (Table 3).

The mean viscosity of formulations were from 253.73±1.88cps to 802.63±1.66cps. The highest viscosity belongs to ME-3 formulation with bicontinueous structure. Multivariate regression was applied for the analysis of correlation between independent variables and MEs viscosity. Linear equation 3 shows all the main effects for viscosity is:

$$\text{Viscosity} = 666 + 21.5\text{S/C} - 14.4(\%\text{oil}) + 19.0(\%\text{water})$$
(Equation 3)

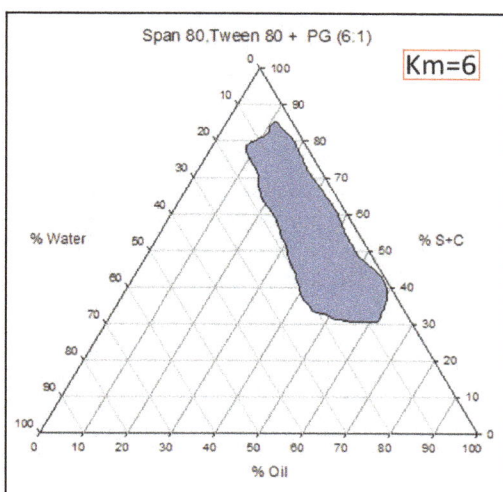

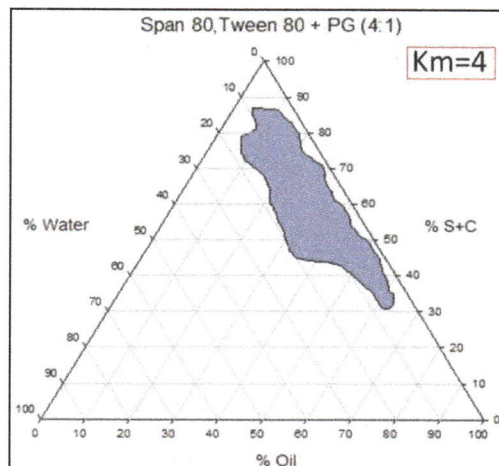

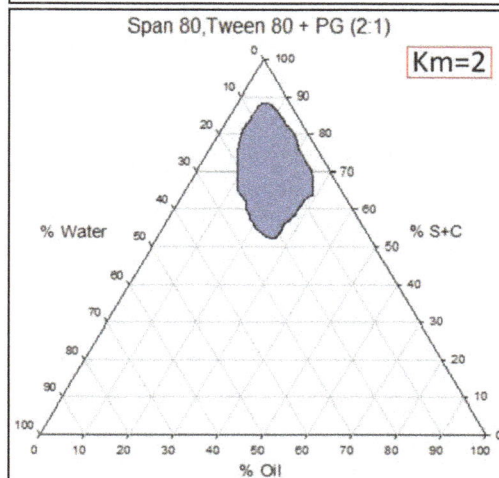

Figure 2. The pseudo-ternary phase diagrams of the oil-surfactant/cosurfactant mixture–water system at the 2:1, 4:1, and 6:1 weight ratio of Span 80 /Tween 80/ Propylene glycol at ambient temperature, dark area show microemulsions zone.

Table 2. Compositions of Selected Microemulsions (% w/w) and Particle Size (mean±SD, n=3)

Formulation	Factorial	S/C	% Oil	% (S+C)	% Water	Particle size (nm)	Polydispersity
ME-1	+ + +	6:1	40	50	10	7.03±0.2nm	0.348±0.012
ME-2	+ + -	6:1	40	55	5	79.8±0.7 nm	0.347±0.025
ME-3	+ - +	6:1	20	70	10	53.6±0.5 nm	0.346±0.016
ME-4	+ - -	6:1	20	74	5	10.3±1.2 nm	0.341±0.021
ME-5	- - -	4:1	20	75	5	21.9±0.6 nm	0.347±0.018
ME-6	- - +	4:1	20	70	10	34.5±1.3 nm	0.348±0.023
ME-7	- + -	4:1	40	55	5	10.3±0.5 nm	0.348±0.021
ME-8	- + +	4:1	40	50	10	11.6±0.3 nm	0.347±0.014
+: high level; - : low level							

Table 3. pH, Refractive index,Conductivity and Zeta potential of selected Naproxen microemulsions (mean±SD, n=3)

Formulation	PH	Refractive index	Zeta potential (mV)	Conductivity (mS/cm)
ME-1	6.60 ± 0.05	1.4460 ± 0.18	0.84	0.136±0.008
ME-2	6.72 ± 0.08	1.4508 ± 0.19	-0.66	0.134±0.002
ME-3	6.85 ± 0.12	1.4531 ± 0.15	-5.34	0.105±0.012
ME-4	6.76 ± 0.09	1.4535 ± 0.20	-10.50	0.077±0.009
ME-5	6.70 ±0.06	1.4561 ± 0.17	-11.50	0.067±0.004
ME-6	6.70 ±0.09	1.4514 ± 0.16	-18.00	0.046±0.018
ME-7	6.89 ± 0.07	1.4505 ± 0.14	-11.80	0.125±0.006
ME-8	6.78 ± 0.10	1.4449 ± 0.19	-15.70	0.067±0.013

The percent of oil had more negative effect on viscosity. There was no significant difference found between the viscosities of free drug and drug loaded MEs (p>0.05).

Figure 3 shows the effect of main factors (S/C,%oil, %water) and their interactions on viscosity of microemulsions. The amount of %water and s/c had more effect on viscosity. Higher amount of %water and s/c ratio performed higher viscosity.

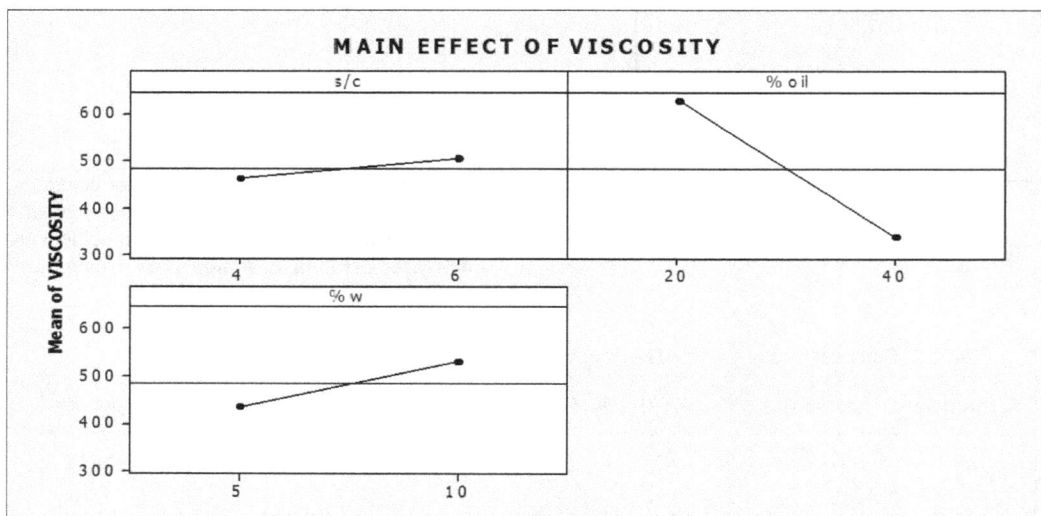

Figure 3. The effect of main effect of independent variables on viscosity

The ME formulations had the zeta potential average (-0.66 to+18.00mv) (Table 3). The highest zeta potential belongs to ME-6 formulation which seems to suggest micellar and bicontinuous structures and the lowest belong to ME-1 which seems to suggest reverse hexagonal and micellar structures. Multivariate regression was used for the analysis of correlation between independent variables and MEs zeta potential. The S/C ratio had more positive effect on zeta potential. There was found significant difference between the zeta potential and S/C ratio. (p<0.05). Linear equation 4 shows all the main effects for zeta potential is:

Zeta Potential=-40.3+5.17(S/C)+0.225(%oil)-0.187(%water)
(Equation 4)

The mean surface tension of formulations was from 44.17±1.46 to 52.17±1.25dynes/cm (Table 4). The surface tension data implies water-in-oil microemulsions because surface tension amounts of MEs is nearby to oil phase surface tension.
Figure 4 shows the release profile of naproxen ME formulations. The cumulative amount of naproxen that had permeated through the cellulose membrane (%) was plotted as a function of time (hours). In this study,

ME-6 and ME-1 have the highest and lowest accumulative release percent, respectively. Table 5 shows release percent and kinetic of release in naproxen ME formulations. Multivariate regression was used for the analysis of correlation between independent variables and MEs release. Analysis of variance is showed no significant correlation between release percentage value of naproxen and independent variables ($p>0.05$). The percent of water and S/C ratio had more negative effect on accumulative release percent. Linear equation 5 shows effect of independent variables on release percent:

$$\%Release=29.2- 3.78S/C-0.086(\%oil)+0.874(\%water)$$
(Equation 5)

Table 4. Surface tension and viscosity of selected microemulsions(mean±SD, n=3)

Formulation	Surface tension (dynes/cm)	Viscosity (cp)
ME-1	44.17 ± 1.46	282.90 ± 1.91
ME-2	47.67 ± 0.85	253.73 ± 1.88
ME-3	46.00 ±1.06	802.63 ± 1.66
ME-4	47.67 ± 1.44	681.13 ± 1.98
ME-5	47.33 ± 0.76	445.60 ± 1.15
ME-6	49.33 ± 1.36	580.83 ± 1.92
ME-7	52.17 ± 1.25	364.17 ± 1.60
ME-8	48.50 ± 1.42	457.90 ± 1.83

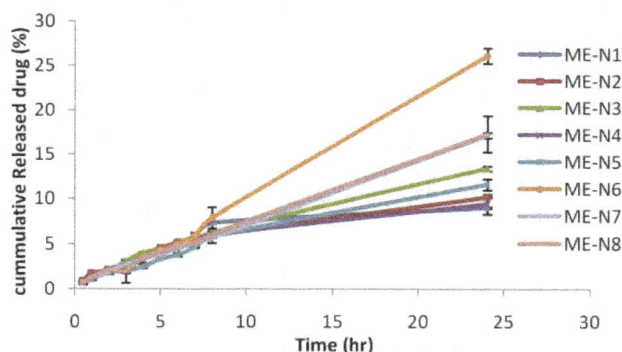

Figure 4. In vitro release profile of MEs formulation of Naproxen.

On the basis of equation 5, it seems that release percent enhanced with decrease in the oil percent and s/c ratio.

In vitro release studies with an artificial hydrophobic membrane can provide information about the diffusion of a drug, which depends on the physico-chemical properties of components, vehicle internal structure, and interaction between drug and vehicle.[18,19]

The release profile of MEs were calculated by fitting the experimental data to equations describing different

kinetic models. Linear regression analyses were made for zero-order ($M_t/M_0 = kt$), first-order ($\ln (M_0–M_t) = kt$), Higuchi ($M_t/M_0 = (kt)1/2$), Log Wagner, Linear wagner, Weibul, Second root of mass, Three-Seconds root of mass, and Pepas kinetics.

Table 5. Percent release and kinetic release of selected microemulsions(mean±SD, n=3)

Formulation	% release	kinetic	R^2	Intercept
1	9.0133	Log Wagner	0.9679	-2.1891
2	10.2128	Higuchi	0.9929	-0.0069
3	13.4262	Weibul	0.9954	-4.3820
4	9.4373	Log Wagner	0.9899	-2.2074
5	11.6378	Pepas	0.9832	-4.5453
6	26.1512	Zero	0.9916	-0.0068
7	17.1690	Zero	0.9983	0.004
8	17.3421	3/2 root of mass	0.9970	0.0023

The amount of naproxen release differ between microemulsion carriers with different internal microstructure. Comparing the amounts of released naproxen after 24 hours as well as the release rate (Figure 3) the slowest release was observed for ME -1 with reverse hexagonal structure and the highest release was observed for ME-6 with bicontinuous and micellar structures.

Table 5 shows kinetic of release in naproxen ME formulations. Multivariate regression was applied for the analysis of correlation between independent variables and MEs kinetic release. Analysis of variance is showed no significant correlation between release kinetic of naproxen microemulsions and independent variables ($p>0.05$).Linear equation 6 shows effect of independent variables on kinetic release:

$$Release \ Kinetic= 3.5-0.25 \ S/C- 0.000(\%oil)+0.1 \ (\% \ water)$$
(Equation 6)

The percent of water and S/C ratio had more positive and more negative effect on kinetic release, respectively, and percent of oil is not effect on the release kinetic of MEs. Three-seconds root of mass kinetic was obtained with increase in percent of water and decrease in s/c ratio whereas zero-order kinetic conversely.

Figure 5 shows the SEM images of ME-1 (with reverse hexagonal structure) and ME-6 (with micellar and bicontinuous structurs), respectively.

The thermal behaviour of water can be a useful and rapid means with which to understand the microstructure of microemulsions.[20] In this context, a small broadened peak at very low temperatures (below -30 ºC) has been suggested to be either internal water or water that is interacting strongly with the surfactants.[21,22] When water is mixed in to a microemulsion system it can be either bound (interfacial) or free (bulk) water depending of its state in the system. In cooling curves of the samples (ME$_1$-ME$_2$-ME$_4$), DSC thermogram showed one exothermic peak at around 0 to -3 °C that indicate the freezing of bulk water in these formulations. The other endothermic peak at around -23 to -27 °C belong to bound water freezing. In cooling curves of ME-3, DSC thermogram showed one exothermic peak at -2 °C (bulk water) and one endothermic peak at -34 °C that indicates bound water that interacts with surfactants

strongly. DSC thermograms of ME-7 and ME-8 showed one exothermic peak at 0 to -1°C (bulk water), also two endothermic at -19 to -21°C (bound water) and -36.5 to -43 °C (the water must be strongly bound or interacts with surfactants). In cooling curves of ME-5 and ME-6, DSC thermogrms showed one exothermic peak of around 0 °C (ME-5) and -4 °C (ME-6), which indicates bulk water. Also, in ME-6 showed one endothermic peak at -41 °C which indicates the water must be strongly bound or interacts with surfactants. Figure 6 shows DSC cooling thermograms of ME-1and ME-6 formulations.

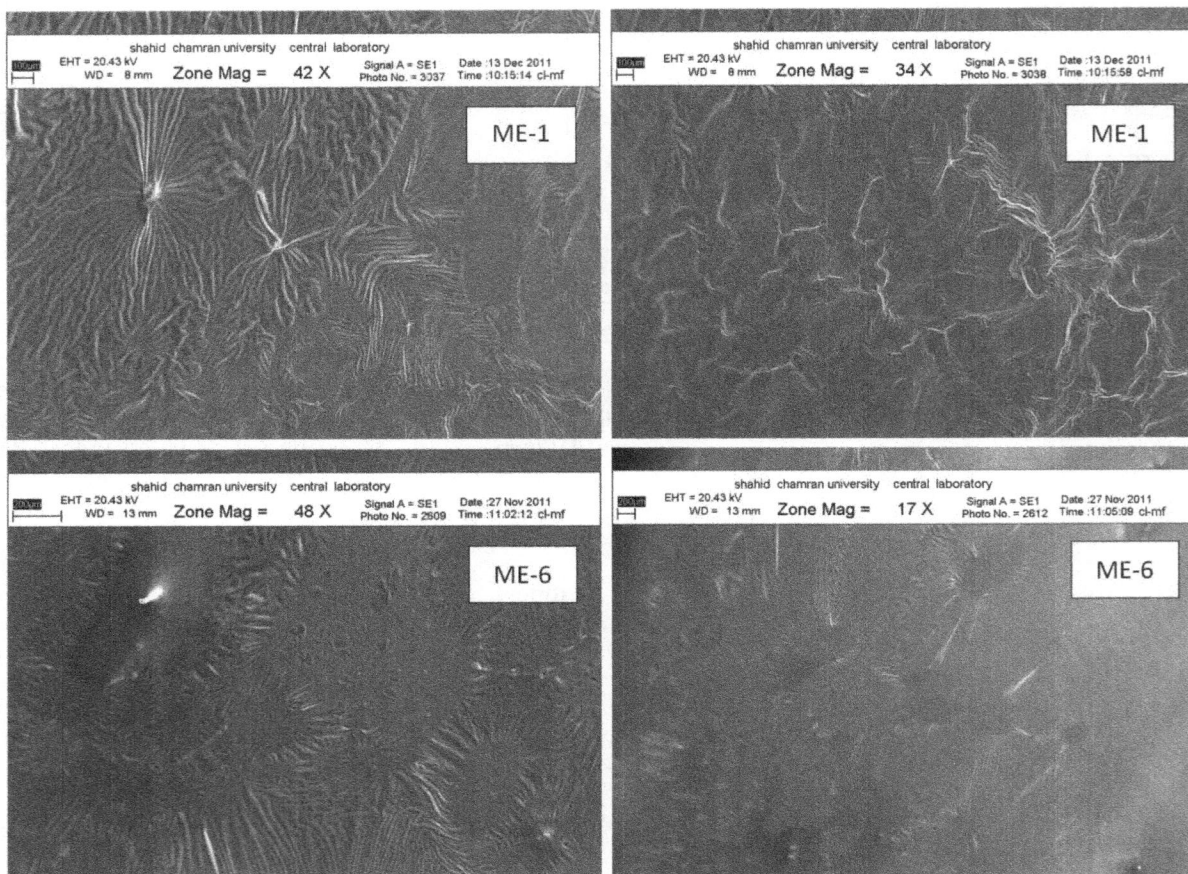

Figure 5. SEM photographs of of ME-2 and ME-6.

The visual inspection experiment was carried out for 3 months by drawing ME sample at weekly interval for the first month and monthly interval for the subsequent months. The visual observation showed no evidence of phase separation or any precipitation or flocculation.

These samples also revealed no sign of phase separation under stress when subjected to centrifugation at 10000rpm for 30 min. The centrifugtion tests showed that microemulsions were remained homogenous without any phase separation throughout the test indicates good physical stability of both preparations.

Conclusion

This study estabilished that physicochemical properties and in vitro release were dependent upon the contents of S/C ratio, oil and water in formulations. Pseudo-ternary Phase diagrams indicated more width microemulsion region with a rise in S/C ratio. With decrease in S/C ratio and oil percent and increase in water percent could be obtained higher in vitro percentage release. The amount of naproxen release differ between microemulsion carriers with various internal microstructures. ME-6 may be preferable for topical naproxen formulation despite that the serious work still needs to be carried out to reveal the mechanisms of drug delivery into the skin.

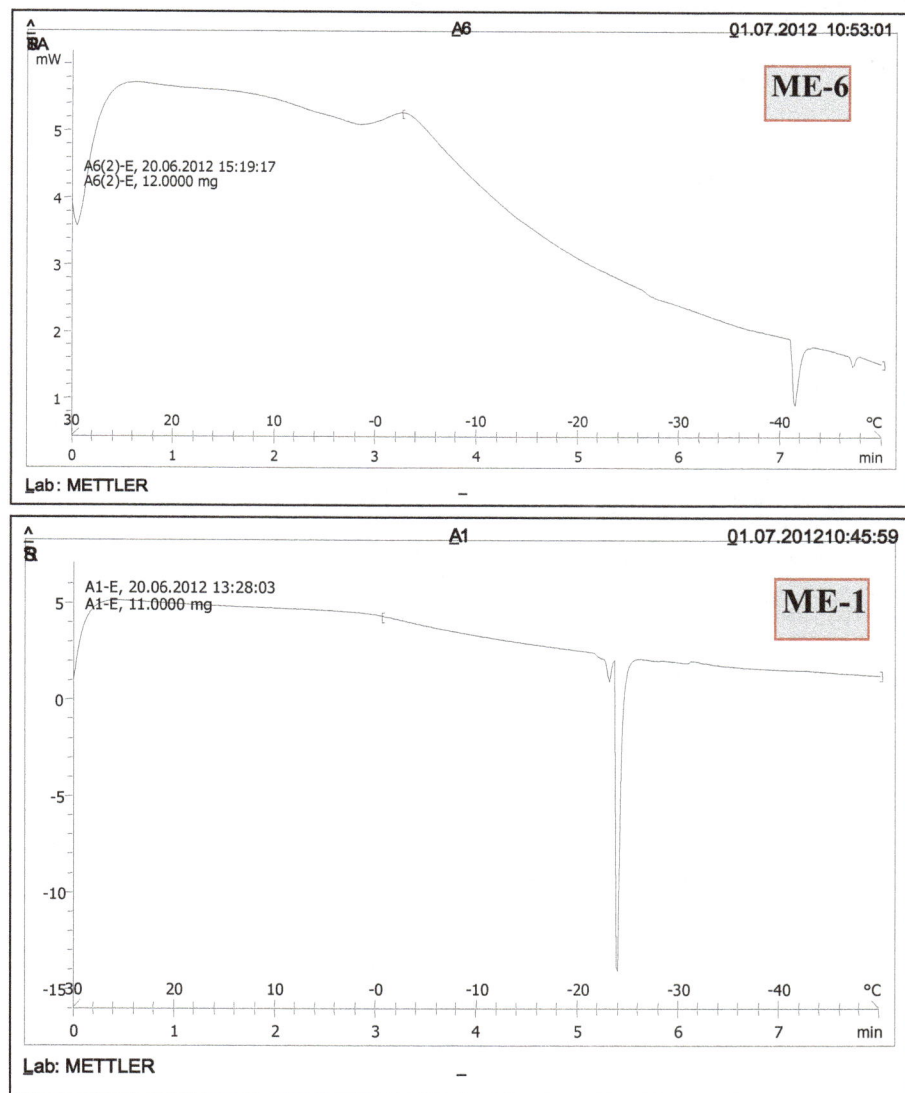

Figure 6. DSC cooling thermograms of ME-1 and ME-6 formulations.

Acknowledgments

This paper is extracted from pharm.D.thesis (Eftekhari,S) and financial support was provided by Ahvaz Jundishapur University of Medical Sciences. The authors are very thankful to Faratin company executive manager (Taheri,M,Iran) for providing gratis sample of Transcutol P, Labrafac PG and Labrafac™ Lipophile WL 1349 from GATTEFOSSE(France) and also GATTEFOSSE company (France).

Conflict of Interest

There is no conflict of interest in this study.

References

1. Schulman JH, Hoar TP. Transparent water-in-oil dispersions: The oleopathic Hydromicelle. *Nature* 1943; 152: 102.

2. Winsor PA. Solvent Properties of Amphiphilic Compounds. London: Butherworth; 1954.

3. Attwood D. Microemulsions. In: Kreuter J, editor. *Colloidal Drug Delivery Systems*. New York: Marcel Dekker; 1994.P.31-71.

4. Raffa RB. The Science and Practice of Pharmacy. In: Gennaro AR, editor. *Remington*. Philadelphia: Lippincott Williams & Wilkins; 2005.P. 1539.

5. Moghimipour E, Salimi A, Leis F. Preparation and Evaluation of tretinoin microemulsion based on pseudo-ternary phase diagram. *Adv Pharm Bull* 2012; 2(2): 141-7.

6. Wilk KA, Zielinska K, Hamerska-Dudra A, Jezierski A. Biocompatible microemulsions of dicephalic aldonamide-type surfactants: Formulation, structure and temperature influence. *J Colloid Interface Sci* 2009;334(1):87-95.

7. Sharif Makhmal zadeh B, Torabi SH, Azarpanah A. Optimization of Ibuprofen Delivery through Rat Skin from Traditional and Novel Nanoemulsion Formulations. *Iran J Pharm Res* 2012; 11(1): 47-58.

8. Langevin D. Microemulsions and liquid crystals. *Mol Cryst Liq Cryst* 1986; 138: 259-305.

9. Eicke HF. The microemulsion concept in nonpolar surfactant solutions. In: Robb ID, editor. *Mikroemulsions*. New York: Plenum; 1982.P. 17-32.

10. Sharif Makhmal zadeh BS, Yazdani M, Rezaai S, Salimi A. The effect of chemical enhancers on Tacrolimus permeation through rat skin. *J Pharm Res* 2010; 5(3): 1309-12.

11. Lapasin R, Grassi M, Coceani N. Effects of polymer addition on the rheology of o/w microemulsions. *Rheol Acta* 2001; 40: 185-92.

12. Ramesh Shah R, Shripal Magdum Ch, Shivagonda Patil Sh, Shanawaj Niakwade N. Preparation and Evaluation of Aceclofenac Topical Microemulsion. *Iran J Pharm Res* 2010; 9(1): 5-11.

13. Djordjevic L, Primorac M, Stupar M. Krajisnik D. Characterization of caprylocaproyl macrogolglycerides based microemulsion drug delivery vehicles for an amphiphilic drug. *Int J Pharm* 2004;271(1-2):11-9.

14. Lv Q, Yu A, Xi Y, Li H, Song Z, Cui J, et al. Development and evaluation of penciclovir-loaded solid lipid nanoparticles for topical delivery. *Int J Pharm* 2009;372(1-2):191-8.

15. Araujo LM, Thomazine JA, Lopez RF. Development of microemulsions to topically deliver 5-aminolevulinic acid in photodynamic therapy. *Eur J Pharm Biopharm* 2010;75(1):48-55.

16. Yue Y, San-ming L, Pan D, Da-fang Z. Physicochemical properties and evaluation of microemulsion systems for transdermal delivery of meloxicam. *Chem Res Chin Univ* 2007; 23(1): 81-86.

17. Peltola S, Saarinen-Savolainen P, Kiesvaara J, Suhonen TM, Urtti A. Microemlsions for topical delivery of estradiol. *Int J Pharm* 2003;254: 99-107.

18. Zvonar A, Rozman B, Bester Rogac M, Gasperlin M. The Influence of Microstructure on Celecoxib Releasefrom a Pharmaceutically Applicable System: Mygliol 812®/Labrasol®/Plurol Oleique®/Water Mixtures. *Acta Chim Slov* 2009; 56: 131-8.

19. Gradzielski M, Hoffmann H. Handbook of Microemulsion Science and Technology. New York: Marcel Dekker; 1999. P. 375.

20. Liu H, Wang Y, Lang Y, Yao H, Dong Y, Li S. Bicontinuous cyclosporin a loaded water-AOT/Tween 85-isopropylmyristate microemulsion: Structural characterization and dermal pharmacokinetics in vivo. *J Pharm Sci* 2009;98(3):1167-76.

21. Podlogar F, Gasperlin M, Tomsic M, Jamnik A, Rogac MB. Structural characterisation of water-tween 40/imwitor 308-isopropyl myristate microemulsions using different experimental methods. *Int J Pharm* 2004;276(1-2):115-28.

22. Podlogar F, Bester Rogac M, Gasperlin M. The effect of internal structure of selected water-tween 40-imwitor 308-ipm microemulsions on ketoprofene release. *Int J Pharm* 2005;302(1-2):68-77.

Targeted Fluoromagnetic Nanoparticles for Imaging of Breast Cancer MCF-7 Cells

Mostafa Heidari Majd[1,2,3], Jaleh Barar[1,4]*, Davoud Asgari[1], Hadi Valizadeh[1], Mohammad Reza Rashidi[1], Vala Kafil[1], Javid Shahbazi[1], Yadollah Omidi[1,4]

[1] Research Center for Pharmaceutical Nanotechnology, Faculty of Pharmacy, Tabriz University of Medical Sciences, Tabriz, Iran.
[2] Faculty of Pharmacy, Zabol University of Medical Sciences, Zabol, Iran.
[3] Student Research Committee, Tabriz University of Medical Sciences, Tabriz, Iran.
[4] Ovarian Cancer Research Center, University of Pennsylvania, Philadelphia, USA.

A R T I C L E I N F O

Keywords:
Magnetic nanoparticles
Folate receptor
Breast cancer
MCF-7 cells
Internalization

A B S T R A C T

Purpose: To achieve simultaneous imaging and therapy potentials, targeted fluoromagnetic nanoparticles were synthesized and examined in human breast cancer MCF-7 cells. *Methods:* Fe_3O_4 nanoparticles (NPs) were synthesized through thermal decomposition of $Fe(acac)_3$. Then, magnetic nanoparticles (MNPs) modified by dopamine-poly ethylene glycol (PEG)-NH_2; finally, half equivalent fluorescein isothiocyanate (FITC) and half equivalent folic acid were conjugated to one equivalent of it. The presence of Fe_3O_4-DPA-PEG-FA/FITC in the folate receptor (FR) positive MCF-7 cells was determined via fluorescent microscopy to monitor the cellular interaction of MNPs. *Results:* FT-IR spectra of final compound confirmed existence of fluorescein on folic acid grafted MNPs. The Fe_3O_4-DPA-PEG-FA/FITC NPs, which displayed a size rang about 30-35 nm using scanning electron microscopy (SEM) and transmission electron microscopy (TEM), were able to actively recognize the FR-positive MCF-7 cells, but not the FR-negative A549 cells. *Conclusion:* The uniform nano-sized Fe_3O_4-DPA-PEG-FA/FITC NPs displayed great potential as theranostics and can be used for targeted imaging of various tumors that overexpress FR.

Introduction

While smart multifunctional nanomedicines and theranostics are becoming robust seamless tools for simultaneous imaging and therapy of cancer, for their effective clinical implementations we need a) to advance technologies for specific targeting of cancer cells, b) to improve imaging/sensing methods, c) to develop biocompatible long circulating bioshuttles for simultaneous delivery of targeting moiety, imaging agent and therapy, and d) to track and control cancerous single cells/bioconvoys to avoid distribution of oncogenic messages, the so called metastasis.[1] Of various advancements holding great promise for improving the sensing/imagining cancerous cells, superparamagnetic/magnetic NPs as effective contrast agents,[2-4] appear to meet such criteria.

MNPs have been used as nanocarriers for specific delivery of chemotherapy agents.[5-7] Possessing unique properties, they can be conjugated with different moieties such as targeting and therapeutics agents. Also MNPs have been used for various purposes such as magnetic bio separation, cell labeling, hyperthermia treatment of solid tumors and contrast agents for magnetic resonance imaging (MRI).[8-10]

In biological micro-compartments such as tumor microenvironment, the surface-modified MNPs ensue to display excellent dispersion characteristics, while the unmodified MNPs have high propensity to form agglomerated macrostructures that can be taken up by mononuclear phagocyte system (MPS) resulting in significant loss of MNPs in blood circulation.[11,12] Surface modification of MNPs with biocompatible polymers (e.g., polyethylene glycol (PEG)) can markedly protect them against immune system clearance providing longer circulation in blood. Further, surface modifications of MNPs were shown to improve their stability, biocompatibility, drug loading potential, and interaction capability with the target cells/tissues.[13,14] MNPs can become stealth through PEGylation, at which they can circumvent the opsonization.[15,16] PEG grafts also provide further conjugation potential with homing devices while keeping them longer in the blood stream and thus providing higher accumulation in the target sites.[11]

Targeted MNPs are often armed with moieties that enable them to detect the disease specific markers such as cancer marker molecules (CMMs), resulting in simultaneous targeted therapy and imaging. Of CMMs, folate receptors were shown to be upregulated in various tumors[17] thus can be targeted by folic acid (FA) which displays extremely high affinity to the folate

*Corresponding author: Jaleh Barar, Ovarian Cancer Research Center, University of Pennsylvania, Philadelphia, USA.
Email: jbarar@mail.med.upenn.edu

receptors. Previously, we have capitalized on synthesis of targeted fluorophoromagnetic nanoparticles conjugated with mitoxantrone (MTX).[18] To pursue the internalization of the FA conjugated MNPs by the FR positive breast cancer MCF-7cells, in the current study, we exploited FA conjugated PEGylated MNPs labeled with Fluorescein isothiocyanate (FITC). Conjugation of FA to the surface of MNPs can combine the passive targeting potential of MNPs with active targeting capabilities, resulting in enhanced permeation and retention (EPR) effects together with increased specific targeting of the tumor cells.[16,19] FITC has widely been used for optical detection of NPs by fluorescence microscopy and flow cytometry, so we functionalized MNPs with an isothiocyanate through reactive group (-N=C=S) that can react with terminal amines.[20]

Materials and Methods

Iron (III) acetylacetonate (Fe(acac)$_3$) and benzyl ether were purchased from Merck chemical company (Hohenbrunn, Germany). Poly Ethylene Glycol (PEG$_{2000}$), triethylamine, N,N, dicyclohexyl-carbodiimide (DCC), and N-hydroxysuccinimide (NHS) were purchased from Merck Chemical Company (Darmstadt, Germany). Oleylamine, bromoacetyl chloride, fluorescein isothiocyanate isomer I (FITC), RPMI 1640 media, MTT and dopamine hydrobromide (DPA) were purchased from Sigma-Aldrich Company (Steinheim, Germany). Folic acid was purchased from Acros Organics Company (New Jersey, USA). N-tert-Butoxycarbonyl-1, 2-ethylenediamine was purchased from Alfa Aesar Company (Lancashire, UK). Penicillin-Streptomycin and Fetal Bovine Serum were purchased from Invitrogen (Paisley, UK). MCF-7 cell lines were purchased from Pastor Cell bank (Iran). All other reagents and solvents were common analytical grade and pure.

Preparation of Fe$_3$O$_4$ Nanoparticles

Fe(acac)$_3$(2.12 g, 6.0 mmol) was dissolved in a mixture of benzyl ether and oleylamine (30 mL: 30 mL) and were stirred by magnetic stirrer.[21-23] The solution was dehydrated at 120 °C for 1h using Dean-Stark apparatus and under flow of argon. After 1 h, temperature was raised quickly to 270 °C for 2 h under argon. The reaction mixture was cooled down to room temperature and then ethanol (80 mL) was added to the dark brown mixture and precipitated with centrifuge at 5000 rpm. The product was re-dispersed in 30 mL n-hexane and stored at 4 °C.[18] Figure 1 Step 1 represents this process. The yield was 1.8 g, i.e. 84.9%.

Synthesis of O-(2'-Boc-Imino-Ethylene-Imino)-O'-(2-Dopamineacetyl) Polyethylene Glycol (DPA-PEG-NHBoc)

For synthesise of DPA-PEG-NHBoc, we conducted three main steps as described previously.[22]

First, polyethylene glycol (PEG$_{2000}$) (10.0 g, 5.0 mmol), bromoacetyl chloride (1.75 mL, 20.0 mmol) and

triethylamine (2.8 mL, 20 mmol) were dissolved in 20 mL dichloromethane. H-NMR result was: δ H (400 MHz; CDCl$_3$) 3.55-3.70 (234 H, -O-CH$_2$-CH$_2$-O-), 4.07 (4H, s, –CH$_2$-Br) and 4.32 (4H, t, –CH$_2$-COO-).

Second, BBrAC-PEG (7.50 g, 3.345 mmol) was dissolved in 250 mL dichloromethane, then dopamine hydrobromide (0.817 g, 3.487 mmol), KI (0.277 g, 1.6725mmol) and K$_2$CO$_3$ (1.615g, 11.707mmol) were added to the solution. H-NMR result was: δ H(400 MHz; CDCl$_3$) 2.69 (2H, t, -CH$_2$-CH$_2$N-), 2.90 (2H, t, –Ph-CH$_2$-CH$_2$-), 3.5-3.7 (234 H, -O-CH$_2$-CH$_2$-O-), 4.0979 (2H, s, –CH$_2$-Br), 4.245 (4H, t, –CH$_2$-COO-), 6.54 (1H, d, Ph) and 6.74 (2H, m, Ph).

Third, DPA-PEG-BrAC (6.00 g, 2.51mmol) and N-tert-butoxycarbonyl-1,2-ethylenediamine (0.475g, 3.012mmol) were dissolved in dichloromethane (250 mL). Then, KI (0.50 g, 3.012mmol) and K$_2$CO$_3$ (1.757 g, 12.552 mmol) were added. H-NMR result was: δ H(400 MHz; CDCl$_3$) 1.409 (9H, s, t-Bu), 2.66 (2H, t, –CH$_2$-CH$_2$N-), 2.80 (2H, t, –Ph-CH$_2$-CH$_2$), 2.90 (2H, t, –CH$_2$-CH$_2$-NHBoc), 3.22 (2H, t, -CH$_2$-NHBoc), 3.5-3.7 (234 H, -O-CH$_2$-CH$_2$-O-), 4.1 (2H, s, Ph-CH$_2$-CH$_2$-NH-CH$_2$- and 2H of –CH$_2$-NH-CH$_2$-CH$_2$- NHBoc), 4.33 (4H, t, - CH$_2$-COO-), 6.53 (1H, d, Ph) and 6.76 (2H, m, Ph).

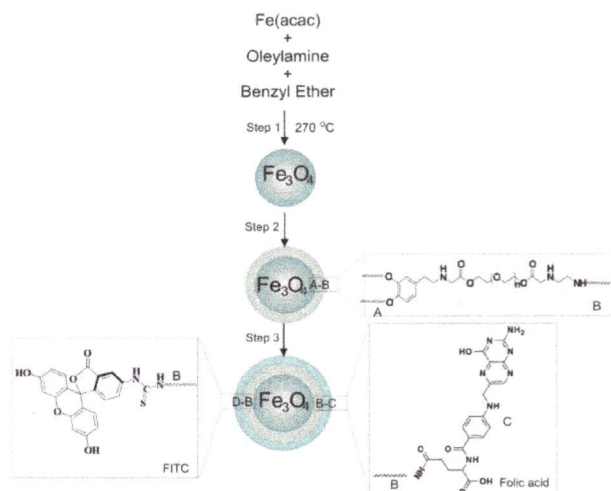

Figure 1. Schematic representation of step-wise synthesis of Fe$_3$O$_4$-DPA-PEG-FA/FITC nanoparticles.

All The solutions were stirred overnight under argon at room temperature (RT) also the insoluble compounds filtered using Buchner vacuum filtration funnel. In three steps for purification of the products, the solvent (dichloromethane) was removed using a rotary vacuum evaporator (Heidolph, Schwabach, Germany) and 30 mL diethyl ether was added for precipitation. Diethyl ether was removed using a rotary evaporator, and then products were redissolved in water/NaCl (35%w/v). Products were extracted from water by the addition of 30 mL dichloromethane and re-precipitation with 30 mL diethyl ether.

DPA-PEG-NHBoc (1.0 g, 0.04 mmol) was dissolved in dichloromethane (20 mL). The solution was stirred using a magnetic stirrer. Then trifluoroacetic acid (1.5 mL) was added and stirred for 1h at RT. Solvent was removed by rotary and product (DPA-PEG-NH$_2$) was washed (3×) with dichloromethane. The final brown color product was precipitated using diethyl ether.

Preparation of Fe$_3$O$_4$-DPA-PEG-NH$_2$ and Conjugation

Fe$_3$O$_4$ (0.5 g, 2.16 mmol) was dispersed in dichloromethane (50 mL).[22] DPA-PEG-NH$_2$ (2.5 g) was added to the solution and stirred overnight under argon blanket at 25 °C. After one night, solutions were sonicated for 15 min and then, Fe$_3$O$_4$-DPA-PEG-NH$_2$ was precipitated using hexane and gathered by centrifugation at 4000 rpm. For purification of modified Fe$_3$O$_4$, the samples were washed (3×) with dichloromethane/hexane (1:5) mixture. Finally, the solid dark-brown color product was re-dispersed in 20 mL ethanol. Figure 1 schematically represents the engineering process.

For conjugation, in the first step, N,N,dicyclohexylcarbodiimide (DCC) (2.95 g, 14.3 mmol), folic acid (3g, 6.8 mmol) and N-hydroxysuccinimide (NHS) (1.643 g, 14.3 mmol) were dissolved in dimethylsulfoxide (DMSO) (30 mL) (2.1:1:2.1mmol).[24] Triethylamine (1.88 mL, 13.6 mmol) was added to the solution while solution was stirred overnight at RT under argon blanket. Then, hexane (40 mL) was added to the flask for precipitation and yellow color product was washed with ether (yield was 1.66 g, 55.33%).

In the second step, modified Fe$_3$O$_4$-DPA-PEG-NH$_2$ (1.00 g) was dispersed in 10 mL DMSO, and then triethylamine (0.17 mL, 1.248 mmol) was added to the solution.[25] FA-NHS (0.0985 g, 0.156 mmol) and fluorescein isothiocyanate (FITC) (0.0607 g, 0.156 mmol) were each dissolved in DMSO (5 mL). The two solutions were added to the reaction flask containing compound and stirred at room temperature overnight under argon blanket. The final product was collected with Invitrogen bead separation system (DYNAL), washed with deionized water (3×) and characterized by FT-IR (Shimadzu FT-IR-8400S spectrophotometer, Shimadzu Scientific Instruments, Japan).

Cell Culture

The FR-positive MCF-7 cell line and the FR-negative lung cancer cell line were used for this study. Both cell lines were cultured at a seeding density of 4.0 × 10^{4}cells/cm^2 onto the cultivation plates/coverslips using normal culture medium (DMEM supplemented with 10% FBS, 100 units/mL penicillin G and 100 µg/mL streptomycin). The cultured cells were kept at 37 °C in a humidified CO2 incubator during cultivation and during experiments.

Fluorescence Microscopy

For fluorescence microscopy, cells were cultivated as described onto the 22-mm^2 coverslips. At 40-50% confluency, they were exposed to a designated concentration of Fe$_3$O$_4$-DPA-PEG-FA/FITC NPs (5 µg/mL) for 1 h at 37 °C in the CO$_2$ incubator. Fixation involved washing the cells (3×) with PBS, followed by 10 min incubation with 2% formaldehyde in PBS at room temperature. After washing cells (3×) with PBS, they were mounted on slides using mounting medium without/with DAPI (50 µM, for 20 min) for nuclear staining. The prepared samples were examined utilizing an Olympus IX81 compound fluorescence microscope equipped with XM10 monochrome camera, Olympus optical Co., Ltd. (Tokyo, Japan) as described previously.

Cellular Impacts

To pursue the cellular impacts of the targeted fluorophoromagnetic nanoparticles, MTT cytotoxicity assay was used. The cultivated cells, at 40-50% confluency, were exposed to Fe$_3$O$_4$-DPA-PEG-FA/FITC NPs (0-5 µg/mL). The media was removed and 150 µL fresh media plus 50 µL MTT solutions (prepared as 2 mg/mL in FBS) were added to each well and incubated for 4 h at 37 °C in a CO$_2$ incubator. The media was removed and the cells were washed (3×), then the formed formazin crystals were dissolved by adding DMSO (200 µL) and Sorenson's buffer (25 µL) to each well plate. The absorbance was read at 570 nm using a spectrophotometer (BioTek Instruments, Inc., Bad Friedrichshall, Germany).

Results

Characterization of Fe$_3$O$_4$ Nanoparticles

The synthesized Fe$_3$O$_4$ nanoparticles at 270°C by thermal decomposition reaction of Fe (acac)$_3$ showed average size about 7 nm (Figure 1, step 1). For removal of water from reaction environment, the reaction mixture was performed using Dean-Stark apparatus at 120 °C. Size of Fe$_3$O$_4$ MNPs was determined using a particle size analyser Zetasizer Nano ZS (Malvern Instruments, UK). As shown in Figure 2A, the surface modification of MNPs with oleylamine layer analysed by FT-IR spectroscopy that revealed the main absorption peaks for oleylamineare: v (NH$_2$) 3435 cm^{-1}, v_{max}/cm^{-1} 3001(=C-H) and 2954s, 2924s, 2852s (C-H); and the explicit absorption peaks related to Fe$_3$O$_4$ are: v_{max}/cm^{-1} 630, 588, 442(Fe-O). Figure 2A shows another important peak at 1523 that represents coordinated bond between Fe (III) of Fe$_3$O$_4$ and NH$_2$ of oleylamine (Fe-N bond).

Characterization of DPA-PEG-NH$_2$

For synthesis of DPA-PEG-NH$_2$, in the first step BBrAC-PEG was synthesized by reacting excess amount of bromoacetyl chloride with PEG in the presence of triethylamine as a base. The FT-IR spectroscopy (Figure 2) validated formation of the BBrAC-PEG, resulting in v_{max}/cm^{-1} 1750 (C=O, PEG-bromoacetyl), 1100 (C-O-C, PEG) and 2880s (CH$_2$). The peak at 1750 cm^{-1} confirms existence of carboxylate in structure of PEG. In the second step, reaction of BBrAC-PEG with one equivalent of dopamine yielded DPA-PEG-BrAc. FT-IR spectrum confirmed existence of phenyl ring in DPA-PEG-BrAcwith v_{max}/cm^{-1} 3100s(=C-H). In the third step, the

DPA-PEG-BrAc was treated with N-tert-butoxycarbonyl-1,2-ethylenediamineto gain DPA-PEG-NHBoc, in which the boc (N-tert-butoxycarbonyl) was removed by trifluoroacetic acid (TFA). The synthesis of DPA-PEG-NH_2 was also confirmed by H-NMR.

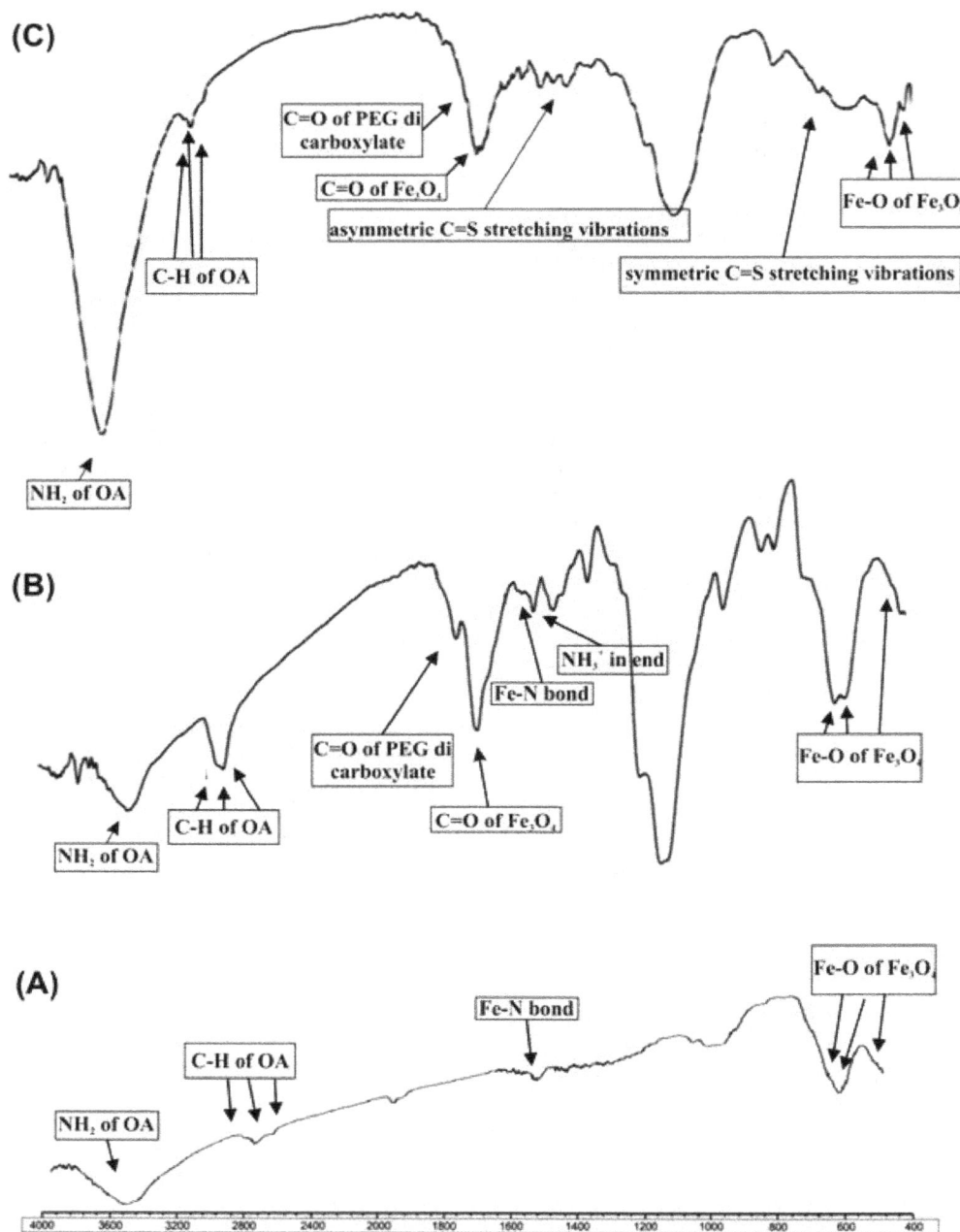

Figure 2. FT-IR spectrophotometer of synthesized Fe_3O_4-DPA-PEG-FA/FITC nanoparticles. A) Fe_3O_4- MNPs. B) Fe_3O_4-DPA-PEG-NH_2, absorption peak in v (1487 cm-1) is related to NH_3^+ available in salt of NH_2TFA. C) Fe_3O_4-DPA-PEG-FA/FITC, the symmetric and asymmetric C=S stretching vibrations at 730 and 1417 cm^{-1} confirmed the formation of thiourea group in the Fe_3O_4- DPA-PEG-FA/FITC.

Characterization of Modified Fe_3O_4

The surface of Fe_3O_4 was modified with DPA-PEG-NH_2 using dopamine moiety. Dopamine has been used as an anchoring agent in DPA-PEG-NH_2 that could replace the oleylamine on surface of Fe_3O_4 MNPs. TEM and SEM micrographs determined the

morphology and size of Fe_3O_4-DPA-PEG-NH_2 with diameter ~13 nm (data not shown). In the FT-IR spectrum of the Fe_3O_4-DPA-PEG-NH_2, in addition to the peaks related to Fe_3O_4 and DPA-PEG, absorption peak at v_{max}/cm^{-1}1487 cm^{-1} is seen that is related to NH_3^+ available in salt of NH_2TFA at the end of the structure of the Fe_3O_4-DPA-PEG-NH_2 (Figure 2B). To quantify the exact amount of the DPA-PEG-NH_2 used to coat the Fe_3O_4 cores, the solvent media of the supernatant was removed using rotary evaporator and the remained DPA-PEG-NH_2 was analyzed.

Characterization of Fluorophor Conjugated-Fe_3O_4 Magnetic Nanoparticles

When half equivalent FITC and half equivalent FA were conjugated to one equivalent of Fe_3O_4-DPA-PEG-NH_2, both moieties (i.e., FA and FITC) were available on FA and FITC grafted MNPs. FA was used to target the FR, while FITC was used to provide a possibility for fluorescence microscopy of cancer cells. FT-IR analysis of FA-MNPs-FITC confirmed conjugation of FITC onto the MNPs (Figure 2C). The symmetric and asymmetric C=S stretching vibrations at 730 and 1417 cm^{-1} confirmed the formation of thiourea group in the Fe_3O_4-MNP-FA/FITC. Furthermore, bond at 3435 cm^{-1} related to NH_2 stretching was detected on surface of MNPs. The TEM and SEM determined the morphology and size (~30 nm) of Fe_3O_4-DPA-PEG-FA/FITC (Figure 3).

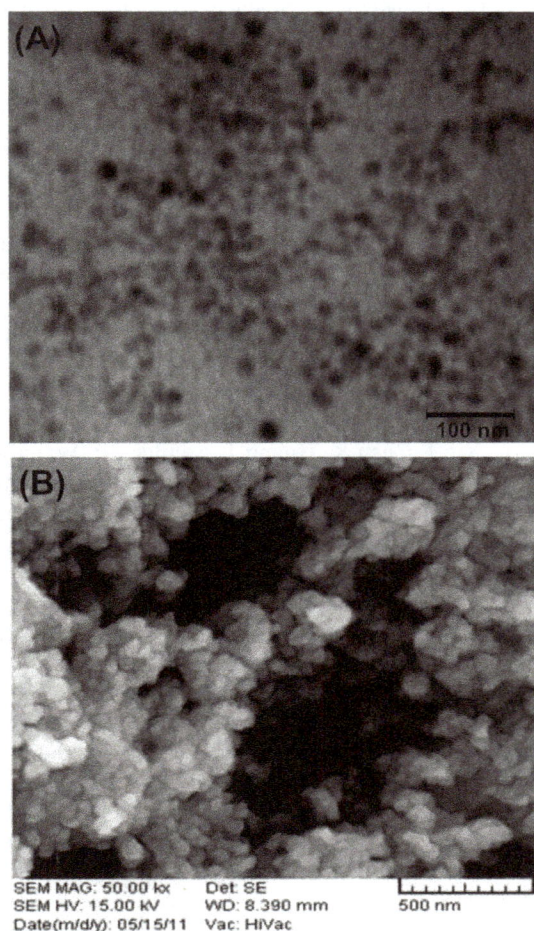

Figure 3. TEM (A) and SEM (B) nano-graph Fe3O4-DPA-PEG-FA/FITC nanoparticles. TEM: transmission electron microscopy. SEM: scanning electron microscopy.

Fluorescence Microscopy and Cellular Impacts

To visualize the cellular interaction of the FR targeted fluoromagnetic NPs, the FR-positive MCF-7 cells and the FR-negative A549 cells were exposed to Fe_3O_4-DPA-PEG-FA/FITC (5 μg/mL) for 1 h. Figure 4 represents the fluorescence microscopy of the MCF-7 cells treated with FR targeted fluoromagnetic NPs. We witnessed substantial binding and/or internalization of the FR targeted fluoromagnetic NPs in the FR-positive MCF-7 cells (Figure 4), but not the FR-negative A549 cells (data not shown), indicating the specificity of these nanosystems toward folate receptor expressing cells.

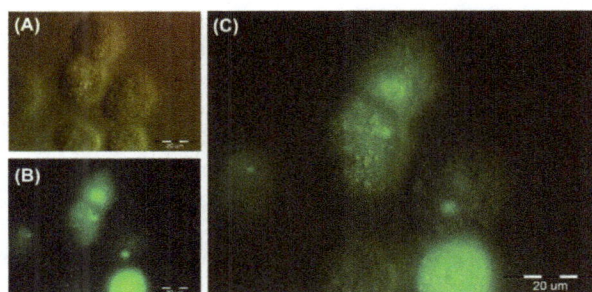

Figure 4. Fluorescence and light microscopy of the MCF-7 cells treated with Fe_3O_4-DPA-PEG-FA/FITC. A) Differential interference contrast (DIC) microscopy image of the MCF-7 cells. B) Fluorescence microscopy (FM) image of the MCF-7 cells treated with fluorophore tagged nanoparticles (MNPs-FA/FITC).C) Superimposed DIC and FM image.

Since these FR targeting fluoromagnetic NPs are used for targeted imaging, we aimed to see their nonspecific toxicity using MTT assay. Figure 5 represents the viability of the treated MCF-7 cells with designated amount of FR targeting fluoromagnetic NPs, which indicate negligible cytotoxicity.

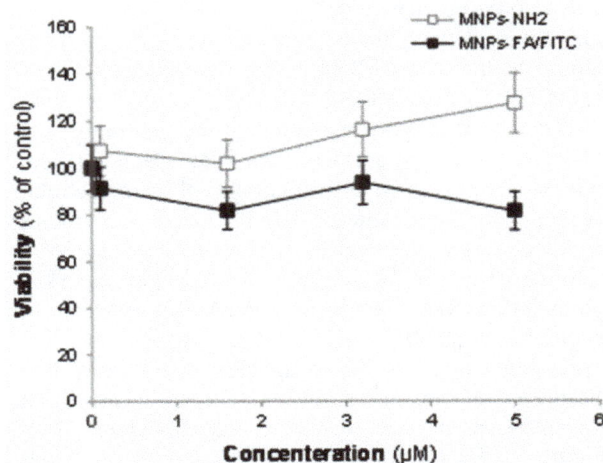

Figure 5. Cellular impacts of Fe_3O_4-DPA-PEG-FA/FITC in MCF-7 cells.

Discussion

Given the fact that nanosized macromolecules are often prone to opsonisation by MPS, the MNPs are PEGylated to become stealth. Such modified MNPs appear to show markedly long circulation in blood and thus high level of extravasation and accumulation in the tumor site. They were seen as clustered inside the various stages of endocytic pathways without damaging cellular organelles where endocytosis mechanism for their entry appears to be a receptor mediated endocytosis,[26] mainly through targeting a CMM such as FR. It should be noted that the absorption of folate is primarily mediated by a membrane transporter with micro-molar affinities for folates, in which the FRs with nanomolar affinities to folate are likely to markedly modulate folate availability for these transporters and functional isoforms of FRs are anchored to the membrane by a glycolipid anchor, the glycosylphosphatidylinositol (GPI) anchor.[27] Further, colocalization of folate and transferrin receptors[28] clearly indicate that the endocytosis of the targeted fluoromagnetic NPs is a receptor mediated process, presumably via calthrin coated pites and/or membranous caveolae. Thus, we aimed to look at the internalization of FR targeting fluoromagnetic NPs in FR-expressing cells.

We synthesized Fe_3O_4 NPs by thermal decomposition reaction of Fe(acac)$_3$ and undertook a series of surface modification steps to achieve FITC and FA conjugated MNPs (Figures 1-3). The synthesized Fe_3O_4 NPs through thermal decomposition reaction of Fe(acac)$_3$ showed average size about 10 nm, similar to previous reports.[22] We used the DPA-PEG-NH$_2$ to coat the Fe_3O_4 NPs to achieve more hydrophilic and stealth MNPs. Further, the DPA-PEG-NH$_2$ modification can provide a versatile platform for further conjugation of MNPs with other functional groups.[29] The PEGylated MNPs (Fe_3O_4-DPA-PEG-NH$_2$) were conjugated with FA and FITC to produce Fe_3O_4-DPA-PEG-FA/FITC NPs. We used FA to actively target the FR, at which these FA armed MNPs can specifically target the FR-positive breast cancer cells.[30]

Our fluorescence microscopy analysis resulted in significant uptake of FR targeting fluoromagnetic NPs by the FR-positive MCF-7 cells (Figure 4). The time-dependency of this process indicate the binding of the MNPs to the cell surface via folate receptor and endocytosis via vesicular trafficking. Following cellular uptake, membrane-encapsulated silicon particles migrated to the perinuclear region of the cell by a microtubule-driven mechanism.[31] Based upon our flow cytometry analysis, the FR targeting MNPs appeared to specifically quantitatively (>95%) detect the FR expressing cells,[18] while no specific cytotoxicity was observed in the treated cells even with high concentration of FR targeting fluoromagnetic NPs (Figure 5). We speculate that they harness the vesicular trafficking pathway(s) for internalization, i.e. the early/late endosomal machineries. Thus, these nanocarriers, if used as drug delivery nanosystem, should be able to escape from demise in the late endsome/lysosome. Lysosomes contain approximately over 40 different hydrolytic enzymes that mediate

controlled intracellular degradation of macromolecules.[32] Thus, due to uniqueness of these trafficking machineries (enzyme composition and pH), targeted MNPs grafted with cytotoxic agents should be engineered in a way to be able to exploit such potential. These FR targeting fluoromagnetic NPs, however, prior to transformation into clinical application, should be fully characterized and tested in appropriate animal models.

Conclusion
The nano-scaled targeted fluoromagnetic theranostics have great potential toward simultaneous imaging and therapy. In this work, we have demonstrated successful synthesis of folic acid/ fluorescein isothiocyanate-PEG conjugated magnetic nanoparticles which could markedly detect the FR expressing cancer cells. Thus, we propose that they can be quantitatively used for specific MRI-based imaging and therapy of various cancers.

Acknowledgments
Authors are thankful to the Research Centre for Pharmaceutical Nanotechnology (RCPN) at Tabriz University of Medical Sciences for the financial support.

Conflict of Interest
The authors declare there is no Conflict of interest in the content of this study.

References
1. Omidi Y. Smart multifunctional theranostics: Simultaneous diagnosis and therapy of cancer. *BioImpacts* 2011;1(3):145-7.
2. Lee N, Hyeon T. Designed synthesis of uniformly sized iron oxide nanoparticles for efficient magnetic resonance imaging contrast agents. *Chem Soc Rev* 2012;41(7):2575-89.
3. Bu L, Xie J, Chen K, Huang J, Aguilar ZP, Wang A, et al. Assessment and comparison of magnetic nanoparticles as mri contrast agents in a rodent model of human hepatocellular carcinoma. *Contrast Media Mol Imaging* 2012;7(4):363-72.
4. Corr SA, Byrne SJ, Tekoriute R, Meledandri CJ, Brougham DF, Lynch M, et al. Linear assemblies of magnetic nanoparticles as mri contrast agents. *J Am Chem Soc* 2008;130(13):4214-5.
5. Yigit MV, Moore A, Medarova Z. Magnetic nanoparticles for cancer diagnosis and therapy. *Pharm Res* 2012;29(5):1180-8.
6. Tietze R, Lyer S, Durr S, Alexiou C. Nanoparticles for cancer therapy using magnetic forces. *Nanomedicine (Lond)* 2012;7(3):447-57.
7. Li C, Li L, Keates AC. Targeting cancer gene therapy with magnetic nanoparticles. *Oncotarget* 2012;3(4):365-70.
8. Ferrari M. Cancer nanotechnology: Opportunities and challenges. *Nat Rev Cancer* 2005;5(3):161-71.

9. Zhou J, Wu W, Caruntu D, Yu MH, Martin A, Chen JF, et al. Synthesis of porous magnetic hollow silica nanospheres for nanomedicine application. *J Phys Chem C* 2007;111(47):17473-7.

10. Robinson I, Tung Le, Maenosono S, Walti C, Thanh NT. Synthesis of core-shell gold coated magnetic nanoparticles and their interaction with thiolated DNA. *Nanoscale* 2010;2(12): 2624-30.

11. Kohler N, Fryxell GE, Zhang M. A bifunctional poly (ethylene glycol) silane immobilized on metallic oxide-based nanoparticles for conjugation with cell targeting agents. *J Am Chem Soc* 2004;126(23):7206-11.

12. Shubayev VI, Pisanic TR, 2nd, Jin S. Magnetic nanoparticles for theragnostics. *Adv Drug Deliv Rev* 2009;61(6):467-77.

13. Bae KH, Kim YB, Lee Y, Hwang J, Park H, Park TG. Bioinspired synthesis and characterization of gadolinium-labeled magnetite nanoparticles for dual contrast t(1)- and t(2)-weighted magnetic resonance imaging. *Bioconjug Chem* 2010;21(3):505-12.

14. Gupta AK, Gupta M. Synthesis and surface engineering of iron oxide nanoparticles for biomedical applications. *Biomaterials* 2005;26(18):3995-4021.

15. Xie J, Xu C, Kohler N, Hou Y, Sun S. Controlled pegylation of monodisperse Fe_3O_4 nanoparticles for reduced non-specific uptake by macrophage cells. *Adv Mater* 2007;19(20):3163-6.

16. Yoo HS, Park TG. Folate-receptor-targeted delivery of doxorubicin nano-aggregates stabilized by doxorubicin-peg-folate conjugate. *J Control Release* 2004;100(2):247-56.

17. Kohler N, Sun C, Wang J, Zhang M. Methotrexate-modified superparamagnetic nanoparticles and their intracellular uptake into human cancer cells. *Langmuir* 2005;21(19):8858-64.

18. Heidari Majd M, Asgari D, Barar J, Valizadeh H, Kafil V, Coukos G, et al. Specific targeting of cancer cells by multifunctional mitoxantrone conjugated magnetic nanoparticles. *J Drug Target* 2013; in press. doi: 10.3109/1061186X.2012.750325.

19. Hu FX, Neoh KG, Kang ET. Synthesis and in vitro anti-cancer evaluation of tamoxifen-loaded magnetite/plla composite nanoparticles. *Biomaterials* 2006;27(33):5725-33.

20. Akça Ö, Ünak P, Medine Eİ, Özdemir Ç, Sakarya S, Timur S. Fluorescein isothiocyanate labeled, magnetic nanoparticles conjugated D-penicillamine-anti-metadherin and in vitro evaluation on breast cancer cells. *Rev Bras Fisica Med* 2011;5(1):99-104.

21. Zhang J, Rana S, Srivastava RS, Misra RD. On the chemical synthesis and drug delivery response of folate receptor-activated, polyethylene glycol-functionalized magnetite nanoparticles. *Acta Biomater* 2008;4(1):40-8.

22. Wang B, Xu C, Xie J, Yang Z, Sun S. Ph controlled release of chromone from chromone-fe3o4 nanoparticles. *J Am Chem Soc* 2008;130(44):14436-7.

23. Moros M, Pelaz B, Lopez-Larrubia P, Garcia-Martin ML, Grazu V, de la Fuente JM. Engineering biofunctional magnetic nanoparticles for biotechnological applications. *Nanoscale* 2010;2(9):1746-55.

24. Sonvico F, Mornet S, Vasseur S, Dubernet C, Jaillard D, Degrouard J, et al. Folate-conjugated iron oxide nanoparticles for solid tumor targeting as potential specific magnetic hyperthermia mediators: Synthesis, physicochemical characterization, and in vitro experiments. *Bioconjug Chem* 2005;16(5):1181-8.

25. Li M, Selvin PR. Amine-reactive forms of a luminescent diethylenetriaminepentaacetic acid chelate of terbium and europium: Attachment to DNA and energy transfer measurements. *Bioconjug Chem* 1997;8(2):127-32.

26. Kumar M, Singh G, Arora V, Mewar S, Sharma U, Jagannathan NR, et al. Cellular interaction of folic acid conjugated superparamagnetic iron oxide nanoparticles and its use as contrast agent for targeted magnetic imaging of tumor cells. *Int J Nanomedicine* 2012;7:3503-16.

27. Sabharanjak S, Mayor S. Folate receptor endocytosis and trafficking. *Adv Drug Deliv Rev* 2004;56(8):1099-109.

28. Yang J, Chen H, Vlahov IR, Cheng JX, Low PS. Evaluation of disulfide reduction during receptor-mediated endocytosis by using fret imaging. *Proc Natl Acad Sci U S A* 2006;103(37):13872-7.

29. Kang SM, Choi IS, Lee KB, Kim Y. Bioconjugation of poly(poly(ethylene glycol) methacrylate)-coated iron oxide magnetic nanoparticles for magnetic capture of target proteins. *Macromol Res* 2009;17(4):259-64.

30. Li K, Jiang Y, Ding D, Zhang X, Liu Y, Hua J, et al. Folic acid-functionalized two-photon absorbing nanoparticles for targeted mcf-7 cancer cell imaging. *Chem Commun (Camb)* 2011;47(26):7323-5.

31. Ferrati S, Mack A, Chiappini C, Liu X, Bean AJ, Ferrari M, et al. Intracellular trafficking of silicon particles and logic-embedded vectors. *Nanoscale* 2010;2(8):1512-20.

32. Barar J, Omidi Y. Cellular trafficking and subcellular interactions of cationic gene delivery nanomaterials. *J Pharm Nutr Sci* 2011;1(1):68-81.

Comparison of Cytotoxic Activity of L778123 as a Farnesyltranferase Inhibitor and Doxorubicin against A549 and HT-29 Cell Lines

Saeed Ghasemi[1], Soodabeh Davaran[1,2], Simin Sharifi[2], Davoud Asgari[1,2], Ali Abdollahi[1], Javid Shahbazi Mojarrad[1,3]*

[1]Department of Medicinal Chemistry, Faculty of Pharmacy, Tabriz University of Medical Sciences, Tabriz, Iran.

[2]Research Center for Pharmaceutical Nanotechnology, Tabriz University of Medical Sciences, Tabriz, Iran.

[3]Tuberculosis and Lung Disease Research Center, Tabriz University of Medical Sciences, Tabriz, Iran.

ARTICLE INFO

Keywords:
Farnesyltransferase inhibitor
MTT assay
Combination therapy
L-778123

ABSTRACT

Purpose: Farnesyltransferase (FTase) is a zinc-dependent enzyme that adds a farnesyl group to the Ras proteins. L778, 123 is a potent peptidomimetic imidazole-containing FTase inhibitor. *Methods*: L778123 was synthesized according to known methods and evaluated alone and in combination with doxorubicin against A549 (adenocarcinomic human alveolar basal epithelial cells) and HT29 (human colonic adenocarcinoma) cell lines by MTT assay. *Results:* L778123 showed weak cytotoxic activity with IC_{50} of 100 and 125 for A549 and HT-29 cell lines, respectively. The combination of doxorubicin and L778123 can decrease IC_{50} of doxorubicin in both cell lines significantly. *Conclusion:* It can be concluded that L778, 123 can be a good agent for combination therapy.

Introduction

The necessity for novel anticancer agents is obvious because of insufficient drugs. The anticancer agents must be effective for cancer therapy, increasing the lifetime and improving quality of life in cancer patients.[1]

Regulation of cellular growth is done by switching between the inactive and the active state of membrane-bound GTP binding proteins (G-proteins). Mutation of the GTP-binding protein Ras that has a key role in cell signaling pathways, can lead to uncontrolled proliferation.

Approximately, 30% of all human cancers are because of mutation of human ras proteins, reaching as high as 90% for pancreas cancer, 50% for colorectal cancer and and 40% for lung. A CAAX tetrapeptide motif exists at their C-terminal of these G-proteins (C: Cys, A: an aliphatic amino acid, X: Ser, Met, Gln, Ala typically Met).[1-6] Ras proteins is undergone a series of modification for their biological functions. Their activation are started by the alkylation (i.e., farnesylation) of cysteine in CAAX motif. Farnesyltransferase (FTase) as a zinc-containing metalloenzyme identify the CAAX tetrapeptide sequence and add the 15 carbon isoprenoid, called a farnesyl group, from farnesyldiphosphate (FPP) to the thiol of cysteine. The farnesylation is an important step for the biological activity of Ras proteins and is a valuable target for chemotherapy.[1,2,7,8] Peptidomimetic

FTase inhibitors are a class of inhibitors which have a thiol moiety. Their thiol moiety could be bound to zinc ion of the FTase enzyme. Replacement of thiol group by another zinc binding moiety such as an imidazole or other heterocyclic rings made non-thiol, non-peptidic, imidazole or non-imidazole containing inhibitors.[9] More than a decade later, researchers reported many groups of imidazole-containing FTase inhibitors which were tested in clinical trials, including L778123 and tipifarnib (Figure 1).

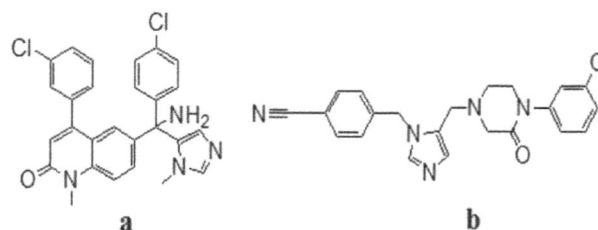

Figure 1. Chemical structures of farnesyltransferase inhibitors: (a) Tipifarnib, (b) L778123.

Doxorubicin is a potent chemotherapy drug which inhibits topoisomerase II. Doxorubicin-containing regimens are used in wide range of cancers include lung, colorectal, breast, esophageal, bladder, ovarian, and head and neck cancers, along with lymphomas and multiple myeloma.[10,11]

*Corresponding author: Javid Shahbazi Mojarrad, Department of Medicinal Chemistry, Faculty of Pharmacy, Tabriz University of Medical Sciences, Tabriz, Iran. Email: jvshahbazi@yahoo.com

In this study, we report synthesis and comparison of cytotoxic activity of L778123 and doxorubicin alone and in combination with each other against A549 (adenocarcinomic human alveolar basal epithelial cells) and HT29 (human colonic adenocarcinoma) cell lines.

Materials and Methods
Chemistry

All reagents and solvents were prepared from Merck and Sigma Aldrich. L-778123 was synthesized was prepared according to known methods described previously.[10] Melting points were measured with an Electrothermal-9100 melting point apparatus and are uncorrected. The IR spectra were recorded on a Shimadzu 4300 spectrophotometer (potassium bromide dicks). ^{1}HNMR and ^{13}CNMR spectra were recorded on a Varian unity 500 spectrometer and chemical shifts (δ) are reported in parts per million (ppm) using tetramethylsilane (TMS) as an internal standard. The mass spectra were run on an Agilent 6410 LC-MS at 70 eV. Merck silica gel 60. F254 plates were used for analytical TLC.

Synthesis of 4-{[5-(hydroxymethyl)-2-mercapto-1H-imidazol-1-yl]methyl-Benzonitrile (1)

A mixture of 4-(Aminomethyl)benzonitrile hydrochloride (4.21 g, 25 mmol), dihydroxyacetone dimmer (DHA) (2.47 g, 27.5 mmol), potassium thiocyanate (KSCN) (3.64 g, 37.5 mmol), acetic acid (3g, 50 mmol) in acetonitrile (24 mL) and water (1.0 mL) were stirred at 55 °C overnight. The mixture was cooled to room temperature and filtered. The precipitate was washed with acetonitrile (25 mL), water (50 mL) and ethylacetate (EtOAc) (25 mL) respectively. The solid was dried at 40 °C overnight to yield 1.
Yield: 73%; m.p = 159-161 °C; IR vmax (KBr)/cm^{-1}: 3120(OH), 2570 (SH), 2230(nitrile), 1620(C=N). ^{1}HNMR (250 MHz, d6-DMSO): δ 12.25 (s, 1H), 7.80 (d, J = 8.5, 2H), 7.37 (d, J = 8.5, 2H), 6.91 (s, 1H), 5.38 (s, 2H), 5.24 (s, 1H), 4.16 (s, 2H).

Synthesis of 4-{[5-(hydroxymethyl)-1H-imidazol-1-yl]methyl} benzonitrile (2)

A solution of sodium nitrite (1.1 g, 16.00 mmol) in water (1.2 mL) was added to a mixture of thioimidazole 1 (1 g, 4.00 mmol) in acetic acid (20 mL) over 30 min at room temperature. Ice (10 g) and then ammonia was added to bring the pH=11 at temperature between 20-30°C. The resulting mixture was stirred for 30 min and filtered. The solid was washed with 2:1 water-methanol (30 mL) respectively. The solid was dried to provide dethionated imidazole 2.
Yield: 85%; mp = 164-166 °C; IR vmax (KBr)/cm^{-1}: 3130(OH), 2230 (nitrile), 1680(C=N); ^{1}HNMR (500 MHz, DMSO-d_6): δ 7.83 (d, J = 8, 2H), 7.72 (s, 1H), 7.3 (d, J = 8, 2H), 6.86 (s, 1H), 5.35 (s, 2H), 5.12 (s, 1H), 4.29 (s, 2H).

Synthesis of 4-{[5-(chloromethyl)-1H-imidazol-1-yl] methyl}benzonitrile Hydrochloride (3)

Oxalyl chloride (1 mL, 11.5 mmol) was added over 30 min to a mixture of DMF (1.78 mL) and acetonitrile (25.6 mL) at temperature below 10 °C to give a white mixture. The mixture was added to a suspension of 2 (2.13 g, 10 mmol) in acetonitrile (17 mL) over 30 min while maintaining the temperature below 6 °C. The mixture was warmed to 25 °C, aged for 3 h and then cooled to 0 °C and aged for 60 min. The solid was filtrated, washed with ice-cold acetonitrile (15 mL) and dried to yield 3.
Yield: 90%; mp = 204-207 °C; IR vmax (KBr)/cm^{-1}: 3100(NH$^+$), 2230 (nitrile), 1610(C=N); ^{1}HNMR (500 MHz, DMSO-d_6): δ 9.50 (d, J=1 Hz. 1H), 7.92 (s, 1H), 7.89 (d, J = 8 Hz, 2H), 7.56 (d, J = 8 Hz, 2H), 5.72 (s, 2H), 4.94 (s, 2H), 4.40 (br s, 1H).

Synthesis of N^1-(3-chlorophenyl)-N^2-(2-hydroxyethyl) glycinamide (4)

To a mixture of 3-chloroaniline (10 g, 78.25 mmol) in isopropyl acetate (90 mL) and potassium bicarbonate (15.62 g, 105.5 mmol) in water (75 mL) was added chloroacetyl chloride (12 g, 105.5 mmol) dropwise over 1 h maintained under 10 °C. The aqueous layer was removed the organic phase containing chloroacetamide was treated with ethanolamine (7.5 mL, 122.78 mmol). The mixture was warmed to 55 °C and aged for 1 h. Water (30 mL) and isopropyl acetate (7.5 mL) were added and the mixture was stirred vigorously at 55 °C for 30 minutes. The organic layer was separated and cooled to 0 °C over 1 h. The precipitate was filtrated, washed with cooled isopropyl acetate (2 × 15 mL) and dried to obtain 4.
Yield: 75%; mp = 103-105 °C; IR vmax (KBr)/cm^{-1} : 3260 (NH), 3200 (OH), 1690 (C=O); ^{1}HNMR (400 MHz, DMSO-d_6): δ 10.10 (br s, 1H), 7.86 (brt, 1H), 7.53 (d, J = 7.4, 1H), 7.33 (t, J = 8.0, 1H), 7.10 (d, J = 7.4, 1H), 4.66 (br s, 1H), 3.48 (t, J = 4.5, 2H), 3.31 (s, 2H), 2.62 (t, J =5.5, 2H); ^{13}CNMR (75 MHz, DMSO-d_6): δ 170.9, 140.1, 133.0, 130.3, 122.9, 118.6, 117.5, 60.3, 52.7, 51.5.

Synthesis of 1-(3-chlorophenyl) piperazine-2-one hydrochloride (5)

Diisopropylazodicarboxylate (DIAD) (5.1 g, 27 mmol) was added over 1.5 h to a mixture of tributylphosphine (5.5 g, 27 mmol) and EtOAc (15 mL) under the nitrogen atmosphere maintained under 0 °C. The mixture was aged at 0 °C for 30 min. The resulting solution was added over 1.5 h to a solution of amide alcohol 4 (4.52 g, 20 mmol) in EtOAc (30 mL) maintained under 0 °C and the mixture was warmed to room temperature over 1 h. Ethanolic HCl (4 M, 5.2 mL, 19.75 mmol) was added to the solution at 40 °C over 2 h. The resulting slurry was cooled to 0 °C and aged at 0 °C for 1 h. The hydrochloride salt was filtered, washed with chilled EtOAc (3 × 10 mL) and dried to afford 5.

Yield: 71%; mp = 232-235 °C; IR vmax (KBr)/cm^{-1}: 3200-2400 (NH$^+$), 1660 (Amide C=O); ^{1}HNMR (400 MHz, DMSO-d_6): δ 10.24 (br s, 2H), 7.50-7.31 (m, 4H), 3.92 (t, J = 4.8, 2H), 3.85 (s, 2H), 3.52 (t, J = 4.8, 2H); ^{13}CNMR (75 MHz, DMSO-d6): δ 162.1, 142.6, 132.9, 130.7, 127.0, 126.0, 124.5, 46.1, 44.9, 39.9.

Synthesis of 4[(5-{[4-(3-chlorophenyl)-3-oxopiperazin-1-yl] methyl}-1Himidazol-1 yl) methyl] benzonitrile (6)

A solution of **5** (4.11 g, 16.5 mmol) in acetonitrile (27 mL), *i*-Pr$_2$NEt (9.30 mL, 52.9 mmol) and **3** (5.00 g, 17.2 mmol) was stirred at 0 °C for 48 h. Water (10 mL) and N,N-*diisopropylethylamine* (*i*-Pr$_2$Net) (0.63 mL) were added. The solution was aged at 0 °C for 30 min and heated to 35 °C. Water (41 mL) was added over 5 min, and the solution was aged for 5- 10 min at 35 °C. Additional water (38 mL) was added over 30 min and the mixture was aged for 30 min at 35 °C. The mixture was cooled at 0 °C for 1 h. The crystals were filtrated and washed with ice-cold 1:5 acetonitrile/H$_2$O (25 mL) and 1:9 acetonitrile/H$_2$O at 5 °C (2 × 30 mL). The solid was dried to yield **6**.

Yield: 80%; mp = 90-92 °C; IR vmax (KBr)/cm^{-1}: 2240(C=N), 1640 (Amide C=O),; ^{1}HNMR (400 MHz, DMSO-d_6): δ 10.24 (br s, 2H), 7.87-6.94 (m, 8H), 5.40 (s, 2H), 3.45 (s, 2H), 3.33 (s, 2H), 3.32 (d, J=5.5,2H), 3.03 (s, 2H), 2.6 (t, J = 5.1, 2H); ^{13}CNMR (75 MHz, DMSO-d6): δ 165.6, 143.9, 143.2, 139.4, 132.8, 132.3, 130.2, 129.1, 127.4, 126.8, 126.1, 125.6, 124.0, 118.5, 109.9, 56.6, 49.1, 48.7, 48.0, 47.3. MS (ESI): 407.19 [M+H].

Growth inhibition assay

Cytotoxicity of L778, 123, doxorubicin and combination of them was examined with MTT assay at 1-200μM concentrations against two human cancer cell lines including A549 (adenocarcinomic human alveolar basal epithelial cells) and HT29 (human colonic adenocarcinoma) cells. Cell suspensions were seeded in 96-well plates with concentrations of 8000-10000 A549 cells and 15000-20000 HT29 cells per well and incubated for 24 h to allow cell attachment. The cells were treated for 72 h with four various concentrations of L778, 123, doxorubicin and combination of them. Culture medium were replaced with 150 μl fresh media plus 50 μl MTT (3-(4, 5-dimethylthiazol- 2-yl)-2, 5-diphenyl tetrazolium bromide) reagent (2mg/mL in PBS). An additional 4 h of incubation at 37 °C were done, and then the medium was discarded. 200 μl dimethyl sulfoxide plus 25μl sorenson buffer (0.1M NaCl, 0.1M glycine, pH: 10.5) was added to each well, and the solution was shacked for 15 min in 37 °C to dissolve the purple tetrazolium crystals. The absorbance of each well was measured by plate reader (SUNRISE TECAN, Austria) at a wavelength of 570 nm. The amount of produced purple formazan is proportional to the number of viable cells. Experiments were performed two times in triplicate for determination of sensitivity to each compound. The IC$_{50}$ was calculated by linear regression analysis, expressed in mean±SD.[12]

Results and Discussion

The synthesis of L778, 123 (Figure 2) was started from 3-chloroaniline and 4-(Aminomethyl) benzonitrile hydrochloride. In one pot, 3-chloroaniline and chloroacetyl chloride in isopropyl acetate at 0 °C were mixed and then ethanolamine was added dropwise at 55°C to give amide alcohol 4 in quantitative yield. Ring closure of the piperazinone was performed with triphenylphosphine and DIAD in ethyl acetate via Mitsunobu reaction at -10 °C to afford 1-(3-Chlorophenyl) piperazine-2-one hydrochloride 5 in 75% overall yield.[5,13,14]

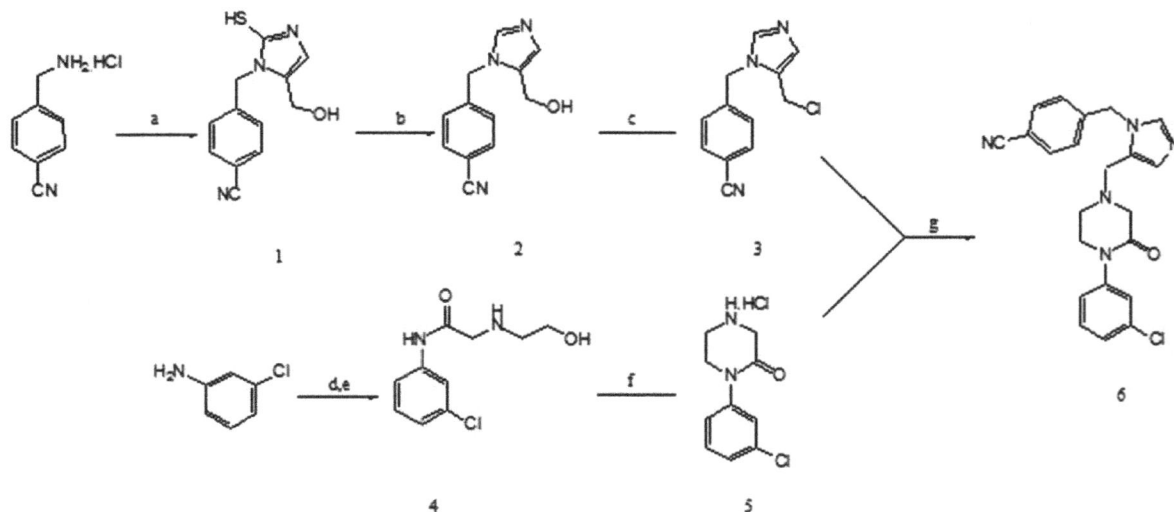

Figure 2. a) DHA, KSCN, CH$_3$CN/H$_2$O, 55 °C, 18h; b) NaNO$_2$, AcOH, H$_2$O, rt, 20 min; c) Oxalyl chloride, DMF/CH$_3$CN, 0 °C to rt, 3h; d) Chloroacetyl chloride, iPrAc, 0 °C to rt, 1h; e) Ethanolamine, iPrAc, 55°C, 2h; f) DIAD, Tributylphosphine, EtOAc, -10 °C to rt, 1h; g) *i*-Pr$_2$NEt, CH$_3$CN/H$_2$O, 0 °C, 39h.

In another pot ring closure of imidazole was performed by dihydroxyacetone, potassium thiocyanate and acetic acid in acetonotrile/H_2O to yield thioimidazole 1. There have been many reports on the dethionation of thioimidazole compounds to their dethionated derivatives using hydrogen peroxide, sodium nitrite and etc.,[5,10,13] but the sodium nitrite as a dethionation reagent has better yield than other reagents.[10] So, the dethionation of thioimidazole was perfomed in water by sodium nitrite at 20-30 °C to afford the dethionated imidazole 2 in 85% yield. The chlorination of the dethionated imidazole 2 was achieved using oxalyl chloride in DMF and acetonitrile to obtain intermediate 3. Finally, the intermediates 3, 5 were reacted in presence of iPrNEt$_2$ in acetonitrile for 48h at 0 °C to yield L778, 123 as free base with 80% yield. Synthesis of L778123 was done in 7 steps with overall yield of 24%.[10]

The results of cytotoxic activity were summarized as IC$_{50}$ (μM) of L778, 123 and doxorubicin alone and in combination with each other by MTT assay in Table 1. The IC$_{50}$ values of L778, 123 against A549 and HT29 cell lines showed that this compound had significant cytotoxic activity at concentrations lower than 100 μM. The IC$_{50}$ values of doxorubicin alone and in combination with L778123 against both cell lines was 3.12, 2.75 μM and 1.72, 1.52 μM respectively. These results showed that however L778, 123 as a farnesyltransferase inhibitor can have a good cytotoxic activity but it is very weak in comparison with doxorubicin as a classic anti-cancer agent (Figure 3). On the other hand, combination of doxorubicin with L778123 can decrease IC$_{50}$ of doxorubicin significantly. It means that combination of doxorubicin and L778123 may generate synergistic effects in both cell lines (Figure 4).

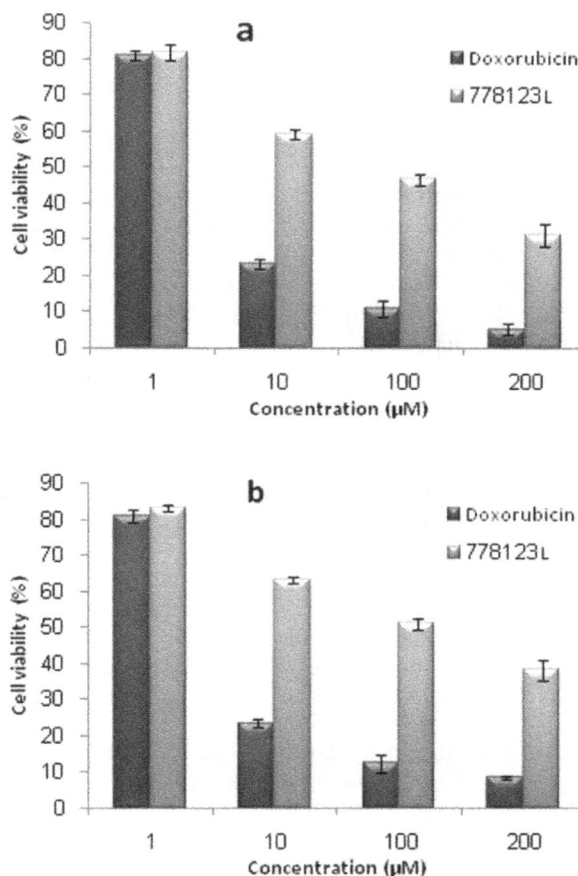

Figure 3. Cell viability of L778123, Doxorubicin and a combination of L778123 and Doxorubicin after 72 h treatment in: a) A549 and, b) HT-29 cell lines.

Table 1. Cytotoxic activity (IC$_{50}$, μM) of L778123 and Doxorubicin (DOX) against HT-29 and A549 cell lines.

	A549	HT29
L778123	100.72±2.16	125.78±2.45
Doxorubicin	3.13±0.11	2.75±0. 15
Combined DOX and L778123	1.72±0.13	1.52±0.16

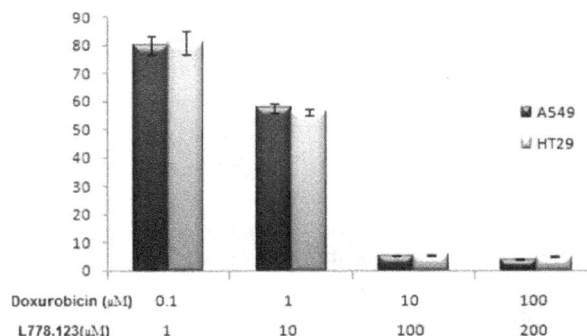

Figure 4. Cell viability of the combination of L778123 and Doxorubicin after 72 h treatment in A549 and HT-29.

Conclusion
In conclusion, L778, 123 was synthesized, characterized by IR, ^{1}HNMR, ^{13}CNMR, LC-Mass and identified as cytotoxic agents. Although this compound showed good potency with IC$_{50}$ equal to 100 μM and 125 μM for A549 and HT29 cell lines respectively, it is very weak in comparison with potent anticancer doxorubicin. L778, 123 can be a good agent for combination therapy with doxorubicin because of synergetic effects.

Acknowledgements
The authors would like to thank the Tuberculosis and Lung Disease Research Center, the Faculty of Pharmacy, and research center for pharmaceutical nanotechnology Tabriz University of Medical Sciences for financial supports. This article was a part of a thesis submitted for PhD degree (No.45) in the Faculty of Pharmacy, Tabriz University of Medical Sciences, Tabriz, Iran.

Conflict of interest
The authors report no conflicts of interest

References
1. Puntambekar DS, Giridhar R, Yadav MR. Insights into the structural requirements of farnesyltransferase inhibitors as potential anti-tumor agents based on 3D-QSAR CoMFA and CoMSIA models. *Eur J Med Chem* 2008;43:142-54.
2. Asoh K, Kohchi M, Hyoudoh I, Ohtsuka T, Masubuchi M, Kenichi Kawasaki, et al. Synthesis and structure–activity relationships of novel benzofuran farnesyltransferase inhibitors. *Bioorg Med Chem Lett* 2009;19:1753-7.
3. Angibaud P, Mevellec L, Meyer C, Bourdrez X, Lezouret P, Pilatte I, et al. Impact on farnesyltransferase inhibition of 4-chlorophenyl moiety replacement in the Zarnestra series. *Eur J Med Chem* 2007;42(5):702-14.
4. Gilleron P, Wlodarczyk N, Houssin R, Farce A, Laconde G, Goossens JF, et al. Design, synthesis and biological evaluation of substituted dioxodibenzothiazepines and dibenzocycloheptanes as farnesyltransferase inhibitors. *Bioorg Med Chem Lett* 2007;17(19):5465-71.
5. Tanaka R, Rubio A, Harn NK, Gernert D, Grese TA, Eishima J, et al. Design and synthesis of piperidine farnesyltransferase inhibitors with reduced glucuronidation potential. *Bioorg Med Chem* 2007;15(3):1363-82.
6. Equbal T, Silakari O, Rambabu G, Ravikumar M. Pharmacophore mapping of diverse classes of farnesyltransferase inhibitors. *Bioorg Med Chem Lett* 2007;17(6):1594-600.
7. Lu A, Zhang J, Yin X, Luo X, Jiang H. Farnesyltransferase pharmacophore model derived from diverse classes of inhibitors. *Bioorg Med Chem Lett* 2007;17(1):243-9.
8. Bolchi C, Pallavicini M, Rusconi C, Diomede L, Ferri N, Corsini A, et al. Peptidomimetic inhibitors of farnesyltransferase with high in vitro activity and significant cellular potency. *Bioorg Med Chem Lett* 2007;17:6192-6.
9. Xie A, Odde S, Prasanna S, Doerksen R. Imidazole-containing farnesyltransferase inhibitors: 3D quantitative structure–activity relationships and molecular docking. *J Comput Aid Mol Des* 2009;23(7):431-48.
10. Maligres PE, Waters MS, Weissman SA, McWilliams JC, Lewis S, Cowen J, et al. Preparation of a clinically investigated ras farnesyl transferase inhibitor. *J Heterocycl Chem* 2003;40(2):229-41.
11. Chisholm-Burns Ma. Pharmacotherapy Principles and Practice. New York: The McGraw-Hill Companies; 2008.
12. Aliabadi A, Shamsa F, Ostad SN, Emami S, Shafiee A, Davoodi J, et al. Synthesis and biological evaluation of 2-phenylthiazole-4-carboxamide derivatives as anticancer agents. *Eur J Med Chem* 2010;45(11):5384-9.
13. Askin D, Lewis S, Weissman SA, inventors; Merck & Co. Inc. assignee. Process for the synthesis of substituted piperazinones via Mitsunobu reaction. USA patent 6160118. 2000.
14. Weissman SA, Lewis S, Askin D, Volante R, Reider PJ. Efficient synthesis of N-arylpiperazinones via a selective intramolecular Mitsunobu cyclodehydration. *Tetrahedron Lett* 1998;39(41):7459-62.

A Unique Report: Development of Super Anti-Human IgG Monoclone with Optical Density Over Than 3

Leili Aghebati Maleki[1,2], Behzad Baradaran[1,2], Jalal Abdolalizadeh[1,2], Fatemeh Ezzatifar[1], Jafar Majidi[1,2]*

[1]Immunology Research Center, Tabriz University of Medical Sciences, Tabriz, Iran.
[2] Tabriz Pharmaceutical Technology Incubator (TPTI).

A R T I C L E I N F O

Keywords:
Monoclonal antibody
Human IgG
Balb/c mice
ELISA

A B S T R A C T

Purpose: Monoclonal antibodies and related conjugates are key reagents used in biomedical researches as well as, in treatment, purification and diagnosis of infectious and non- infectious diseases. *Methods:* Balb/c mice were immunized with purified human IgG. Spleen cells of the most immune mouse were fused with SP2/0 in the presence of Poly Ethylene Glycol (PEG). Supernatant of hybridoma cells was screened for detection of antibody by ELISA. Then, the sample was assessed for cross-reactivity with IgM & IgA by ELISA and confirmed by immunoblotting. The subclasses of the selected mAbs were determined. The best clone was injected intraperitoneally to some pristane-injected mice. Anti-IgG mAb was purified from the animals' ascitic fluid by Ion exchange chromatography and then, mAb was conjugated with HRP. *Results:* In the present study, over than 50 clones were obtained that 1 clone had optical density over than 3. We named this clone as supermonoclone which was selected for limiting dilution. The result of the immunoblotting, showed sharp band in IgG position and did not show any band in IgM&IgA position. *Conclusion:* Based on the findings of this study, the conjugated monoclonal antibody could have application in diagnosis of infectious diseases like Toxoplasmosis, Rubella and IgG class of other infectious and non- infectious diseases.

Introduction

Monoclonal antibodies can be produced in specialized cells through a method now popularly known as hybridoma technology.[1] Hybridoma technology was first invented by two scientists, Georges Kohler and Cesar Milstein. From 1975, Köhler and Milstein successfully fused antibody- producing mouse spleen cells with mouse myeloma cells, the fusion of somatic cells has been carried out for many years with a variety of different aims and this technique quickly became one of immunology´s key technologies.[2] Using hybridoma technology, monoclonal antibodies have been prepared against a wide range of antigens including growth factors, growth factor receptors, viruses, bacterial products, hormones and differentiated antigens.[3]

In fact, monoclonal antibodies (mAbs) have been widely applied in various fields such as diagnosis applications, purification, disease monitoring, identifying prognostic markers and therapy.[4] For most research, diagnostic and therapeutic purposes, monoclonal antibodies derived from a single clone and thus specific for a single epitope, are preferable.[5]

In most diagnostic kits of the infectious diseases, for instance, Rubella, H.pylor Toxoplasmosis and etc, the conjugated monoclonal antibodies against human IgG carry out as a key role. Due to in this need, generation of mAb seems invaluable. To approach these goals, generation and characterization of a highly specific mAb against human IgG was investigated.

The prim aim of this study including: production and application of mabs against human IgG for development of diagnostic kits and large scale, semi-industrial production and standardization of this product towards self-sufficiency of the country.

Materials and Methods

Immunization Procedure and Screening of Immunized Animals

Four female Balb/c (6-8 weeks old) mice were used for purified human IgG (Affinity Purified Human IgG, Sigma) immunization. Each mouse was immunized 4 times with an interval of two-three weeks subcutaneously. The first Immunization was performed using Freund's complete adjuvant (Sigma-Aldrich Co. Louis, USA). Incomplete Freund's adjuvant (Sigma-Aldrich Co. Louis, USA) was used for the 2nd, 3rd and 4th immunization. For the first immunization, 50 µg of purified human IgG was mixed with an equal volume

*Corresponding author: Jafar Majidi, Immunology Research Center, Tabriz University of Medical Sciences, Tabriz, Iran.
Email: jmajidiz@yahoo.com

of Freund's complete adjuvant. For the subsequent immunizations 50 µg purified human IgG were injected with Freund's incomplete adjuvant. Three days before the cell fusion, 50 µg of antigen (without any adjuvant) was injected intravenously.

A week after the second injection, blood was taken from each mouse by a vertical incision of the tail vein and the antibody response was measured by ELISA. The mouse with the highest serum antibody titre was selected as the spleen donor. Sera collected from non-immunized and immunized mice served as negative and positive controls.

Cell Fusion and Hybridoma Production
Three days after final immunization, spleen of the immunized mouse was aseptically removed and fused with SP2/0 myeloma cell line at a ratio of 1:5 (1 SP2/0 and 5 spleen cells) by PEG (polyethyleneglycol, MW 1450, Sigma) as fusogen. Selective HAT medium (Gibco) was added to the fused cells and cells were seeded into five 96-well microtitre plates (Nunc) containing feeder layer. The cells were incubated at 37 °C with 5% CO2 for 2-3 days. Cell growth and colony formations were examined daily. Colonies were appeared after 5-7 days. Once the colony diameter reached to 1 mm the presence of antibody against the immunized antigen was determined by ELISA method. Then, positive hybridomas were selected for further studies.

Cloning of Hybridoma Cells by Limiting Dilution Assay
After screening, the clones with high absorbance were selected for cloning by Limiting Dilution (L.D) method. The cells were diluted so that contained only one cell in each 10 µl. Twelve days after L.D, the supernatants of monoclones were screened for production of antibody. Suitable monoclones possessing high absorbance were selected for further characterization and considered for mass production.

Assessment of Anti-IgG Cross-Reactivity with other Classes of Immunoglobulins by a Sandwich ELISA
In order to determine the cross reactivity with IgM & IgA, the micro titer plates were coated with each class of the purified immunoglobulins (5µg/ml in coating buffer, 100µl/well) and incubated for 1.5 hour at 37 °c. Plates were saturated with 2% BSA at 37 °C for 1.5 hr. Wells were then washed 3 times with PBS containing 0.05% Tween 20 (PBS-T) for 5 min. At the next step, Hybridoma culture supernatants with distinct dilution was added to the wells and incubated as described above. Then, 100 µl of 1:4000 dilution of HRP-conjugated rabbit anti-mouse IgG (Sigma-Aldrich Co. Louis, USA) was added to the wells and incubation was continued for 1.5 hrs at 37 °C. After washing, 100 µl of Tetramethylbenzidine (TMB) substrate was added to each well and the plate was incubated at room temperature in a dark place. After 15 min, the reaction

was stopped by adding 100 µl of stopping solution (0.16 M H_2SO_4) to each well. The Optical Density (OD) of the reactions was measured at 450 nm by an ELISA reader (STAT FAX 303+). In the end of the reaction and by reading their absorbance, cross reactivity of the monoclonal antibodies with IgM & IgA was determined.

Isotype Determination
The class and subclass of the mAbs were determined by an ELISA with a mouse monoclonal sub isotyping kit containing rabbit anti-mouse IgG1, IgG2a, IgG2b, IgG3, IgM and IgA, following the procedure provided by the manufacturer (Thermo, USA).

Production of Ascitic Fluids
Hybridoma cells producing IgG mAbs were grown in $RPMI_{1640}$ supplemented with 10% fetal bovine serum, harvested and washed twice in PBS (pH 7.2).Ten days after pristane injection, 6-8 weeks old Balb/c mice were injected intraperitoneally with $2-3\times10^6$ hybridoma cells suspended in 0.5 ml PBS (pH 7.2). Fluid was collected from the peritoneal cavity 8 to 10 days after the injection of the cells, by using of needle 19. Ascitic fluid was kept at 4 °C for 1 h and centrifuged at 5000 g for 15 min. Supernatant was collected and stored at -20 °C until used.

Antibody Purification
The monoclonal antibodies were purified from ascitic fluid by Ion exchange chromatography based on its isotype. Briefly, ascitic fluids were filtered through 45 µm filter and were diluted 1 to 2 with PBS and fractionated with 40% saturated ammonium sulfate. After several times of washing with 40% ammonium sulfate, the fraction was centrifuged for 15 minutes in 5000g. The precipitated fraction was dialyzed against 0.05 M phosphate buffer pH 7.4 containing 0.05 M Nacl. The final dialyze was exchanged against the column washing buffer (Tris 40 mM). Purification of ascitic fluid was done by Ion exchange chromatography (DEAE-Sepharose 6B) which is a simple and economical method. At first, the column was eluted with washing buffer (Tris 40 mM, pH 8.1) in order that the pH of the external buffer to be the same as the pH of internal buffer. Then the dialyzed sample in 60 mg/3ml concentration was run to the column with dimensions of 1.6×15cm. Distinct antibody was eluted from the column through washing buffer containing 50 mM Nacl, and the fractions were collected in 5 ml/20 ml. Finally, the purified fractions were kept for conjugation with Peroxidase.

SDS-PAGE Gel Electrophoresis
Confirmation of the mAb purity was monitored by SDS-PAGE in reduced and non-reducing condition. In addition, to check the result of cross reactivity with IgM & IgA by ELISA method this technique was used. The samples (purified mAb, purified IgG, IgM&IgA)

were mixed with sample buffer, then boiled for 2 - 5 min and cooled on ice. Electrophoresis was done in a 12.5% SDS-PAGE gel with a mini- PROTEAN electrophoresis instrument (Bio- Rad Laboratories, Hercules, CA, USA) 100 mA for 1 hr. The gel was stained with Coomassie Brilliant Blue R-250 (Sigma).

Western Blotting

Western blotting technique was used for confirming the result of ELISA and to see pattern of specificity and cross -reactivity of anti-IgG monoclonal antibody.

Briefly, the nitrocellulose membrane and several thicknesses of Whatman chromatography papers were soaked in the transfer buffer (25 mM Tris, 192 mM glycine, 20% V/V methanol, pH 8.3). The wet nitrocellulose membrane was overlaid on the wet Whatman sheets by taking precaution to avoid bubbles. Then, the gel of SDS-PAGE was placed on the wet nitrocellulose membrane and then several wet Whatman papers were placed on it. Transfer of the proteins from gel to nitrocellulose membrane was done in 100V for 3 hours. Then, non- specific sites were blocked with 2% BSA solution. After three times of washing, the membrane was cut into strips and incubated for 2 hours at 37 °C with the supernatants of suitable clones. Again, after five times of washing, the strips were incubated for 2 hours at 37 °C with Rabbit Anti- Mouse IgG conjugate (1/2000 dilution). The strips were washed and detected by ECL (Amersham Phamacia Biotech Inc, USA) hyperfilm after exposure for 5 min.

Labelling of Monoclonal Antibody with Horseradish Peroxidase Enzyme (HRP)

For conjugation, the Nakan and Periodate methods were used. Briefly, 4 mg of HRP was dissolved in 1 ml of distillated water. Then 0.2 ml freshly prepared sodium Periodate solution (0.1M) was added to the enzymatic solution and incubated on shaker for, 20 minutes at room temperature. The solution was dialyzed against acetate buffer (pH 4.4), overnight at 4 °c. 8 mg of the purified monoclonal antibody was dissolved in 1 ml sodium carbonate (10 mM, pH 9.5).The pH of the dialyzed enzyme was reached to 9 and immediately the solution containing monoclonal antibody was added to it and shaked for 2 hours at room temperature. Then 0.1 ml of the freshly prepared sodium brohydrate was added and incubated for 30 minutes at room temperature. The final solution was precipitated with ammonium sulfate and then was dialyzed against PBS buffer.

Results

Among the five immunized Balb/c mice against human IgG, the serum of the immune mouse at 1/32000 dilution, indicated the highest absorbance in reaction with human IgG using ELISA method. So the immune mouse was selected for the fusion. The final result of the successful fusion of the immune mouse spleen cells with myeloma SP2/0 cells were about 50 wells containing positive clones with high absorbance in reaction with IgG that 1 clone had optical density over than 3. We named this clone as supermonoclone (Figure 1) and was selected for cloning by limiting dilution (L.D) method. The yield of limiting dilution was many clones with absorbance over than 3 and about 2 at 0.01 dilutions which did not show any cross-reactivity with IgM and IgA by ELISA method (Table l).

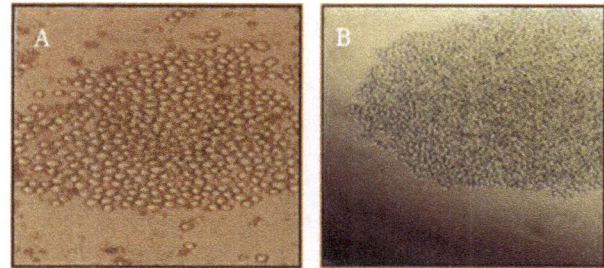

Figure 1. Proliferated suitable mono clone (supermonoclone) selected for injection into the peritoneum of mice. Supermonoclone in the growing form (Mag.10X) (A), Supermonoclone in the highly proliferated form (Mag.4X) (B).

Table 1. Comparison of the mean absorbance of supernatant of the supermonoclone at 450 nm.

	IgG	IgM	IgA
SP2/0 (N.C)	0.05	0.07	0.06
Mouse Serum (N.C)*	0.1	0.08	0.09
Immune mouse serum (P.C)**	1.1	0.2	0.2
Super monoclone	>3	0.21	0.18
Supermonoclone(1/100 dilution)	2	0.11	0.1
*negative control with 1/32000 dilution, **positive control with 1/32000 dilution			

Isotype of this mAb was identified as IgG1and k light chain (Table 2). For large scale production of monoclonal antibody, super monoclone related hybridoma cells were injected into the peritoneum of the Balb/c mice, which have previously been primed with 0.5ml pristane. After 7-10 days, approximately 5 ml ascitic fluid was harvested from the peritoneum of each mouse. Ascitic fluid purified with Ion exchange chromatography, and conjugated with HRP. There was 30 mg protein in ascitic fluid that reduced to 7.5 mg antibody after purification step. The result of purification confirmed with SDS-PAGE and PAGE. In SDS PAGE, two bands of 50 kDa and 25 kDa were appeared that demonstrator heavy and light chains. In PAGE, only one 150 kDa band was appeared that demonstrator of purified antibody (Figure 2). The specificity and cross reactivity of the anti-IgG was also confirmed by an Immunoblotting procedure (data not show). The titer of mAb in ascitic fluid was examined by ELISA method and the results showed that its

1/100,000 dilution has high absorbance with IgG (above 1) but has no absorbance with IgM & IgA (Table 3).Also, the results of conjugation indicated that

1/64000 dilution of conjugate had high absorbance with IgG (above 1) and didn't show any cross reactivity with IgM & IgA (Table 3).

Table 2. Results of subclass isotyping of mouse mAb at 450 nm.

	IgG1	IgG2a	IgG2b	IgG3	IgA	IgM	Kappa	Lambda
Mouse anti-human IgG	1.101	0.131	0.154	0.168	0.117	0.136	1.692	0.138

Figure 2. SDS- PAGE of purified monoclonal antibody. In reduced form (A), two bands were seen in 50 & 25 kDa but in non-reduced condition (B), only one band was seen in about 150 kDa.

Table 3. Comparison of the mean absorbance and cross reactivity of ascitic fluid and anti- human IgG conjugate at 450 nm.

	IgG	IgM	IgA
SP2/0 (N.C)	0.05	0.07	0.06
Mouse Serum (N.C)*	0.1	0.08	0.09
Immune mouse serum (P.C)**	1.1	0.18	0.12
Ascitic fluid (1/100000 dilution)	1.2	0.09	0.08
Mouse anti- human IgG conjugate (1/64000 dilution)	1.4	0.07	0.06
*negative control with 1/32000 dilution, **positive control with 1/32000 dilution			

Discussion

Hybridoma technology has been rapidly and successfully applied to a wide variety of biological problems of both theoretical and practical importance.[6] MAbs are therefore of enormous utility in applications such as experimental biology, medicine, biomedical research, diagnostic testing, and therapy.[7] More importantly, each antibody is highly specific for a particular antigen; this characteristic feature of antibodies has led to their routine usage in diagnostic kits.[8]

IgG antibodies are involved in predominantly the secondary immune response.[9] The presence of specific IgG, in general, corresponds to maturation of the antibody response. In addition, in chronic condition of infectious diseases; the class of the produced antibody against pathogen is IgG.[10] Therefore monoclonal anti-human IgG is very important, significant and as a key reagent for its recognition. Accordingly, production of monoclonal antibody without any cross reactivity with homologous molecules such as other classes of immunoglobulins can be used in diagnostic kits of infectious diseases.[11]

When mAbs are produced, it is important to consider antigen features, which include the quality and quantity of the antigen and the antigen preparation. The specificity of the immune response obtained depends on the purity of the antigen applied.[12] Therefore in this study, purified human IgG immunoglobulins were used to immunize Balb/c mice. Upon such procedure, we observed high immunologic response in the immunized mouse, whose serum resulted in absorbance above 1 with 1/32000 dilution and the most immune mouse was selected for the fusion.

In similar previous study, Majidi et al produced monoclonal antibody against human IgE which could be used in designing ELISA kits. Purified IgE was used for immunization, in order to produce mAb.[13]

In a study, YÜCEL et al produced hybridomas against Hepatitis B virus (HBV) by fusing spleen cells from hyper immunized mice with SP2/0 mouse myeloma cell. HBsAg proteins were used for immunization then; they concluded that these mAbs were valuable for diagnosis of hepatitis B surface antigen in human serum.[1] In all of these studies, native proteins purified from the natural source were preferred for its most likely to produce useful antibodies and high concentrations of mAbs produced.

In the present study, the best clone designated as supermonoclone, was injected intraperitoneally to pristane-injected mice. The production of monoclonal antibody in the ascitic fluid is commercially cost effective also; a rapid, reproducible method for large-scale production in comparison with expensive and time-consuming culture methods.[14] Anti-IgG mAb was purified from the animals' ascitic fluid by Ion exchange chromatography .The purity of the sample was tested by SDS-PAGE. Immunoblotting and ELISA were done and the results showed that the harvested antibody recognizes human IgG and there was no cross-reactivity with other classes of immunoglobulins. Furthermore, anti-IgG mAb was interacted with human IgG with a very high specificity and affinity. These mAbs with high affinity are useful tools for quantitation of human IgG subclass levels in various diseases. So, this mAb could be a useful tool for use in the development of diagnostic kits based on sandwich ELISA. Taking all together, the conjugated monoclonal antibody could have application in diagnosis of infectious diseases like Toxoplasmosis, Rubella, H.Pylori and IgG class of other infectious and non-infectious diseases. Importantly, production of purified monoclonal antibody and HRP conjugated IgG could be consider another step toward Iran self-sufficiency.

Acknowledgements

We would like to thank for Tabriz Pharmaceutical Technology Incubator (TPTI) and Immunology Research Center (IRC) for kind assistance, respectively. This work was supported by a grant from Tabriz Pharmaceutical Technology Incubator (TPTI).

Conflict of Interest

The authors report no conflicts of interest.

References

1. Yucel F, Manav A, Basalp A. Production and characterization of monoclonal antibodies against hepatitis B viruses and application of a quick sandwich ELISA. *Hybrid Hybridomics* 2003;22(3):173-7.
2. Modjtahedi H. Monoclonal Antibodies as Therapeutic Agents: Advances and Challenges. *Iran J Immunol* 2005;2(1):3-21.
3. Kohler G, Milstein C. Continuous cultures of fused cells secreting antibody of predefined specificity. *Nature* 1975;256(5517):495-7.
4. Guan M, Su B, Ye C, Lu Y. Production of extracellular domain of human tissue factor using maltose-binding protein fusion system. *Protein Expr Purif* 2002;26(2):229-34.
5. Daginakatte GC, Chard-Bergstrom C, Andrews GA, Kapil S. Production, characterization, and uses of monoclonal antibodies against recombinant nucleoprotein of elk coronavirus. *Clin Diagn Lab Immunol* 1999;6(3):341-4.
6. Sangdokmai A, Pimpitak U, Buakeaw A, Palaga T, Komolphis K. Production and Characterization of Monoclonal Antibodies Against Aflatoxin M1. International Conference on Environmental, Biomedical and Biotechnology; Singapoore: IACSIT Press; 2011.
7. Fraser PD, Misawa N, Sandmann G, Johnson J, Schuch W, Bramley PM. Production and characterisation of monoclonal antibodies to phytoene synthase of Lycopersicon esculentum. *Phytochemistry* 1998;49(4):971-8.
8. Lang AB, Schuerch U, Cryz SJ Jr. Optimization of growth and secretion of human monoclonal antibodies by hybridomas cultured in serum-free media. *Hybridoma* 1991;10(3):401-9.
9. Chevrier MC, Chateauneuf I, Guerin M, Lemieux R. Sensitive detection of human IgG in ELISA using a monoclonal anti-IgG-peroxidase conjugate. *Hybrid Hybridomics* 2004;23(6):362-7.
10. Hajighasemi F, Khoshnoodi J, Shokri F. Development of two murine monoclonal antibodies recognizing human nG1m(a)-like isoallotypic markers. *Hybridoma (Larchmt)* 2008;27(6):473-9.
11. Hussain A, Pankhurst T, Goodall M, Colman R, Jefferis R, Savage CO, et al. Chimeric IgG4 PR3-ANCA induces selective inflammatory responses from neutrophils through engagement of Fcgamma receptors. *Immunology* 2009;128(2):236-44.
12. Baradaran B, Hosseini AZ, Majidi J, Farajnia S, Barar J, Saraf ZH, et al. Development and characterization of monoclonal antibodies against human epidermal growth factor receptor in Balb/c mice. *Hum Antibodies* 2009;18(1-2):11-6.
13. Majidi J, Zavaran Hosseini A, Hassan ZM, Alimohamadian MH. Production of monoclonal antibody against human Immunoglobulin E. *Iran J Allergy Asthma Immunol* 2000;1(2):81-7.
14. Aghebati Maleki L, Majidi J, Baradaran B, Abdolalizadeh J, Kazemi T, Aghebati Maleki A, et al. Large Scale Generation and Characterization of Anti-Human CD34 Monoclonal Antibody in Ascetic Fluid of Balb/c Mice. *Adv Pharm Bull* 2013;3(1):211-6.

Simultaneous Determination of Loratadine, Desloratadine and Cetirizine by Capillary Zone Electrophoresis

Gabriel Hancu[1]*, **Camelia Câmpian**[1], **Aura Rusu**[1], **Eleonora Mircia**[2], **Hajnal Kelemen**[1]

[1] *Department of Pharmaceutical Chemistry, Faculty of Pharmacy, University of Medicine and Pharmacy, Târgu Mureş, Romania.*

[2] *Department of Organic Chemistry, Faculty of Pharmacy, University of Medicine and Pharmacy, Târgu Mureş, Romania.*

ARTICLE INFO

Keywords:
Antihistamines
Loratadine
Desloratadine
Cetirizine
Capillary electrophoresis
Separation

ABSTRACT

Purpose: The aim of the study was the development of a simple and rapid analytical procedure for the determination of the most frequently used antihistamine derivatives.
Methods: A capillary zone electrophoretic method was developed for the simultaneous separation of loratadine, desloratadine and cetirizine. Efforts were focused primarily on the optimisation of the experimental parameters: buffer composition and concentration, buffer pH, applied voltage, temperature, injection pressure and time.
Results: The optimised parameters for the separation were: 25 mM buffer electrolyte, buffer pH 2.5, voltage + 25 kV, temperature 25 °C, injection pressure 50 mbar, injection time 3 seconds, capillary 48 cm (effective length 40 cm) x 50 μm, detection at 240 nm. Under these conditions, the analysis time was below 5 minutes, the order of migration being: desloratadine, cetirizine and loratadine. The developed method was validated in terms of linearity, limits of detection and quantification, intra- and inter-day precision, selectivity and robustness.
Conclusion: Capillary zone electrophoresis proved to be a suitable method for the simulatneous determination of the three studied antihistamine derivatives.

Introduction

An H1 receptor antagonist is a histamine antagonist of the H1 receptor used in therapy to reduce or eliminate effects mediated by histamine, an endogenous chemical mediator released during allergic reactions.[1]

Second-generation H1 antihistamines are newer drugs that are much more selective for peripheral H1 receptors as opposed to the H1 receptors of the central nervous system (CNS) and cholinergic receptors. This selectivity significantly reduces the occurrence of adverse drug reactions, such as sedation, while still providing effective relief of allergic conditions. The reason for their peripheral selectivity is that most of these compounds are zwitterionic at physiological pH; consequently, they are polar compounds, meaning that they do not cross the blood–brain barrier and act mainly outside the CNS.[1]

Loratadine(LOR) (ethyl 4-(8-chloro-5,6-dihydro-11H-benzo[5,6]cyclohepta[1,2-b]pyridin-11-ylidene)-1-piperidinecarboxylate) is a second generation long acting H1 histamine antagonist drug, structurally related with tricyclic antidepressants. LOR undergoes extensive first pass metabolism in the liver, forming an active metabolite, **desloratadine (DSL)** (8-chloro-6,11-dihydro-11-(4-piperdinylidene)-5H-benzo[5,6]cyclohepta[1,2-b]pyridine), which retains its antihistaminic activity.[1,2]

LOR and DSL are selective peripheral H1 receptor antagonists, which produce no substantial effect on the CNS. DSL exhibits similar pharmacodynamic activity with a relative potency of two to three-fold greater than LOR probably due to a higher affinity for histamine H1 receptors.[1,3]

Cetirizine (CET) ((±)-[2-[4-[(4-chlorophenyl)phenylmethyl]-1-piperazinyl]ethoxy]acetic acid) is also a second generation long acting H1 antihistamine drug, the primary metabolite of the anxiolytic drug, hydroxizine. CET is zwitterionic and relatively polar and thus crosses only slightly the blood-brain barrier, exhibiting minimal effects on the CNS. The levorotatory enantiomer (R-enantiomer) of CET, levocetirizine is the more active form; and is marketed also as pure enantiomer.[1,3]

The chemical structures of the studied H1 antihistamines are presented in Figure 1.

In the literature several methods have been decribed for the simultaneous determination of different antihistamines from complex mixtures including thin layer chromatography,[4] high performance liquid chromatography,[5] and capillary electrophoresis.[6,7]

The simultaneous determination of LOR and DSL was also reported using liquid chromatography.[8,9] Capillary electrophoresis was used for the determination of LOR

---

*Corresponding author: Gabriel Hancu, Faculty of Pharmacy, University of Medicine and Pharmacy Târgu Mureş, GhMarinescu 38, 540000 Târgu Mureş, Romania, Email: g_hancu@yahoo.com

and its related impurities,[10] but there are no reports regarding the simultaneous electrophoretic determination of LOR and DSL.

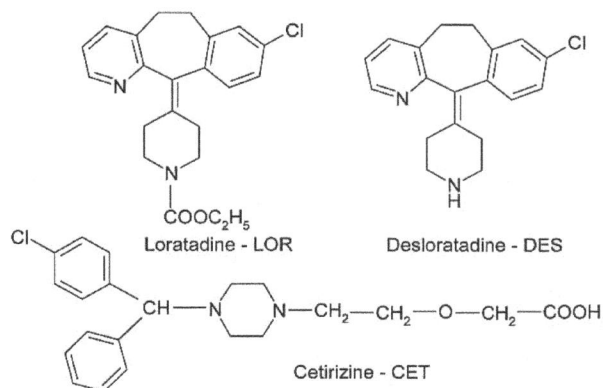

Figure 1. The chemical structures of the studied H1 antihistamines

In the last decade, capillary electrophoresis (CE) has proven to be an attractive alternative to high performance liquid chromatography because of its good selectivity and high separation efficiency in combination with short analysis times, low operational costs and fast method development.[11]

The aim of our work was the development of a simple and rapid procedure for the simultaneous separation of the three studied antihistamine derivatives and also the optimization of the analytical conditions in order to obtain a good separation resolution and a short analysis time.

Materials and Methods

The analyzed antihistamines were purchased from different distributors: loratadine (Tonira Pharma Limited, India), desloratadine (Morepen Laboratories, India) and cetirizine (RA Chem Pharma Limited, India). All substances were of pharmaceutical grade.

For the determinations from pharmaceutical products we used the following commercial preparation: Symphoral tablets (Gedeon Richter, Romania) containing 10 mg LOR, Aerius tablets (Schering Plough, USA) containing 5 mg DESL, Zyrtec tablets (UCB Pharma, Germany) containing 10 mg CET.

The following reagents of analytical grade were used: phosphoric acid 85%, sodium tetraborate, disodium hydrogenophosphate, sodium didydrogenophosphate (Merck, Germany), methanol, sodium hydroxide (Lach Ner, Czech Republic). Purified water was provided by a Milli-Q Plus water purification system (Millipore, USA). The separation was performed on an Agilent 6100 CE system (Agilent, Germany) equipped with a diode array UV detector. The separation was carried out on an uncoated fused-capillaries of 48 cm (effective length 40 cm) x 50 μm I.D. The electropherograms were recorded and processed by Chemstation 7.01 (Agilent, Germany). The pH of the buffer solutions was determined with the Terminal 740 pH–meter (Inolab, Germany).

Stock solutions containing 100 μg/ml of each compound were prepared in methanol and later were diluted conveniently for the analysis. The samples were introduced in the system at the anodic end of the capillary by hydrodynamic injection. All samples and buffers were filtered through a 0.45 μm syringe filter and degassed by ultrasound for 5 minutes before use.

To determine the studied antihistamines from tablets, twenty tablets from the same batch product were weight and pulverized in a mortar, and an amount of powder equivalent to the average weight of a tablet was accurately weighed and used. The powder was dissolved in methanol, and then the solution was diluted to the appropriate concentration sonicated for 10 minutes and filtered through 0.45 μm syringe filter. The samples was centrifuged at 3500 rpm for 10 minutes, the supernatant was diluted; further the same procedures were followed as for the preparation of standard solutions for the CE separation.

The capillaries were conditioned before use with 0.1 M sodium hydroxide for 30 minutes and with the background electrolyte used in the analysis for 30 minutes. The capillary was rinsed for 1 minute with 0.1M sodium hydroxide and buffer solutions before each electrophoretic separation.

Results and Discussion
Preliminary analysis

Electrophoretic mobilities and ionization behavior of analytes are the key factors driving separations in capillary zone electrophoresis (CZE). In CZE, the selectivity of the method is fundamentally based on charge-to-volume ratios, as separation occurs due to the differences between the own electrophoretic mobilities of the analytes. Knowledge of these basic physicochemical properties of analytes gives valuable information about their nature and makes it easier to choose appropriate experimental conditions for their separation.

In order to find the suitable conditions for the separation a series of preliminary experiments were conducted at different pH and buffer compositions. In the preliminary analysis we used 25 mM phosphoric acid (pH –2.1), 25 mM disodium hydrogenophosphate – 25 mM sodium didydrogenophosphate (pH – 7) and 25 mM sodium tetraborate (pH – 9.3) background electrolytes (BGEs) respectively and we adjusted the pH of the buffer by adding a 0.1M sodium hydroxide solution.

We applied some "standard" electrophoretic conditions for a CZE analysis: temperature 20 °C, applied voltage + 20 kV, injection pressure/time 50 mbar/3 sec, sample concetration 10 μg/ml. We recorded previously the UV spectra of three antihistamines in methanol and found absorption maximum at 232 nm for LOR, at 244 nm for DSL and 250 nm for CET; consequently an intermediate value of 240 nm was elected as detection wavelength in the CE separations.

The pKa value of LOR is 5 while the pKa values for DSL are 4.2 corresponding to the pyridine functional group and 9.7 corresponding to the piperidine functional group.[12] CET has three ionizable moieties resulting in pKa values of 2.2, 2.9 and 8.0, and depending on the pH it predominantly exists as a zwitterion. CET will be negatively or positively charged depending on the pH of the environment, as it posses two basic and one acidic functions, offering the possibility of using either an acidic or an alkaline running buffer for its determination.[13] This was one of the main reasons why CET was elected in this separation, as a substance whose electrophoretic behavior is in contrast with the ones of LOR and DSL.

Optimization of the electrophoretic separation
Selectivity in CZE can be controlled by background electrolyte (BGE) concentration, pH, organic modifiers, applied voltage, temperature, injection parameters and capillary length. All these parameters were varied and results are summarized below.

The first optimization step involved selecting the optimal buffer solution and buffer pH for the separation. Using the previously selected BGEs we conducted a systematic study over a pH range between 2-11, in which the charge of the analytes changes, as indicated by the pKa values presented above, and the electroosmotic flow (EOF), thus influencing the ionic mobilities of the analytes. Figure 2 shows the migration times of the studied antihistamines over the studied pH range. We may observe that LOR can be determined over a pH range 2-5, while DSL and CET can be detected on the whole studied pH range. Over the pH range 7-9 CET migrates very close or even with the EOF. The migration times of the analyzed substances increased over the pH range 2-5, were almost similar over the pH range 5-9, and decreased over the pH range 9-11. Buffer concentration ranging from 25 mM to 100 mM were tested, higher buffer concentrations increased migration times of the analytes, without significant influence on the separation. A buffer containing 25 mM phosphoric acid at a pH of 2.5 was elected as optimum for the separation.

At such a low pH, the ionisation of the acidic silanol groups on the capillary surface is slight and, therefore, the EOF flow rate and its influence on the separation is not significant. Consequently the separation is based only on the differences between the own electrophoretic mobilities of the analytes.

We used methanol and acetonitrile as organic modifiers but the results indicated that the addition of these modifiers had a detrimental effect on the separation.

Migration times and the resolution of the separation are influenced by the applied voltage and the system temperature. A higher voltage leads to more efficient separation and a shorter analysis time, but high currents can be a limiting factor for the separation, the limit depending on the system's ability to dissipate heat generated during electrophoresis. An increase in temperature causes a slight decrease in migration times because of the decrease in the viscosity of the buffer. Basically it is essential to establish a balance between the applied voltage and the temperature of the system. The optimum voltage was set at + 25 kV while the optimum temperature was set at 20 °C, in order to obtain a good resolution and a short analysis time.

A high injection pressure and a fast injection time may improve selectivity of the separation and also the shape and amplitude of the peaks. The optimum injection parameteres were set at a 50 mbar injection pressure and a 2 seconds injection time.

Using buffer solution containing 25 mM phosphoric acid, at a pH of 2.5, applying a voltage of + 25 kV at a temperature of 20 °C, we achieved the simultaneous separation of the studied antihistamines in approximately 5 minutes, the order of separation being: DES, CET, LOR (Figure 3).

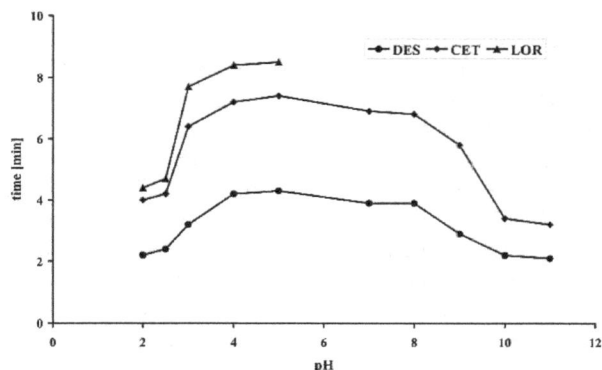

Figure 3. Electropherogram of the separation of the studied antihistamines using the optimized analytical conditions

Analytical performance
The optimized separation method was evaluated on the basis of precision (migration times and peak areas), linearity, robustness, limit of detection (LOD) and limit of quantification (LOQ).

Very similar migration times and peak areas and heights were obtained for six repeated measurements of the three analytes, the RSD values being smaller than 1% (Table 1).

The individual linear regression equations for each antihistamine was calculated according to six concentrations in a specific range (2.5 - 50 µg/mL) and

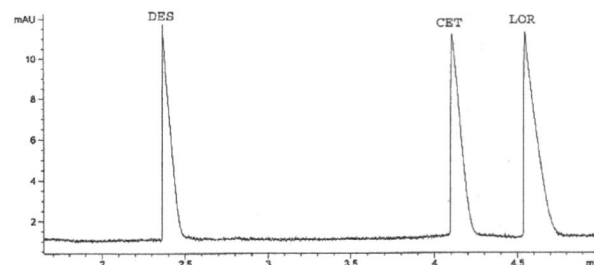

Figure 2. Effect of buffer pH on the separation of the studied antihistamines

three replicates per concentration (Table 2). The linear regression coefficients were always above 0.99.

LOD and LOQ were estimated as: standard deviation of regression equation/slope of the regression equation multiplied by 3.3 and 10, respectively (Table 2).

Table 1. Analytical parameters of the studied antihistamines separation (n = 6, sample concentration = 10 µg/mL)

Substance	Migration time (min)	RSD (%)		
		RSD (%) migration time	RSD (%) peak area	DSR (%) peak height
DES	2.275	0.027	0.804	0.675
CET	3.925	0.061	0.906	0.659
LOR	4.308	0.058	0.874	0.798

Table 2. Linearity regression data for the separation of the studied antihistamines (n=3, concentration range=2.5-50 µg/mL)

Substance	Regression equation	Correlation coefficient	LOD (µg/ml)	LOQ (µg/ml)
DES	y = 1.9195x + 2.622	0.993	1.25	3.50
CET	y = 1.8798 + 1.9175	0.998	1.35	3.90
LOR	y = 2.3931x + 4.3726	0.993	1.30	3.70

The intra-day (average of 6 measurements taken on the same day) and inter-day precision (average of 6 measurements taken over 5 days) at three different concentrations (2.5, 5, 10 µg/mL) was also determined. Precision, expressed as relative standard deviations (RSD%) and accuracy expressed a relative error, were lower than 2.5% for all analytes (Table 3). This indicates the ability of the developed method to be used for the analysis of the studied substances in pharmaceutical preparations.

Table 3. Intra and inter-day precision of the studied antihistamines separation

Substance	precision		
	Day 1 (n=6)	Day 3 (n=6) RSD (%)	Day 5 (n=6)
DES	0.25	1.14	1.66
CET	0.60	1.57	2.05
LOR	0.55	1.44	2.12

The robustness of the method was examined by analyzing a mixture of the analytes (n = 3) by making slight changes to the following parameters: buffer pH (2.5-3.0), buffer concentration (25-30 mM), applied voltage (22-25 kV) and injection pressure (40-50 mbar), taking in consideration the variation of migration times. The slight variation of these parameter does not significantly modify the migration times (RSD<2.5%).

The optimized procedure was applied to the analysis of the studied individual antihistamines found in pharmaceutical preparations. Ten samples of each pharmaceutical formulation were analysed, and three injections were done to obtain the average values of the drug concentration. All the label claims were in the range of 95.5–101.5%, and the results were in agreement with the contents declared by the manufactures. The peaks obtained from the samples

prepared from tablets were very similar with those obtained from standard and there were no noticeable interference from the matrix. It is important that tablets excipients do not interfere in the determination of the studied antihistamines, since they allow direct injections, thus involving minimum handling.

Conclusion

A CZE procedure with UV detection has been developed for the determination of the three most frequently used H1 antihistamine derivatives (DES, LOR, CET). Discussions have been focused on the optimization of the separation conditions by considering the following experimental parameters: buffer composition, buffer pH, voltage, temperature, pressure injection and time; under the criteria of maximum resolution and minimum analysis time. The proposed method was validated according to ICH guidelines. All the values were good enough for the method to be used in routine analysis.

The method proved to be robust, precise, simple and specific and is suitable for the practical determination of the studied antihistamines from pharmaceuticals and maybe also from biological samples.

Conflict of Interest

The authors declare that they have no conflict of interest.

References

1. Sweetman SC. Martindale: The Complete Drug Reference. 37th ed. London: Pharmaceutical Press; 2011.
2. European Pharmacopoeia. 7th ed. Strasbourg: Council of Europe; 2010.
3. Block JH, Beale JM. Wilson and Gisvold's textbook of Organic Medicinal and Pharmaceutical Chemistry. 11th ed. Philadelphia: Lippincott Williams and Wilkins; 2004.

4. Czerwinska K, Wyszomirska E, Mazurek AP. Identification and determination of selected histamine antagonists by densitometric method. *Acta Pol Pharm* 2013;70(1):19-26.

5. Kountourellis JE, Markopoulo C, Georgakopoulos P. An HPLC method for the separation and simultaneous determination of antihistamines, sympathomimetic amines and dextromethorphan in bulk drug material and dosage forms. *Anal Lett* 1990;23(5):883-91.

6. Capella-Peiro ME, Bossi A, Esteve-Romero J. Optimization by factorial design of a capillary zone electrophoresis method for the simultaneous separation of antihistamines. *Anal Biochem* 2006;352(1):41-9.

7. Rambla-Alegre M, Peris-Vicente J, Esteve-Romero J, Capella-Peiro ME, Bose D. Capillary electrophoresis determination of antihistamines in serum and pharmaceuticals. *Anal Chim Acta* 2010;666(1-2):102-9.

8. El-Sherbiny DT, El-Enany N, Belal FF, Hansen SH. Simultaneous determination of loratadine and desloratadine in pharmaceutical preparations using liquid chromatography with a microemulsion as eluent. *J Pharm Biomed Anal* 2007;43(4):1236-42.

9. Vlase L, Imre S, Muntean D, Leucuta SE. Determination of loratadine and its active metabolite in human plasma by high-performance liquid chromatography with mass spectrometry detection. *J Pharm Biomed Anal* 2007;44(3):652-7.

10. Fernandez H, Ruperez FJ, Barbas C. Capillary electrophoresis determination of loratadine and related impurities. *J Pharm Biomed Anal* 2003;31(3):499-506.

11. Singh Sekhon B. An overview of capillary electrophoresis: pharmaceutical, biopharmaceutical and biotechnology applications. *J Pharm Educ Res* 2011;2(2):2-36.

12. Popovic G, Cakar M, Agbaba D. Acid-base equilibria and solubility of loratadine and desloratadine in water and micellar media. *J Pharm Biomed Anal* 2009;49(1):42-7.

13. Geiser L, Henchoz Y, Galland A, Carrupt PA, Veuthey JL. Determination of pKa values by capillary zone electrophoresis with a dynamic coating procedure. *J Sep Sci* 2005;28(17):2374-80.

Thermal Analysis of Some Antidiabetic Pharmaceutical Compounds

Ali Kamal Attia*, Magda Mohamed Ibrahim, Mohamed Abdel Nabi El-Ries

National Organization for Drug Control and Research, P.O. Box 29, Cairo, Egypt.

ARTICLEINFO

Keywords:
Antidiabetics
Thermal analysis
Decomposition
Activation energy

ABSTRACT

Purpose: Thermal behavior of some antidiabetic drugs such as pioglitazone hydrochloride (PTZ), rosiglitazone maleate (RGZ), glibenclamide (GBD) and glimepiride (GMP) has been studied. *Methods:* Thermogravimetric analysis (TGA), derivative thermogravimetry (DTG) and differential thermal analysis (DTA) techniques were used to study the thermal behavior of the drugs under investigation. *Results:* Thermal analysis technique was used to obtain quality control parameters such as melting point 193.13 °C, 122.42 °C, 173.75 °C and 208 °C for PTZ, RGZ, GBD and GMP, respectively. The values of melting point of gave satisfactory results in comparison to that obtained by using the official method. Non-isothermal methods were employed to determine the activation energy values of the first stage of thermal decomposition. Comparison of the activation energy values suggests the following sequence of thermal stability: GMP > GBD > RGZ > PTZ. *Conclusion:* The results obtained are useful for the identification of these compounds and permitted interpretations concerning their thermal decomposition. Thermal stability of pharmaceutical compounds can be studied and compared by using thermal analysis techniques.

Introduction

Thermal analysis is a technique in which a physical property of a substance and/or its reaction products is measured as a function of temperature. Thermal analysis can measure weight loss on heating, melting points, heat and energy transitions and change in the substance form. Thermal analysis techniques are widely used in the pharmaceutical sciences for the characterization and quality control of drugs, stability, drug-excipient interactions and purity studies of raw materials and pharmaceutical products.[1-5]
Several methods have been reported for the determination of the studied drugs including chromatographic,[6-9] electrochemical,[10] and titrimetric methods.[11,12] The use of thermal analysis for antidiabetic drugs has been very limited; compatibilities of some commonly used pharmaceutical excipients with glimepiride and glibenclamide have been described.[13,14] Therefore, the main objective of this study is to investigate and compare the thermal behavior of some antidiabetic drugs such as PTZ, RGZ, GBD and GMP using the TGA, DTG and DTA techniques.
PTZ is an oral antidiabetic agent used in the treatment of type 2 diabetes. After administration, PTZ decreases insulin resistance in the periphery and liver resulting in increased insulin dependent glucose disposal and decreased hepatic glucose output.[15,16] RGZ is a thiazolidinedione antihyperglycemic agent that works by increasing insulin sensitivity in target tissues, as well as decreasing hepatic gluconeogenesis.[17] Oliveira et al studied isothermal thermogravimetric studies and compatibility between GBD and some pharmaceutical excipients using thermoanalytical techniques (TGA/DSC).[13] Cides et al studied the thermal behavior, compatibility study and decomposition kinetics of glimepiride by using isothermal and non-isothermal methods. The activation energy values are 123 and 150 KJ.mol[-1] using isothermal method and Onawa method, respectively.[14]
GBD and GMP are the potent second generation oral sulfonylurea antihyperglycemic agents that widely used for the treatment of type 2 diabetes mellitus.[18,19]

Materials and methods

Pioglitazone hydrochloride and rosiglitazone maleate were obtained from Unipharma and Apex Pharmaceutical Company, Egypt, respectively; glibenclamide and glimepiride were supplied from Aventis Pharmaceutical Company, Egypt. All the used drugs have high purity (more than 99%).

Methods

Thermogravimetric analysis, derivative thermogravimetry and differential thermal analysis measurements were made by using simultaneous DTA-TGA thermal analyzer apparatus (Shimadzu DTG-

*Corresponding author: Ali Kamal Attia, National Organization for Drug Control and Research, P.O. Box 29, Cairo.
Email: alikamal1978@hotmail.com

60H). The weight of samples is ranging from 4 to about 7 mg, using a platinum pan. Measurements were carried out from ambient to 900 °C in dynamic nitrogen atmosphere with the flow rate of 30 ml min^{-1} and heating rate of 10 °C min^{-1}.

The activation energies of the used drugs for the first stage of decomposition were obtained from TGA curves by using Coats-Redren method,[20] and Horowitz-Metzger method.[21]

Coats-Redfern method
The Coats-Redfern method equation can be represented as follows:

$$\log\left(\frac{\log\left[\frac{W_f}{W_f - W}\right]}{T^2}\right) = \log\left[\frac{AR}{\phi E^*}\left(1 - \frac{2RT}{E^*}\right)\right] - \frac{E^*}{2.303\,RT}$$

Where ϕ was the heating rate. Since $1 - 2RT/E^* \cong 1$, the plot of the left-hand side of equation against $1/T$ would give a straight line. E^* was then calculated from the slope and the Arrhenius constant (A) was obtained from the intercept.

Horowitz and Metzger method
The Horowitz-Metzger equation can be represented as follows:

$$\log.[\log\frac{W_f}{W_f - W}] = \frac{\theta.E^*}{2.303\,RT_s^2} - \log 2.303$$

Where W_f was the mass loss at the completion of the decomposition reaction, W was the mass loss up to temperature T, R was the gas constant, T_s was the DTG peak temperature and $\theta = T - T_s$. A plot of log [log W_f / (W_f - W)] against θ would give a straight line and E^* could be calculated from the slope.

Results and Discussion
Thermal analysis behavior of PTZ
The TGA, DTG and DTA curves of PTZ are shown in Figure 1. The DTG curve shows four stages of decomposition: At the first stage (145-225.9 °C); PTZ exhibits a weight loss of 9.53% due to the loss of HCl molecule. A weight loss of 57.09% observed between 225.9 °C and 327.73 °C which may be attributed to the loss of $C_{10}H_8NO_3S$. Beyond 389.34 °C, the drug decomposed in two stages due to the loss of C_4H_9 at 389.34-468 °C (weight loss of 14.71%) and the loss of C_5H_3N at 468-551.55 °C (weight loss of 19.47%).

The DTA curve (Figure 1) shows a small endothermic peak at 193.13 °C due to the melting of PTZ which is acceptable to the values of the reported melting temperature,[22] and the melting temperature that determined by melting point apparatus (Table 1). An exothermic peak is observed at 270.75 °C corresponding to the second decomposition stage. Another abroad endothermic peak appears between

327.73 °C and 389.34 °C. Two sharp exothermic peaks are observed at 444.47 °C and 498.20 °C corresponding to the third and fourth decomposition stages in the DTG curve, respectively. The results obtained from TGA, DTG and DTA indicate that PTZ melts with decomposition. Thermal degradation pattern of PTZ was shown in Figure 2.

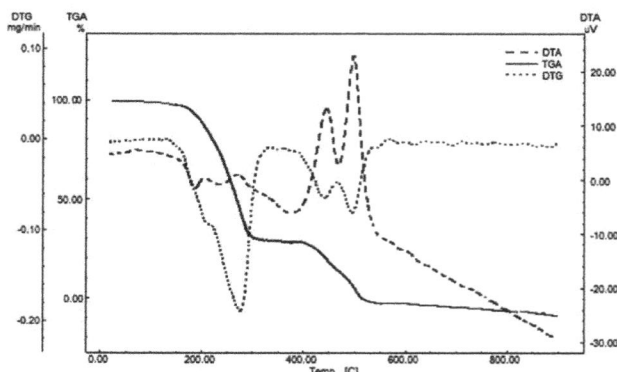

Figure 1. Thermal analysis curves (TGA, DTG and DTA) of PTZ.

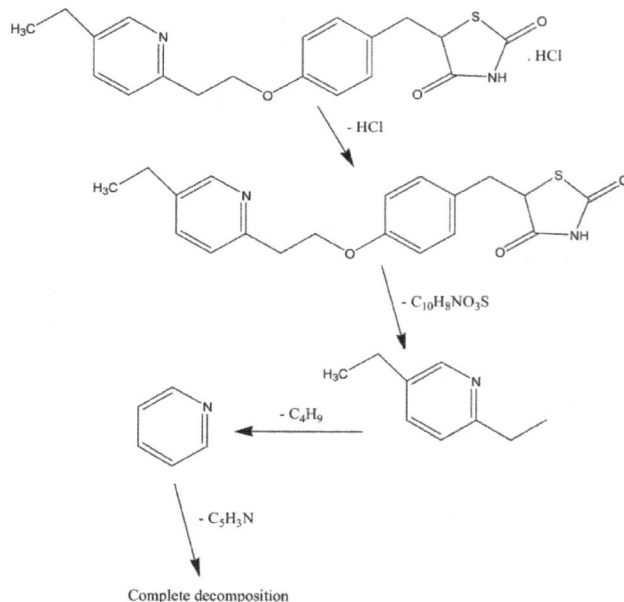

Figure 2. Thermal degradation pattern of PTZ.

Thermal analysis behavior of RGZ
Figure 3 represents TGA, DTG and DTA curves of RGZ. The TGA curve shows four stages of decomposition. The DTG curve represents the stages of decomposition: the first one begins at 150.61 °C and ends at 231.43 °C with a mass loss of 24.50% due to the loss of $C_4H_4O_4$ molecule, the second stage between 231.43 °C and 317 °C shows weight loss of 24.50% due to the loss of $C_3H_2NO_2S$. RGZ continues to decompose in a third stage (317-481°C) showing a mass loss of 22.39% due to the loss of C_7H_6O and fourth and last stage (481-644.58 °C) with a mass loss of 28.51% which may be ascribed to the loss of $C_8H_{11}N_2$.

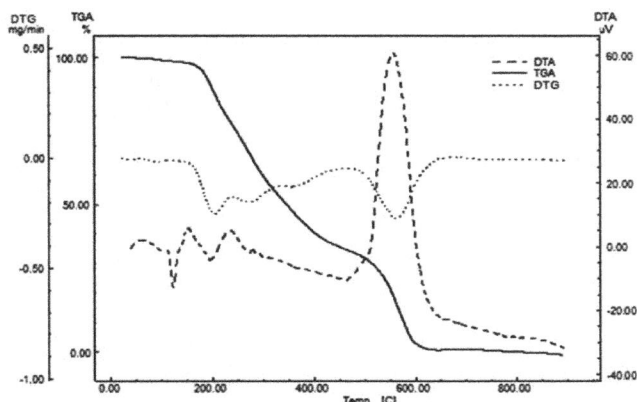

Figure 3. Thermal analysis curves (TGA, DTG and DTA) of RGZ.

The DTA curve in Figure 3 shows an endothermic peak at 122.42 °C attributed to the melting of the compound which agrees to the reported melting temperature,[22] and the melting temperature that determined by melting point apparatus. The results were shown in Table 1. One endothermic peak is found at 192.75 °C corresponding to the first decomposition stage. Broad endothermic peak presented from 231.43 °C to 481 °C which corresponds to the second and third stages of decomposition. A very strong and sharp exothermic peak is showed at 556.49 °C which may be attributed to the last decomposition stage. Thermal degradation pattern of RGZ was shown in Figure 4.

Table 1. The melting points values and the activation energies for the first stage of decomposition of PTZ, RGZ, GBD and GMP.

Drug	Melting point (°C)			Activation energy E^* (KJ.mol^{-1})	
	DTA Method	Apparatus	Literature[22]	Coats-Redfern method	Horowitz-Metzger method
PTZ	193.13	194.00	193.00-194.00	77.44	88.19
RGZ	122.42	123.00	122.00-123.0	102.29	111.72
GBD	173.75	174.00	172.00-174.00	114.23	126.73
GMP	208.00	206.00	207.00	125.79	142.62

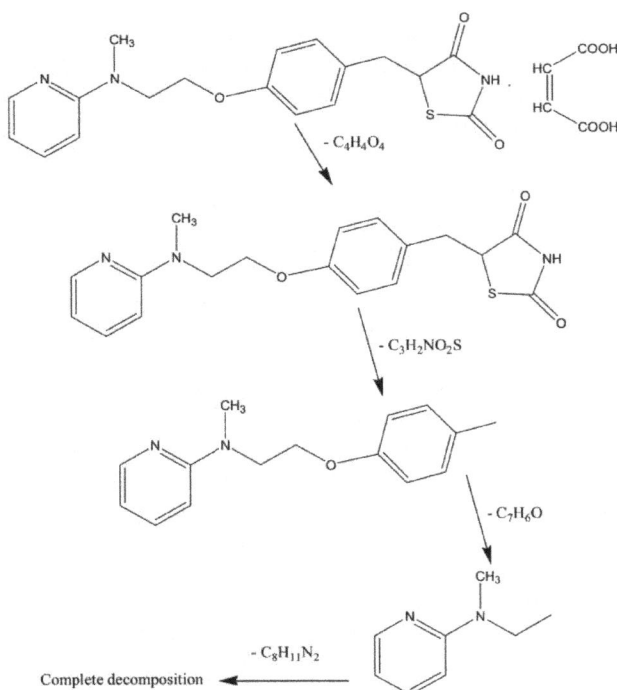

Figure 4. Thermal degradation pattern of RGZ.

mass of 43.13% which corresponds to the loss of $C_{10}H_{11}NClO_2$ and the third and final stage (392.36-677.53 °C) involves a mass loss of 28.34% which corresponds to the loss of $C_6H_4SO_2$.

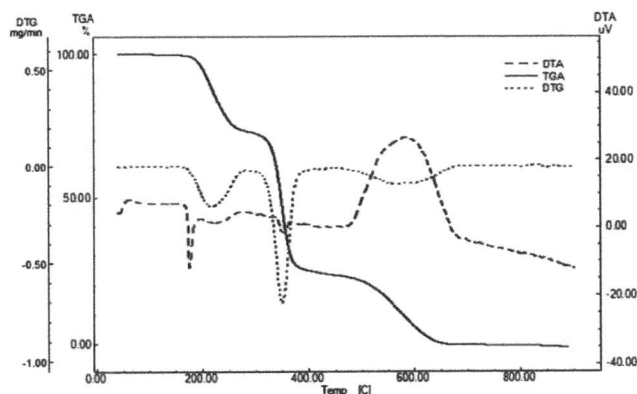

Figure 5. Thermal analysis curves (TGA, DTG and DTA) of GBD.

The DTA curve shows a sharp endothermic peak at 173.75 °C due to the melting of the GBD which is in agreement with the values obtained from literature,[22] and by using melting apparatus (Table 1); this peak is followed by a small and flattened endothermic peak from 196 °C to 286.60 °C which corresponds to the first decomposition stage. At 350.81 °C the DTA curve shows a small endothermic peak which corresponds to the second decomposition stage and a strong and broad exothermic peak at 580 °C which is due to the last decomposition stage of the drug. Thermal degradation pattern of GBD was shown in Figure 6.

Thermal analysis behavior of GBD

The TGA, DTG and DTA curves in Figure 5 show that GBD is thermally stable up to 185 °C. The TGA and DTG curves indicate mass losses in three well defined stages between 185 °C and 677.53 °C. The mass loss 28.54% for the first stage (185-286.60 °C) suggests the elimination of $C_7H_{13}N_2O$. The second stage of decomposition (286.60-392.36 °C) involves a loss in

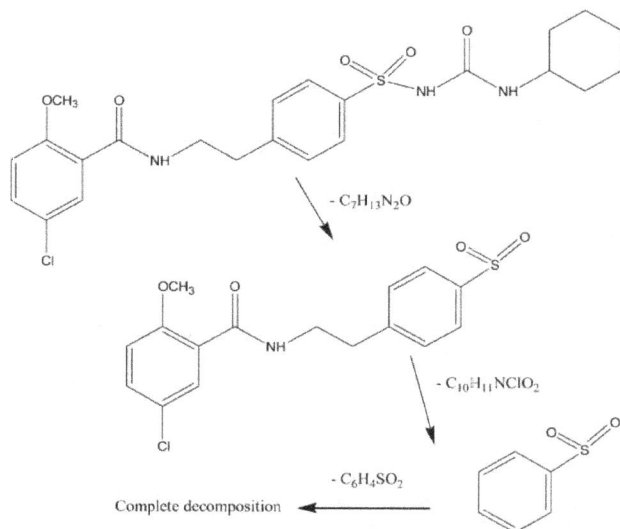

Figure 6. Thermal degradation pattern of GBD.

Thermal analysis behavior of GMP

The TGA and DTG curves in Figure 7 show that GMP is thermally stable up to about 198 °C and then decomposes in the first stage up to 269.31 °C with a mass loss of 31.75% which suggests the loss of $C_8H_{15}N_2O$. GMP continues to decompose from 269.31 °C to 369 °C in the second stage of decomposition showing a mass loss of 39.66% due to the loss of $C_{10}H_{15}N_2O_2$ and the third and last stage in the temperature range of 369-690 °C (28.54%) is ascribed to the loss of $C_6H_4SO_2$.

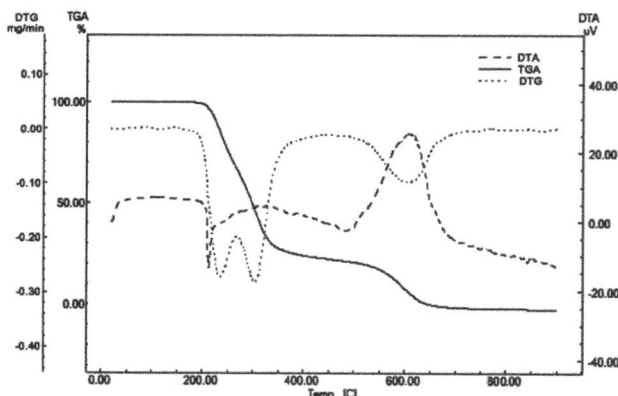

Figure 7. Thermal analysis curves (TGA, DTG and DTA) of GMP.

The DTA curve of GMP (Figure 7) shows a sharp endothermic peak at 208 °C that corresponds to melting followed by a broad flat exothermic peak between 220 °C and 480 °C which is corresponding to the first and second stages of decomposition of GMP followed by a strong and broad exothermic peak at 607 °C corresponding to the third decomposition stage of GMP. Thermal degradation pattern of GMP was shown in Figure 8.

The previous results show that PTZ, RGZ, GBD and GMP start to decompose at 145 °C, 150.61 °C, 185 °C

and 198 °C, respectively. These results suggest increasing thermal stability in the same order. Kinetic studies were conducted to investigate these results through calculation and comparison of the activation energies obtained from the first stage of decomposition of these drugs.

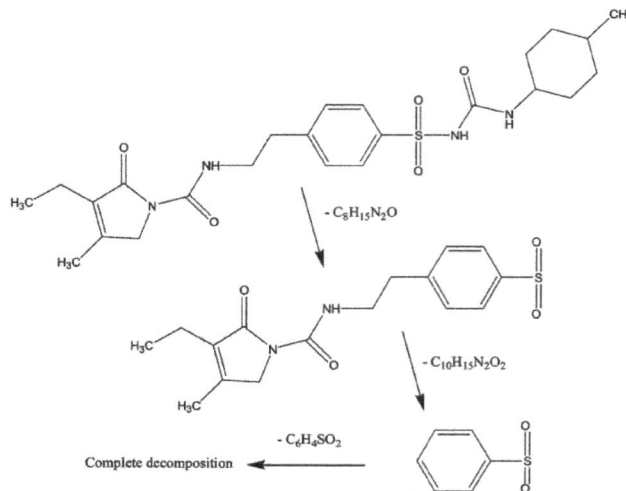

Figure 8. Thermal degradation pattern of GMP.

Determination of activation energies

For the first order kinetic process, the activation energy (E^*) values for the first stages of decomposition of PTZ, RGZ, GBD and GMP were determined by using Coats-Redfern and Horowitz-Metzger methods. The results are shown in Figure 9 and Figure 10. The activation energy values of GMP are 123 and 150 KJ.mol^{-1} using isothermal method and Ozawa's method, respectively.[14] These results are in agreement with the values obtained from Coats-Redfern and Horowitz-Metzger methods, and this is an important experimental finding. The results were listed in Table 1. It is clear that the obtained values of activation energies of the used drugs are in reasonably good agreement. The activation energies obtained for the first stage of decomposition of these drugs show different values, suggesting the following sequence of thermal stability: GMP > GBD > RGZ > PTZ.

Conclusion

Thermal analysis methods are widely used in the fields of pharmaceutical sciences. The TGA, DTG and DTA curves permitted interpretations of some antidiabetic agents such as PTZ, RGZ, GBD and GMP concerning their thermal decomposition. Thermal stability of pharmaceutical compounds can be studied and compared by using thermal analysis techniques. The results justify the use of DTA as a routine technique for the identification of these drugs through the melting point. Kinetic results demonstrated differences in thermal stability between the four drugs and suggested the following sequence of stability: GMP > GBD > RGZ > PTZ.

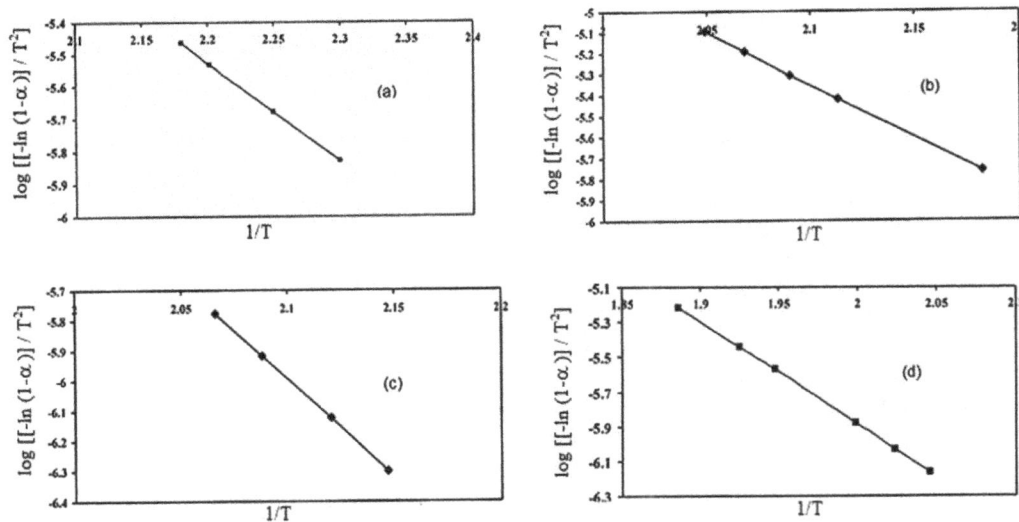

Figure 9. Coats-Redfern plots of PTZ (a), RGZ (b), GBD (c) and GMP (d), α = W / W$_f$.

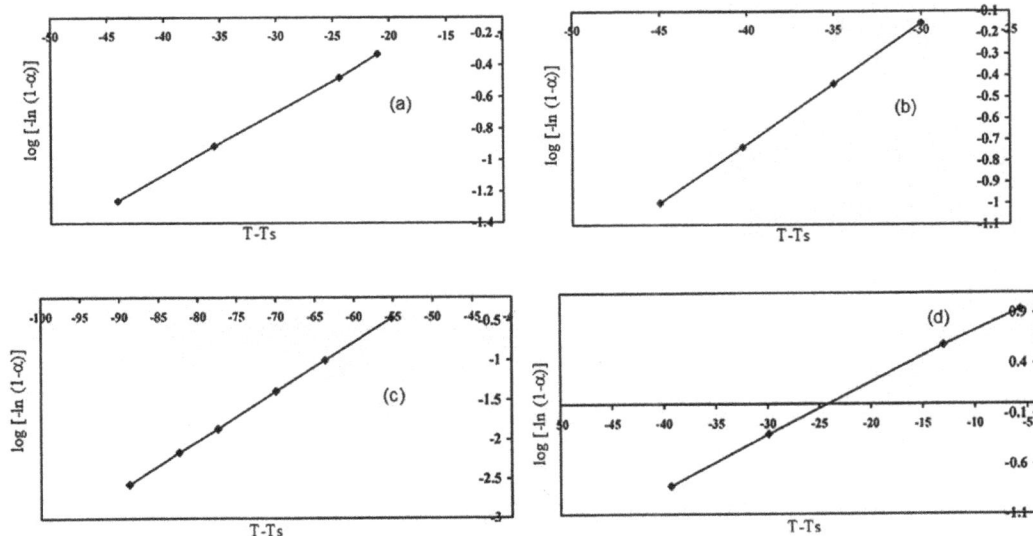

Figure 10. Horowitz-Metzger plots of PTZ (a), RGZ (b), GBD (c) and GMP (d), α = W / W$_f$.

Conflict of Interest
The authors report no conflicts of interest.

References
1. Al-Nahary TT, El-Ries MA, Sultan M, Mabkhot YN, Al-Hussam AM. Thermal stability of anti-rheumatic pharmaceutical drugs parecoxib sodium and valdecoxib. *J Saudi Chem Soc* 2012;16(2):177-82.
2. Kenawi IM, Barsoum BN, Youssef MA. Drug-drug interaction between diclofenac, cetirizine and ranitidine. *J Pharm Biomed Anal* 2005;37(4):655-61.
3. Radha S, Gutch PK, Ganesan K, Vijayaraghavan R, Suman J, Subodh D. Thermal analysis of interactions between an oxime and excipients in some binary mixtures by differential scanning calorimetry and thermagravimetric analysis. *J Pharm Res* 2010;3(3):590-5.
4. Abou-Sekkina M, El-Ries MA, Molokhia A, Rabie N, Wassel A. γ-Induced thermal stability and thermal studies on timolol β-Blocker. *J Therm Anal Calorim* 2002;68(3):1017-23.
5. Haung Y, Cheng Y, Alexander K, Dalimore D. The thermal analysis study of the drug captopril. *Thermochim Acta* 2001;367-8:43-58.
6. Lakshmi KS, Rajeh T, Shrinivas S. Simultaneous determination of metformin and pioglitazone by reversed phase HPLC in pharmaceutical dosage forms. *Int J Pharm Pharm Sci* 2009;1(2):162-6.
7. Rathinavel G, Uma NU, Valarmathy J, Samueljoshua L, Selvin TC, Ganesh M, et al. RP-

HPLC method for the simultaneous estimation of rosiglitazone and gliclazide in tablets. *E-J Chem* 2009;6(4):1188-92.

8. Reddy BP, Boopathy D, Bibin M, Prakash M, Perumal P. Method development and validation of simultaneous determination of pioglitazone and glimepiride in pharmaceutical dosage form by RP-HPLC. *Int J Chem Tech Res* 2010;2(1):50-3.

9. Rudy B, Araujo MBD, Salgado HRN. Development and validation of an UV-derivative spectrophotometric method for determination of glimepiride in tablets. *J Braz Chem Soc* 2011;22(2):292-9.

10. Badawy WA, El-Ries MA, Mahdi IM. Electrochemical determination of some antidiabetic drugs for type 2 diabetic patients. *Talanta* 2010;82(1):106-12.

11. British pharmacopoeia. London: Her Majesty's stationary office; 2009.

12. United States Pharmacopeia 33/National Formulary 28. Rockville, MD, USA: United States Pharmacopeial Convention; 2010.

13. Oliveira GGG, Ferraz HG, Matos JSR. Thermoanalytical study of glibenclamide and excipients. *J Therm Anal Calorim* 2005;79(2):267-70.

14. Cides LCS, Araujo AAS, Filho MS, Matos JR. Thermal behaviour, compatibility study and decomposition kinetics of glimepiride under isothermal and non-isothermal conditions. *J Therm Anal Calorim* 2006;84(2):441-5.

15. Hofmann CA, Edwards CW, 3rd, Hillman RM, Colca JR. Treatment of insulin-resistant mice with the oral antidiabetic agent pioglitazone: evaluation of liver GLUT2 and phosphoenolpyruvate carboxykinase expression. *Endocrinology* 1992;130(2):735-40.

16. Kletzien RF, Foellmi LA, Harris PK, Wyse BM, Clarke SD. Adipocyte fatty acid-binding protein: regulation of gene expression in vivo and in vitro by an insulin-sensitizing agent. *Mol Pharmacol* 1992;42(4):558-62.

17. Sweetman SC. Martindale, The complete drug reference. 36th ed. London: Pharmaceutical Press; 2009.

18. Turner RC, Cull CA, Frighi V, Holman RR. Glycemic control with diet, sulfonylurea, metformin, or insulin in patients with type 2 diabetes mellitus: progressive requirement for multiple therapies (UKPDS 49). UK Prospective Diabetes Study (UKPDS) Group. *JAMA* 1999;281(21):2005-12.

19. Graham SDG, Aronson JK. Oxford textbook of clinical pharmacology and drug therapy. 3rd ed. New York: Oxford University Press; 2002.

20. Coats AW, Redfern JP. Kinetic parameters from thermogravimetric data. *Nature* 1964;201(4914):68-9.

21. Horowitz HH, Metzger G. A new analysis of thermogravimetric traces. *Anal Chem* 1963;35(10):1464-8.

22. Neil MJO. The Merck index, an encyclopedia of chemicals, drugs and biological. 14th ed. New Jersey: Merck research laboratories, Whitehouse station; 2006.

Impact of Caffeine on Weight Changes Due to Ketotifen Administration

Bohlool Habibi Asl[1], Haleh Vaez[1,2]*, Turan Imankhah[3], Samin Hamidi[2,3]

[1] *Department of Pharmacology, Faculty of Pharmacy, Tabriz University of Medical Sciences, Tabriz, Iran.*

[2] *Student Research Committee, Faculty of Pharmacy, Tabriz University of Medical Sciences, Tabriz, Iran.*

[3] *Faculty of Pharmacy, Tabriz University of Medical Sciences, Tabriz, Iran.*

ARTICLE INFO

Keywords:
Ketotifen
Caffeine
Appetite
Weight changes
Mice

ABSTRACT

Purpose: Prescription of ketotifen as an effective antihistamine in asthma and allergic conditions is associated with side effect of weight gain. Caffeine is an agent which increases thermogenesis and improves energy expenditure and also effective in asthma. The aim of current study was to evaluate caffeine impact in reducing weight gain side effect of ketotifen.

Methods: Male mice at the weight limit of 20-30 gr in 8 groups were randomly chosen and injected following drug dosages for 45 days intraperitoneally: control group (normal saline 10 ml/kg), three groups of ketotifen (4, 8, 16 mg/kg), three groups of caffeine (4, 8, 16 mg/kg) and one group of ketotifen (4 mg/kg) in combination with caffeine (4 mg/kg). Weight changes have been recorded and assessed every 3 days for 45 days.

Results: The results showed that in all dosages of the two drugs, significant weight loss occurred in comparison with the control group.

Conclusion: The effect of caffeine on weight loss according to our results, matches with human studies, while ketotifen contradictory to our assumption, resulted in weight loss which probably was related to the difference in metabolic pathways in mice and humans, or maybe the used doses of ketotifen in this study were insufficient to reduce TNF-α production or influence in serotonin release and be effective on appetite or weight gain.

Introduction

According to World Health Organization (WHO) report in 2013, overweight and obesity are the fifth leading risk for global deaths, as there is a strong scientific agreement that obesity significantly increases the risk of serious chronic diseases like hypertension and cardiovascular disease, diabetes, obstructive sleep apnea and some forms of cancer and finally contributes to overall mortality.[1,2] Weight gain occurrence, due to genetic predisposition or result from lifestyle and intake of calories more than needed or as a side effect of some medications; interventions should be done to combat this epidemic problem.

Ketotifen, is a safe anti-histamine with low dose and long-lasting effects, which inhibits release of mediators involved in asthma and allergies. Its primary pharmacological roles are histamine receptor antagonism, phosphodiesterase inhibition and prevention of calcium flux in smooth muscles. Distinctive anti-asthmatic properties of ketotifen which make it a suitable and effective treatment in asthma include: preventative effect on airway hyperreactivity associated with activation of platelets by PAF (Platelet Activating Factor) or caused by sympathomimetic drugs or the exposure to allergen; inhibition of eosinophils and platelets in the airways; suppression of the influx of eosinophils into inflammatory local and antagonism of bronchoconstriction due to leukotrienes.[3] Ketotifen, like most antihistamines not only sedates and slows down body metabolism, but also can stimulate appetite and induce weight-gain.[4,5] Specially ketotifen causes a significant weight gain in children with asthma,[6] maybe as a chronic state of this disease and the long duration of drug use in asthma. Besides the prolonged use, the other effective factor in weight gain of these patients is the simultaneous use with corticosteroids which are prescribed in asthma and have weight gain effect due to their induced edema and mechanism of action. Thereby the weight gain incidence practically is higher in ketotifen-received asthmatic patients and it is tried to overcome this side effect by use of different agents as like as essential oils.[7] Considering this effect of ketotifen few studies performed to make use of this side effect in a positive way in catechia. As a result of these studies, it is concluded that, ketotifen could be useful in the management of HIV-associated malnutrition by inhibition of release of TNF-alpha from stimulated peripheral blood mononuclear cells.[8] Also due to this side effect, in some researches it has been used as an agent to induce weight gain.[7,9]

*Corresponding author: Haleh Vaez, Department of Pharmacology, Faculty of Pharmacy, Tabriz University of Medical Sciences, Tabriz, Iran.
Emails: vaezh@tbzmed.ac.ir ; haleh.vaez@gmail.com

Caffeine is a methyl-xanthine with brain stimulant effect which unlike ketotifen increases alertness and concentration, and is considered as a stimulant of energy expenditure which can increase thermogenesis and fat oxidation,[10] and can alter the energy balance by improving energy consumption. Clinical applications of caffeine have been reviewed in 1995.[11] There is some evidence suggesting a positive effect of methyl-xanthine especially caffeine, in several diseases such as parkinsonism,[12,13] asthma,[14] apnea,[15] cancer,[16] diabetes[17] and in migraine as an adjunctive analgesic in combination with ergotamine.[18,19] Furthermore, it may be added to a variety of analgesics and some antiviral drugs.[20] Different studies regarding the effects of caffeine-induced weight loss and energy expenditure are available.[21-30] As it was pointed by Curatolo et al., caffeine appeared to be safe in regular used dosages, and can be considered as a useful agent to induce thermogenesis and lose weight.[31,32] Thereby, Epidemiological data suggest that increasing caffeine consumption may lead to a small reduction in long-term weight gain.[29,33,34]

Combinations of different drugs as a multi-ingredient formulation are prepared to improve drug effects or to prevent exacerbation of side effects of drugs. In this study with considering both of these roles, the impact of caffeine (an effective agent in asthma which is a bronchodilator and also reduces respiratory muscle fatigue)[35,36] in reducing body weight, individually and in co-administration with ketotifen (an effective agent in asthma and allergies), has been investigated in mice model.

Materials and Methods
Animals
Male mice at the weight limit of 20-30 g divided in 8 groups (n=8 in each group) randomly and maintained with free access to standard mice food and tap water. All steps of experiment performed accordance with the Guide for the Care and Use of Laboratory Animals (National Institutes of Health Publication No 85-23, revised 1985).

Drugs
Pure powders of ketotifen fumarate and caffeine in anhydrate form were purchased from Darupaksh Pharmaceutical Company, Tehran, Iran. Sodium chloride solution (0.9 %) was used as solvent of the drugs and determined doses were injected intraperitoneal (i.p.) to the mice.

Experimental protocols
Animals treated for 45 days in one control group and seven groups of treatment with different doses of drugs. Control group received normal saline 10 ml/kg, i.p. and in drug receiving groups, there were three groups of ketotifen in concentration of 4, 8, 16 mg/kg, i.p. and three groups of caffeine in concentration of 4, 8, 16 mg/kg, i.p. and one group of caffeine 4mg/kg, i.p. in

combination with ketotifen 4 mg/kg, i.p. injection. Required dose of drugs for each mouse was calculated based on its body weight and injected intraperitoneally for 45 consecutive days. Weight changes were recorded as body weight (BW) and assessed every three days over 45 days of experiment and the dose of drugs were adjusted every three day based on the new recorded weight of each mouse.

Statistics analysis
Data was expressed as Means± SEM for each group in each time of BW measurement. To compare group means and determine significant differences between different groups, the analysis of variance (ANOVA) was used and assessed by Tukey test. Differences were considered as significant for $P<0.05$.

Results
Weight changes due to different doses of ketotifen (4, 8, 16 mg/kg)
According to Figure 1, comparison of weight changes in ketotifen 4 mg/kg and control group of receiving normal saline during 45 days of experiment, showed that there were significant differences on days of 24, 28, 36, 40 and 45 ($P<0.05$). For the dose of 8 mg/kg of ketotifen, there were significant differences on days of 40 and 45 of experiment ($P<0.05$). Also in dose of 16 mg/kg of ketotifen there was a statistically significant difference on days of 32 ($P<0.01$) and 24, 28, 40 and 45 of experiment ($P<0.001$).

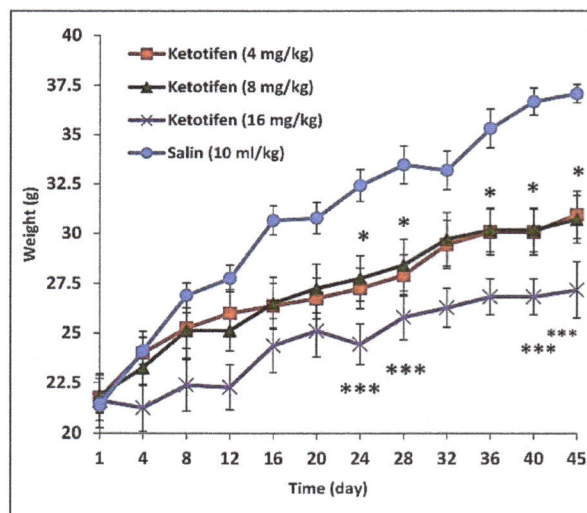

Figure 1. Weight changes due to different doses of ketotifen (4, 8, 16 mg/kg) in mice for 45 days. Values represent the Mean± SEM of 8 animals for each group. Significantly different from the control group; *p<0.05, **p<0.01, ***p<0.001.

Weight changes due to different doses of caffeine (4, 8, 16 mg/kg)
Comparison of weight change in groups receiving various doses of caffeine compared to control group, showed that there were significant differences, for 4 mg/kg of caffeine on 40 and 45th day of experiment

(P<0.05) and in dose of 8 mg/kg of caffeine in 24 and 40th day (P<0.05) and 45th day (P<0.01) of the study. For higher dose of caffeine (16 mg/kg) there were statistically significant differences on days of 28, 32 (P<0.05) and 36, 40 and 45th of the study (P<0.01) (Figure 2).

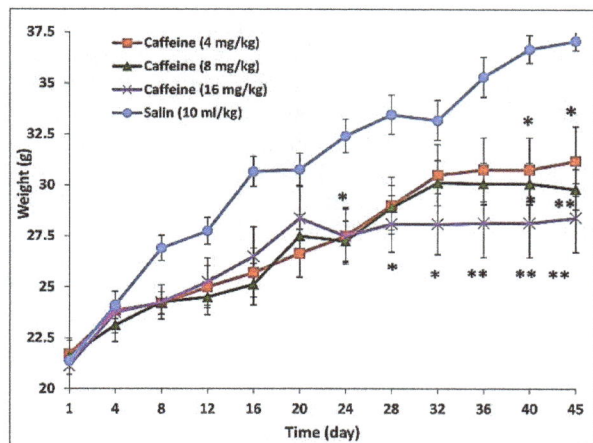

Figure 2. Weight changes due to different doses of caffeine (4, 8, 16 mg/kg) in mice for 45 days. Values represent the Mean± SEM of 8 animals for each group. Significantly different from the control group; *p<0.05, **p<0.01.

Weight changes due to co-administration of ketotifen (4 mg/kg) and caffeine (4 mg/kg)

Weight changes due to co-administration of ketotifen (4 mg/kg) and caffeine (4 mg/kg) in comparison with control group (normal saline 10 ml/kg) showed significant differences, on days of 28, 36, 40 (P<0.01) and 32 and 45 of experiment (P<0.05) (Figure 3). However the effect of co-administration is not significantly different with either single drug of ketotifen or caffeine in dose of 4 mg/kg.

Weight changes due to administration of same dose of the two drugs of ketotifen and caffeine

According to the diagrams in Figure 4 which compare weight changes in same dose of ketotifen and caffeine, there was no significant difference in any doses of 4, 8 and 16 mg/kg. However each dose of ketotifen and caffeine in comparison with control group had caused significant weight loss.

Discussion

The results of present study show that, the injection of different doses of ketotifen and caffeine induced significant weight loss in comparison with control group. To interpret the result obtained from this study, we should concentrate on mechanism of action of these drugs.

Caffeine (1,3,7-trimethylxanthine), is the major pharmacologically active methylxanthine in coffee and tea.[37] The predominate mechanism of its action is by blocking the action of adenosine as a competitive inhibitor of A_1 and A_{2a} adenosine receptor due to the

similarity in its molecular structure to the nucleotide adenosine. Consistent with this effect on adenosine receptors, caffeine also releases norepinephrine, dopamine and serotonin in the brain and increases circulating catechol amines, following stimulation of central nervous system and energy metabolism in the peripheral tissues.[38,39] A small amount of caffeine inhibits presynaptic adenosine receptors and increases release of catecholamine neurotransmitters. Also in larger quantities (>10 μmol/lit), inhibition of phosphodiesterase and increase in cAMP concentration ultimately leads to increase in calcium influx into cells and in doses higher than 100 μmol/lit, caffeine disrupt calcium retention through reticulum sarcoplasmic in cells.[40]

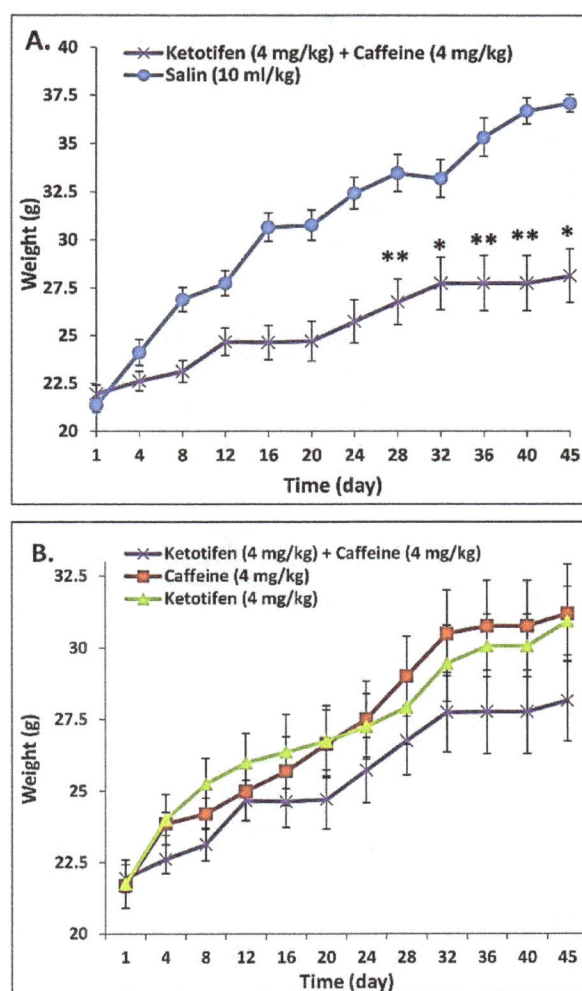

Figure 3. Weight changes due to co-administration of ketotifen (4 mg/kg) and caffeine (4 mg/kg) in mice for 45 days, in comparison with control group (A) and in comparison with separate dose of ketotifen (4 mg/kg) and caffeine (4 mg/kg) (B). Values represent the Mean± SEM of 8 animals for each group. Significantly different from the control group; *p<0.05, **p<0.01.

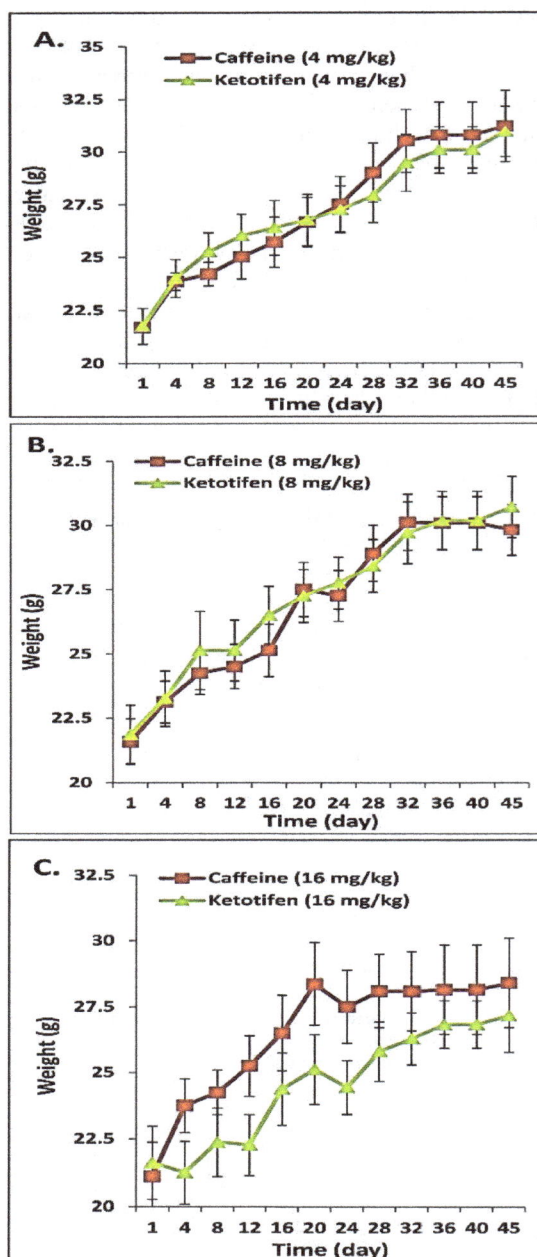

Figure 4. Weight changes due to administration of ketotifen (4 mg/kg) and caffeine (4 mg/kg) (A), ketotifen (8 mg/kg) and caffeine (8 mg/kg) (B), ketotifen (16 mg/kg) and caffeine (16 mg/kg) (C) in mice for 45 days. Values represent the Mean± SEM of 8 animals for each group.

Caffeine alone has several important metabolic effects. Caffeine stimulates fat utilization in muscle tissue during exercise.[41] In addition, a dose-dependent increase in basal energy expenditure with caffeine is reported by Astrup et al., which exerted through an increase in lactate and triacylglycerol production and increased vascular smooth muscle tone.[42] Increase in lipid turnover and lipid oxidation by interference in Cori-cycle and the FFA-triglyceride cycle and acting as a thermogenesis agent can be added to the mechanism of action of caffeine.[43-45] Effect of caffeine

on thermogenesis regulation accomplished through an inhibitory effect on the enzyme phosphodiesterase , and results in increasing of cyclic adenosine mono phosphate (cAMP) content; and later, synaptic nerve system activity amplified and activated hormone-sensitive lipase, which promotes lipolysis.[43,46] Another probable mechanism of weight loss caused by caffeine is through diuretic and natriuretic effect, which is induced by blockage of hepatic adenosine-mediated sensory nerves and a hepatorenal reflex.[47] There is evidence that moderate caffeine intake might be useful in preventing obesity by inhibiting proliferative activity in white adipose tissue.[48] It is suggested also, that the anti-obesity effect of caffeine is due to the additive and/or synergistic inhibitory activity of caffeine on intracellular lipid accumulation.[49] The usual amount of caffeine increases circulating cortisol concentrations, but does not have short term effects on appetite, energy intake, glucose metabolism, and inflammatory markers.[50] All of the mentioned mechanisms suggest a beneficial effect of caffeine as a weight loosing agent and as a good factor to combine with some drugs with side effect of weight gain. In the same way, in this study, with use of different doses of caffeine in comparison with the control group, significant weight loss was observed, which may be due to the effect of caffeine in inducing diuresis, increasing lipolysis and basal metabolism, enhancement in mobility and reduction of feeling fatigue.

The other studied drug, ketotifen is a second-generation noncompetitive H1-antihistamine and mast cell stabilizer which besides its anti-histaminic activity, also function as a leukotriene antagonist and a phosphodiesterase inhibitor. However, appetite stimulation and weight gain are its common side effects in human.[51,52] A probable mechanism of ketotifen on weight gain and appetite is attributed to inhibitory effect on production of TNF-α which has been confirmed in human studies.[8] It has been evidenced that TNF-α plays a key role in regulating energy metabolism[53] and can act directly on adipocytes to regulate the release of leptin.[54] Leptin acts on receptors in the hypothalamus of the brain, where it inhibits appetite.[55] Ketotifen by inhibitory effect on production of TNF-α can reduce leptin level and thereby decreased the inhibition of leptin on appetite and finally result in weight gain. In addition to mentioned appetite enhancing mechanism of ketotifen, this drug by influence in 5-hydroxytryptamine regulation, could involve in central serotonin disinhibition,[56] leading to decrease serotonin level and as the fact of suppressant effect of serotonin on appetite, ketotifen caused an increase in food intake tendency and appetite.

In the present study, different doses of ketotifen not only did not cause significant weight gain but also induced significant weight loss compared to the control group. The results may be due to the difference in metabolic pathways in mice and humans, or maybe the used doses of ketotifen in this study were not in the range of doses to reduce TNF-α production or influence serotonin release and be effective on appetite or weight gain, which require further studies and measuring the level of TNF-α. This contradictory effect of ketotifen is also reported in other studies. As an example, in an evaluation of combining ketotifen and oxymetholone on weight gain and performance status in human immunodeficiency virus (HIV) patients with chronic cachexia, addition of ketotifen did not result in weight gain[57] or in another study of evaluation of co-administration of ketotifen and cyproheptadine, the injection of different doses of ketotifen showed different results in mice, while the high doses of ketotifen caused a significant weight gain, compared to the control group, but the low doses resulted in a significant weight loss[9] which amplify the importance of doses used in research and indicate the probability of the different mechanism of different doses in variant patients.

Conclusion

According to this study and determining the separate and also combined prescription of ketotifen and caffeine on weight changes in mice, further study in exact mechanism of weight gain and effect of these drugs in these processes should be done to find the causes of weight loosing effect of ketotifen in low doses. And also measurement of the consumed food and water by animals is recommended to assess the impact of these drugs on appetite. Therefor to clarify the issue arising from different results of this study and previous works, and to attribute a new application of these drugs in the form of co-administration, it is suggested to study more in this field, maybe with higher doses or different protocol and time range. It means that maybe with higher doses of ketotifen and inducing weight gain, the combination of caffeine and ketotifen will be effective in reducing this side effect and also by the means of this combination in asthmatic patients the efficacy of ketotifen in controlling the disease symptoms can be enhanced.

Acknowledgements

The authors thank the Faculty of Pharmacy of Tabriz University of Medical Sciences, for providing technical support for this study.

Conflict of Interest

The authors declare that they have no conflict of interest.

References

1. Haslam DW, James WP. Obesity. *Lancet* 2005;366(9492):1197-209.
2. Saito Y, Kita T, Mabuchi H, Matsuzaki M, Matsuzawa Y, Nakaya N, et al. Obesity as a risk factor for coronary events in Japanese patients with hypercholesterolemia on low-dose simvastatin therapy. *J Atheroscler Thromb* 2010;17(3):270-7.
3. Thomson, Micromedex. Drug Information for the Health Care Professional. 24th ed. Greenwood Village: United States Pharmacopeial Convention, Inc; 2004.
4. Couluris M, Mayer JL, Freyer DR, Sandler E, Xu P, Krischer JP. The effect of cyproheptadine hydrochloride (periactin) and megestrol acetate (megace) on weight in children with cancer/treatment-related cachexia. *J Pediatr Hematol Oncol* 2008;30(11):791-7.
5. Ali AH, Yanoff LB, Stern EA, Akomeah A, Courville A, Kozlosky M, et al. Acute effects of betahistine hydrochloride on food intake and appetite in obese women: a randomized, placebo-controlled trial. *Am J Clin Nutr* 2010;92(6):1290-7.
6. Craps LP. Immunologic and therapeutic aspects of ketotifen. *J Allergy Clin Immunol* 1985;76(2 Pt 2):389-93.
7. Asnaashari S, Delazar A, Habibi B, Vasfi R, Nahar L, Hamedeyazdan S, et al. Essential oil from Citrus aurantifolia prevents ketotifen-induced weight-gain in mice. *Phytother Res* 2010;24(12):1893-7.
8. Ockenga J, Rohde F, Suttmann U, Herbarth L, Ballmaier M, Schedel I. Ketotifen in HIV-infected patients: effects on body weight and release of TNF-alpha. *Eur J Clin Pharmacol* 1996;50(3):167-70.
9. Nemati M, Habibi B, Sharifi K. Effect of ketotifen and cyproheptadine on appetite and weight changes in mice. *Iran J Pharm Sci* 2006;2(3):123-8.
10. Dulloo AG, Geissler CA, Horton T, Collins A, Miller DS. Normal caffeine consumption: influence on thermogenesis and daily energy expenditure in lean and postobese human volunteers. *Am J Clin Nutr* 1989;49(1):44-50.
11. Sawynok J. Pharmacological rationale for the clinical use of caffeine. *Drugs* 1995;49(1):37-50.
12. Carey RJ. Antiparkinsonian effects of caffeine depend upon pavlovian drug conditioning processes. *Brain Res* 1990;518(1-2):186-92.
13. Schwarzschild MA, Chen JF, Ascherio A. Caffeinated clues and the promise of adenosine A(2A) antagonists in PD. *Neurology* 2002;58(8):1154-60.
14. Tilley SL. Methylxanthines in asthma. *Handb Exp Pharmacol* 2011(200):439-56.
15. Henderson-Smart DJ, De Paoli AG. Prophylactic methylxanthine for prevention of apnoea in preterm infants. *Cochrane Database Syst Rev* 2010(12):CD000432.
16. Ohta A, Sitkovsky M. Methylxanthines, inflammation, and cancer: fundamental mechanisms. *Handb Exp Pharmacol* 2011(200):469-81.
17. Kempf K, Herder C, Erlund I, Kolb H, Martin S, Carstensen M, et al. Effects of coffee consumption on subclinical inflammation and other risk factors for type 2 diabetes: a clinical trial. *Am J Clin Nutr* 2010;91(4):950-7.

18. Yancey JR, Dattoli G. Caffeine as an analgesic adjuvant for acute pain in adults. *Am Fam Physician* 2013;87(1):11.

19. Nieber K. [Does caffeine enhance the analgesic efficacy?]. *Dtsch Med Wochenschr* 2013;138(8):352.

20. Jankiewicz K, Chroscinska-Krawczyk M, Blaszczyk B, Czuczwar SJ. [Caffeine and antiepileptic drugs: experimental and clinical data]. *Przegl Lek* 2007;64(11):965-7.

21. Striegel-Moore RH, Franko DL, Thompson D, Barton B, Schreiber GB, Daniels SR. Caffeine intake in eating disorders. *Int J Eat Disord* 2006;39(2):162-5.

22. Dulloo AG. Herbal simulation of ephedrine and caffeine in treatment of obesity. *Int J Obes Relat Metab Disord* 2002;26(5):590-2.

23. Hackman RM, Havel PJ, Schwartz HJ, Rutledge JC, Watnik MR, Noceti EM, et al. Multinutrient supplement containing ephedra and caffeine causes weight loss and improves metabolic risk factors in obese women: a randomized controlled trial. *Int J Obes (Lond)* 2006;30(10):1545-56.

24. Greenway FL, De Jonge L, Blanchard D, Frisard M, Smith SR. Effect of a dietary herbal supplement containing caffeine and ephedra on weight, metabolic rate, and body composition. *Obes Res* 2004;12(7):1152-7.

25. Boozer CN, Nasser JA, Heymsfield SB, Wang V, Chen G, Solomon JL. An herbal supplement containing Ma Huang-Guarana for weight loss: a randomized, double-blind trial. *Int J Obes Relat Metab Disord* 2001;25(3):316-24.

26. Tremblay A, Masson E, Leduc S, Houde A, Després J-P. Caffeine reduces spontaneous energy intake in men but not in women. *Nutr Res* 1988;8(5):553-8.

27. Pasman WJ, Westerterp-Plantenga MS, Saris WH. The effectiveness of long-term supplementation of carbohydrate, chromium, fibre and caffeine on weight maintenance. *Int J Obes Relat Metab Disord* 1997;21(12):1143-51.

28. Westerterp-Plantenga MS, Lejeune MP, Kovacs EM. Body weight loss and weight maintenance in relation to habitual caffeine intake and green tea supplementation. *Obes Res* 2005;13(7):1195-204.

29. Lopez-Garcia E, Van Dam RM, Rajpathak S, Willett WC, Manson JE, Hu FB. Changes in caffeine intake and long-term weight change in men and women. *Am J Clin Nutr* 2006;83(3):674-80.

30. Hursel R, Viechtbauer W, Westerterp-Plantenga MS. The effects of green tea on weight loss and weight maintenance: a meta-analysis. *Int J Obes (Lond)* 2009;33(9):956-61.

31. Curatolo PW, Robertson D. The health consequences of caffeine. *Ann Intern Med* 1983;98(5 Pt 1):641-53.

32. Westerterp-Plantenga MS. Green tea catechins, caffeine and body-weight regulation. *Physiol Behav* 2010;100(1):42-6.

33. Dalbo VJ, Roberts MD, Stout JR, Kerksick CM. Effect of gender on the metabolic impact of a commercially available thermogenic drink. *J Strength Cond Res* 2010;24(6):1633-42.

34. Hursel R, Westerterp-Plantenga MS. Thermogenic ingredients and body weight regulation. *Int J Obes (Lond)* 2010;34(4):659-69.

35. Welsh EJ, Bara A, Barley E, Cates CJ. Caffeine for asthma. *Cochrane Database Syst Rev* 2010(1):CD001112.

36. Bara AI, Barley EA. Caffeine for asthma. *Cochrane Database Syst Rev* 2000(2):CD001112.

37. Nehlig A. Coffee, tea, chocolate, and the brain. Boca Raton, Florida: CRC Press; 2004.

38. Benowitz NL. Clinical pharmacology of caffeine. *Annu Rev Med* 1990;41:277-88.

39. Nehlig A, Daval JL, Debry G. Caffeine and the central nervous system: mechanisms of action, biochemical, metabolic and psychostimulant effects. *Brain Res Brain Res Rev* 1992;17(2):139-70.

40. Snyder SH. Adenosine receptors and the actions of methylxanthines. *Trends Neurosci* 1981;4(0):242-4.

41. Spriet LL, Maclean DA, Dyck DJ, Hultman E, Cederblad G, Graham TE. Caffeine ingestion and muscle metabolism during prolonged exercise in humans. *Am J Physiol* 1992;262(6 Pt 1):E891-8.

42. Astrup A, Toubro S, Cannon S, Hein P, Breum L, Madsen J. Caffeine: a double-blind, placebo-controlled study of its thermogenic, metabolic, and cardiovascular effects in healthy volunteers. *Am J Clin Nutr* 1990;51(5):759-67.

43. Acheson KJ, Gremaud G, Meirim I, Montigon F, Krebs Y, Fay LB, et al. Metabolic effects of caffeine in humans: lipid oxidation or futile cycling? *Am J Clin Nutr* 2004;79(1):40-6.

44. Westerterp-Plantenga M, Diepvens K, Joosen AM, Berube-Parent S, Tremblay A. Metabolic effects of spices, teas, and caffeine. *Physiol Behav* 2006;89(1):85-91.

45. Diepvens K, Westerterp KR, Westerterp-Plantenga MS. Obesity and thermogenesis related to the consumption of caffeine, ephedrine, capsaicin, and green tea. *Am J Physiol Regul Integr Comp Physiol* 2007;292(1):R77-85.

46. Cornelis MC, El-Sohemy A, Campos H. Genetic polymorphism of the adenosine A2A receptor is associated with habitual caffeine consumption. *Am J Clin Nutr* 2007;86(1):240-4.

47. Ming Z, Lautt WW. Caffeine-induced natriuresis and diuresis via blockade of hepatic adenosine-mediated sensory nerves and a hepatorenal reflex. *Can J Physiol Pharmacol* 2010;88(11):1115-21.

48. Bukowiecki LJ, Lupien J, Follea N, Jahjah L. Effects of sucrose, caffeine, and cola beverages on obesity, cold resistance, and adipose tissue cellularity. *Am J Physiol* 1983;244(4):R500-7.

49. Nakabayashi H, Hashimoto T, Ashida H, Nishiumi S, Kanazawa K. Inhibitory effects of caffeine and its metabolites on intracellular lipid accumulation in

murine 3T3-L1 adipocytes. *Biofactors* 2008;34(4):293-302.

50. Gavrieli A, Yannakoulia M, Fragopoulou E, Margaritopoulos D, Chamberland JP, Kaisari P, et al. Caffeinated coffee does not acutely affect energy intake, appetite, or inflammation but prevents serum cortisol concentrations from falling in healthy men. *J Nutr* 2011;141(4):703-7.

51. Phillips MJ, Meyrick Thomas RH, Moodley I, Davies RJ. A comparison of the in vivo effects of ketotifen, clemastine, chlorpheniramine and sodium cromoglycate on histamine and allergen induced weals in human skin. *Br J Clin Pharmacol* 1983;15(3):277-86.

52. Katzung BG. Basic & clinical pharmacology. 9th ed. Katzung BG, editor. New York: Lange Medical Books/McGraw Hill; 2004.

53. Sethi JK, Hotamisligil GS. The role of TNF alpha in adipocyte metabolism. *Semin Cell Dev Biol* 1999;10(1):19-29.

54. Kirchgessner TG, Uysal KT, Wiesbrock SM, Marino MW, Hotamisligil GS. Tumor necrosis factor-alpha contributes to obesity-related hyperleptinemia by regulating leptin release from adipocytes. *J Clin Invest* 1997;100(11):2777-82.

55. Henry BA, Goding JW, Alexander WS, Tilbrook AJ, Canny BJ, Dunshea F, et al. Central administration of leptin to ovariectomized ewes inhibits food intake without affecting the secretion of hormones from the pituitary gland: evidence for a dissociation of effects on appetite and neuroendocrine function. *Endocrinology* 1999;140(3):1175-82.

56. Aguilera A, Selgas R, Codoceo R, Bajo A. Uremic anorexia: a consequence of persistently high brain serotonin levels? The tryptophan/serotonin disorder hypothesis. *Perit Dial Int* 2000;20(6):810-6.

57. Hengge UR, Baumann M, Maleba R, Brockmeyer NH, Goos M. Oxymetholone promotes weight gain in patients with advanced human immunodeficiency virus (HIV-1) infection. *Br J Nutr* 1996;75(1):129-38.

21

Microwave Assisted Synthesis of 1-[5-(Substituted Aryl)-1*H*-Pyrazol-3-yl]-3,5-Diphenyl-1*H*-1,2,4-Triazole as Antinociceptive and Antimicrobial Agents

Shantaram Gajanan Khanage[1]*, Popat Baban Mohite[1], Ramdas Bhanudas Pandhare[2], S. Appala Raju[3]

[1] *Department of Pharmaceutical Chemistry and PG studies, M.E.S. College of Pharmacy, Sonai, Ahmednagar, Maharashtra, India-414105.*

[2] *Department of Pharmacology, M.E.S. College of Pharmacy, Sonai, Tq-Newasa, Dist.-Ahmednagar, Maharashtra, India-414105.*

[3] *Department of Pharmaceutical chemistry, H.K.E. 'S College of Pharmacy, Sedam road, Gulbarga, Karnataka, India-585105.*

ARTICLE INFO

Keywords:
Microwave
Antinociceptive
Antimicrobial
Hot plate method
MIC
Chalcones

ABSTRACT

Purpose: An efficient technique has been developed for microwave assisted synthesis of 1-[5-(substituted aryl)-1H-pyrazol-3-yl]-3,5-diphenyl-1H-1,2,4-triazole as antinociceptive and antimicrobial agents.

Methods: The desired compounds (S_1-S_{10}) were synthesized by the microwave irradiation via cyclization of formerly synthesized chalcones of 3,5-diphenyl-1*H*-1,2,4-triazole and hydrazine hydrate in mild acidic condition. All newly synthesized compounds were subjected to study their antinociceptive and antimicrobial activity. The analgesic potential of compounds was tested by acetic acid induced writhing response and hot plate method. The MIC values for antimicrobial activity were premeditated by liquid broth method.

Results: The compounds S_1, S_2, S_4, S_6 and S_{10} were found to be excellent peripherally acting analgesic agents when tested on mice by acetic acid induced writhing method and compounds S_3, S_6 and S_1 at dose level of 100 mg/kg were exhibited superior centrally acting antinociceptive activity when tested by Eddy's hot plate method. In antimicrobial activity compound S_{10} found to be broad spectrum antibacterial agent at MIC value of 15.62 µg/ml and compound S_6 was exhibited antifungal potential at 15.62 µg/mL on both fungal strains.

Conclusion: Some novel pyrazoles clubbed with 1,2,4-triazole derivatives were synthesized and evaluated as possible antimicrobial, centrally and peripherally acting analgesics.

Introduction

Triazole derivatives have always attracted the attention of medicinal chemists because of their many therapeutic applications. 1,2,4-triazoles and related fused heterocyclic derivatives are of great biological interest such as anticancer,[1,2] antimicrobial,[3-6] anticonvulsant,[7] anti-inflammatory, analgesic,[8,9] antidepressant,[10] antitubercular,[11,12] antimalarial[13] and hypoglycemic[14] activities.

The pyrazole ring system is a five membered heterocyclic ring structure composed of two nitrogen atoms and used in the synthesis of pharmaceuticals. The pyrazole moiety is a versatile lead molecule in pharmaceutical development and has a wide range of biological activities. In the past few years, the therapeutic interest of pyrazole derivatives in pharmaceutical and medicinal field has been given a great attention to the medicinal chemist. Literature survey reveals that pyrazole derivatives are well known

to have anti-inflammatory, analgesic, antipyretic,[15] antibacterial,[16,17] anticancer,[18,19] antituberculine,[20] antimalarial[21] activities. This stimulated our interest to synthesize some novel pyrazoles derivatives containing triazole moiety of biological importance.

In addition to previously synthesized compounds 1-(3,5-diphenyl-1H-1,2,4-triazol-1-yl)-3-(substituted aryl) prop-2-en-1-one[22,23] some new analogues of titled nucleus were synthesized and evaluated for antinociceptive and antimicrobial activity. The structures of the compounds were confirmed by FTIR, NMR and mass spectroscopy studies, their antinociceptive activity was evaluated by chemical nociception model of acetic acid induced writhing response and hot plate method on mice. The antimicrobial activity was studied by (Minimum Inhibitory Concentration) MIC.

In continuation of our previous work on 3,5-disubstituted 1,2,4-triazole and related clubbed heterocycles,[22,23] in

---

*Corresponding author: Shantaram Gajanan Khanage, M.E.S. College of Pharmacy, Sonai, At post-Sonai, Tq-ewasa, Dist.-Ahmednagar, Maharashtra-414105, India. Email: 1982@gmail.com

this article the efforts have been made to synthesize and explore the antinociceptive and antimicrobial activity of some novel 1-[5-(substituted aryl)-1H-pyrazol-3-yl]-3,5-diphenyl-1H-1,2,4-triazole derivatives.

Materials and Methods
Chemicals
The melting points were determined in open tube capillary using Thermonik precision apparatus and are uncorrected. The purity of compounds was checked by TLC on silica gel G plates. IR spectra were recorded on PERKIN ELMER 8201 PC IR spectrophotometer. ^{1}HNMR spectra were recorded in DMSO on BRUKER DRX NMR spectrometer (400 MHz). Mass spectra (FAB-MS) of the compounds were recorded on 70V on JEOL D-300 spectrophotometer (Jeol Ltd., Tokyo, Japan). Microwave assisted reactions were carried out in a Catalysts Microwave synthesizer. Elemental analysis for C, H and N were performed on a PERKIN ELMER 240 elemental analyzer. The reaction time of animals on hot plate were studied on digital analgesiometer. The standard drugs Ibuprofen, Pentazocine, Ampicilline, Ciprofloxacine and Fluconazole were obtained as gift sample from Wockhardt Ltd., Aurangabad, India. Sabouraud Dextrose broth (SDB), Sabouraud Dextrose Agar (SDA), Peptone water and solvents used for the experimental work were commercially procured from E. Merck Ltd., Mumbai, India and Qualigens Ltd., Mumbai, India.

Animals and microbial cultures
Adult mice (Swiss strain 25-30 g) were used for evaluation of antinociceptive activity. The animals were housed under standard environmental conditions (light period of 12 h/day, temperature 25-27 °C and relative humidity 30-70%) with access to food and water *ad libitum*. The experiment was performed according to Committee for the Purpose of Control and Supervision of Experiments on Animals (CPCSEA) guidelines and the experimental protocol was approved by the Institutional Local Animal Ethical Committee. The microbial cultures of gram positive bacteria *B. subtillis* (NCIM 2063), gram negative bacteria *E. coli* (NCIM 2065), yeast *C. albicans* (NCIM 3471) and mold *A. niger* (NCIM 1196) were procured from National Centre for Industrial Microorganisms (NCIM), Pune, India.

Synthesis of 1-[5-(substituted aryl)-1H-pyrazol-3-yl]-3,5-diphenyl-1H-1,2,4-triazole derivatives (S_1-S_{10})
The desired compounds (S_1-S_{10}) were synthesized by the cyclization of 1-(3,5-diphenyl-1H-1,2,4-triazol-1-yl)-3-(substituted aryl) prop-2-en-1-one (Chalcones, 0.01 mol) and hydrazine hydrate (0.01 mol) in presence of small amount of glacial acetic acid. The reaction mixture was subjected to microwave irradiation for 10 minutes at 280 w. After the completion of reaction, the precipitate of product obtained was washed with cold water and dried. The crude product was recrystallized from ethanol water mixture (1:1). All the compounds were obtained in good yield. Physical and spectral data of the compounds S_1-S_{10} are mentioned in Figure 1 and Table 1.

Figure 1. Physical and analytical data of compounds S_1-S_{10}.

Compound	Ar	Molecular Formula	M.P. (°C)	Yield (%)	Elemental Analysis (found)		
					%C	%H	%N
S_1	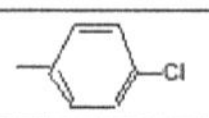 —⬡—Cl	$C_{23}H_{16}ClN_5$	155-157	89	69.43 (69.23)	4.05 (4.13)	17.60 (17.36)
S_2	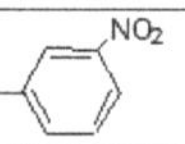 ⬡—NO₂	$C_{23}H_{16}N_6O_2$	150-152	79	67.64 (67.77)	3.95 (3.99)	20.58 (20.66)
S_3	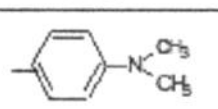 —⬡—N(CH₃)₂	$C_{25}H_{22}N_6$	149-151	83	73.87 (73.89)	5.46 (5.19)	20.67 (20.47)
S_4	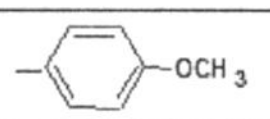 —⬡—OCH₃	$C_{24}H_{19}N_5O$	158-159	91	73.27 (73.12)	4.87 (4.86)	17.80 (17.89)
S_5	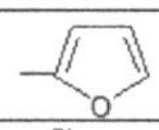 —⬡O	$C_{21}H_{15}N_5O$	142-144	93	71.38 (71.30)	4.28 (4.28)	19.82 (19.70)
S_6	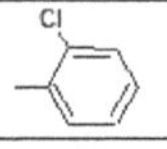 —⬡ (Cl)	$C_{23}H_{16}ClN_5$	160-162	87	69.43 (69.19)	4.05 (4.09)	17.60 (17.63)
S_7	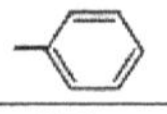 —⬡	$C_{23}H_{17}N_5$	155-157	76	76.01 (76.22)	4.71 (4.77)	19.27 (19.45)
S_8	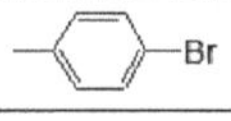 —⬡—Br	$C_{23}H_{16}BrN_5$	179-181	72	62.46 (62.32)	3.65 (3.69)	15.83 (15.77)
S_9	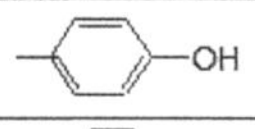 —⬡—OH	$C_{23}H_{17}N_5O$	165-167	74	72.81 (72.77)	4.52 (4.60)	18.46 (18.74)
S_{10}	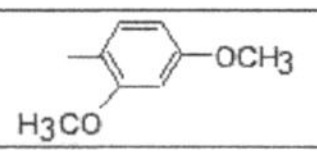 —⬡—OCH₃ (H₃CO)	$C_{25}H_{21}N_5O_2$	170-172	85	70.91 (70.43)	5.00 (4.92)	16.54 (16.53)

Table 1. Spectral data of compound S_1-S_{10}.

Compound	IR(KBr) cm^{-1}	^{1}H-NMR (δ ppm)	MS (FAB, positive ion mode) m/z [M+1]$^+$
S_1	3071 (Ar-CH), 1620 (C=N, triazole),785(-Cl),3291 (NH, pyrazole)	7.45-8.49 (14H, m, Ar-H), 6.12 (1H, s, NH of pyrazole), 3.23 (1H, s, CH of pyrazole)	398
S_2	3077 (Ar-CH), 1623 (C=N, triazole),1557 (-NO2), 3285 (NH, pyrazole)	7.48-8.20 (14H, m, Ar-H), 6.27 (1H, s, NH of pyrazole), 3.30 (1H, s, CH of pyrazole)	408
S_3	3070 (Ar-CH), 1628 (C=N, triazole), 3153, 3149 (-NCH3), 3273 (NH, pyrazole)	7.40-8.41 (14H, m, Ar-H), 6.31 (1H, s, NH of pyrazole), 3.29 (1H, s, CH of pyrazole), 3.16 (6H, s, -N(CH$_3$)2)	406
S_4	3074 (Ar-CH), 1626 (C=N, triazole), 1157 (-OCH3), 3246(NH, pyrazole)	7.36-8.31 (14H, m, Ar-H), 6.25 (1H, s, NH of pyrazole), 3.33 (1H, s, CH of pyrazole), 3.82 (3H, s, OCH$_3$),	393
S_5	3068 (Ar-CH), 1625 (C=N, triazole), 1226 (C-O-C), 3259 (NH, pyrazole)	6.89-8.48 (13H, m, Ar-H), 6.16 (1H, s, NH of pyrazole), 3.35 (1H, s, CH of pyrazole)	353
S_6	3075 (Ar-CH), 1627 (C=N, triazole), 779 (-Cl), 3297 (NH, pyrazole)	7.22-8.53 (14H, m, Ar-H), 6.26 (1H, s, NH of pyrazole), 3.24 (1H, s, CH of pyrazole)	398
S_7	3079, 3072 (Ar-CH), 1623 (C=N, triazole),3267 (NH, pyrazole)	6.45 -8.59 (15H, m, Ar-H), 6.33 (1H, s, NH of pyrazole), 3.37 (1H, s, CH of pyrazole)	363
S_8	3069 (Ar-CH), 1621 (C=N, triazole),696 (-Br), 3270 (NH, pyrazole)	7.35-8.44 (14H, m, Ar-H), 6.28 (1H, s, NH of pyrazole), 3.31 (1H, s, CH of pyrazole)	442
S_9	3077 (Ar-CH), 1625(C=N, triazole), 3359(-OH).	7.43-8.29 (14H, m, Ar-H), 6.13 (1H, s, NH of pyrazole), 3.35 (1H, s, CH of pyrazole), 10.27 (s, 1H, Ar-OH)	379
S_{10}	3081 (Ar-CH), 1628 (C=N, triazole,1153 (-OCH3), 3278 (NH, pyrazole)	7.41-8.47 (13H, m, Ar-H), 6.31 (1H, s, NH of pyrazole), 3.32 (1H, s, CH of pyrazole), 3.79 (6H, s, OCH$_3$)	423

Evaluation of antinociceptive activity

Study protocol was approved by the Institutional Animal Ethics Committee for the purpose of control and supervision of experiments on animals (IAEC, Approval No.1211/ac/08/CPCSEA) before experiment. Swiss strain albino mice of either sex weighing 25–30 g were used for this study. The test compounds were administered intraperitoneally in 10% v/v Tween 80 suspension. The antinociceptive activity was evaluated using acetic acid induced writhing (abdominal constriction test) test and Hot plate method.

Acute toxicity study

The acute toxicity for the test compounds was determined by the Miller and Tainter method administering the compounds intraperitoneally. LD$_{50}$ of the test compounds calculated by Miller and Tainter (1944) method,[24] initially least tolerated (smallest) dose (100% mortality) and most tolerated (highest) dose (0% mortality) were determined by hit and trial method. For the antinociceptive activity the LD$_{50}$ of the test compounds was measured at 100 mg/kg (Table 2).

Table 2. Determination of LD$_{50}$ mg/kg values of test compounds by Miller and Tainter method.

compound	Least tolerated Dose with 100% mortality	Most tolerated Dose with 0% mortality	LD$_{50}$ mg/kg with 50% mortality
S_1.S_{10}	25	200	100

Acetic acid induced writhing method (Abdominal Constriction Test)[25]

The animals were divided into 12 groups of six mice each. The control group of animals was administered with 10% v/v Tween 80 (0.5 ml) suspension. The animals of another group were injected intraperitoneally with standard drug Ibuprofen (10 mg/kg). After 20 min of the administration the test compounds, all the groups of mice were given with the writhing agent 3% v/v aqueous acetic acid in a dose of 2 ml/kg intraperitoneally. The writhing produced in these animals was counted visually for 15 min and the numbers of writhings produced in treated groups were compared with control group. The results of analgesic activity are recorded in Table 3. Analgesic activity in percent was calculated by using following formula.

$$\text{rotection} = 100 - [\{(\text{No. of writhes in treated mice})/(\text{No. of writhes in untreated mice})\} \times 100]$$

Table 3. Evaluation of analgesic activity by acetic acid induced writhing method.

Sr. No.	Treatment	Dose (mg/kg)	Writhing episodes in 15 min (Mean ± S.E.M.)	Percent protection
1	Control	-	39.42±0.4247	-
2	Ibuprofen	10	11.56±0.3458**	71
3	S_1	100	13.23±0.5647**	66
4	S_2	100	15.56±0.4475**	61
5	S_3	100	16.14±0.5895**	59
6	S_4	100	13.09±0.7858**	67
7	S_5	100	18.36±0.3256**	53
8	S_6	100	14.89±0.5358**	62
9	S_7	100	22.68±0.3874**	42
10	S_8	100	20.47±0.4578**	48
11	S_9	100	16.78±0.6544**	57
12	S_{10}	100	14.47±0.7478**	63

** $P < 0.01$ represent significant difference when compared with control groups.

Hot plate method

The analgesic activity measured by central analgesia of hot plate method.[26] The temperature of a metal surface in the hot plate test was set at 55±1.0 °C. The time taken by the animals to lick the fore or hind paw or jump out of the place was taken as the reaction time. Latency to the licking paws or jumping from plate was determined before and after treatment. The latency was recorded at the time of 0 (just before any treatment) and 15, 30 and 60 min after intraperitoneal administration of test compounds. A latency period of 15 sec was defined as complete analgesia as cut off time to prevent damage to mice. The reference compound Pentazocine was administered in a dose of 5 mg/kg. The time course of hot plate latency was expressed as the percentage of the maximum possible effect (%MPE) according to the following formula:

$$\%MPE = \frac{(\text{post drug latency}) - (\text{pre drug latency})}{(\text{cut off time}) - (\text{pre drug latency})} \times 100$$

After the treatment of test and reference compounds, the pain thresholds of the animals were observed and presented in Table 4.

Table 4. Evaluation of analgesic activity by Hot plate method.

Treatment	Average Reaction Time in seconds before treatment (Mean ± S.E.M.)	Reaction time in seconds after treatment (Mean ± S.E.M.)			%MPE
		15 min	30 min	60 min	
Control	4.75±0.1547	4.75±0.1683	4.75±0.2663	4.75±0.4541	-
Pentazocine	4.70±0.5012**	7.70±0.5611**	9.67±0.4602**	11.81±0.5254**	69.02
S_1	4.66±0.5521**	7.65±0.6346**	9.83±0.5645**	11.67±0.4369**	67.79
S_2	4.63±0.4985**	7.60±0.5234**	9.87±0.4865**	11.54±0.4356**	66.44
S_3	4.67±0.4123**	7.52±0.6532**	9.92±0.5433**	11.79±0.4156**	68.92
S_4	4.61±0.5374**	7.55±0.5585**	9.72±0.5658**	11.47±0.5541**	66.02
S_5	4.69±0.4374**	6.45±0.5418**	8.36±0.6256**	9.27 ±0.5454**	44.42
S_6	4.65±0.4969**	7.42±0.4769**	9.79±0.5169**	11.71±0.5075**	68.21
S_7	4.56±0.5154**	6.70±0.4559**	8.49±0.5474**	9.37±0.5525**	46.07
S_8	4.43±0.4541**	7.52±0.5585**	9.77±0.5456**	10.82±0.6084**	60.65
S_9	4.56±0.46735**	7.39±0.4646**	9.53±0.5136**	10.53±0.6359**	57.18
S_{10}	4.68±0.5548**	7.56±0.6636**	9.59±0.5552**	10.37±0.4427**	55.13

** $p<0.01$ represent the significant difference when compared with control group.

Statistical analysis

Data were presented as arithmetic mean±SEM. Statistical analysis was performed by one way variance (ANOVA) followed by Dunnett's test. ''p'' value of less than 0.05 was considered as statistically significant.

Antimicrobial Activity

Determination of Minimum Inhibitory Concentration (MIC): The Minimum Inhibitory Concentration (MIC) of the test compounds against *Bacillus subtillis* (NCIM 2063), *Escherichia coli* (NCIM 2065), *Candida albicans* (NCIM 3471) and *Aspergillus niger* (NCIM 1196) was determined by liquid broth method of two fold serial dilution technique.[27] In this assay, the minimum concentration of each test compound required to inhibit the growth of microorganism was determined. The final concentration of test compounds ranged from 250 to 7.81µg/ml. Ampiciline and Ciprofloxacine were used as a standard antibacterial drug and Fluconazole was used as a standard antifungal drug. All the standard drugs were tested at concentrations ranging from 100 to 3.12 µg/ml respectively. The tubes were inspected visually to determine the growth of the organism as indicated by turbidity. MIC values of each tested compound recorded in Table 5 and 6.

Table 5. Antibacterial activity data of 1-[5-(substituted aryl)-1H-pyrazol-3-yl]-3,5-diphenyl-1H-1,2,4-triazole derivatives.

Comp	Concentration in µg/ml against B. Subtillis						MIC µg/ml	Concentration in µg/ml against E. Coli						MIC µg/ml
	250	125	62.5	31.25	15.62	7.81		250	125	62.5	31.25	15.62	7.81	
S$_1$	-	-	-	-	+	+	31.25	-	-	-	-	+	+	31.25
S$_2$	-	-	-	-	+	+	31.25	-	-	-	-	+	+	31.25
S$_3$	-	-	-	+	+	+	62.5	-	-	+	+	+	+	125
S$_4$	-	-	-	-	+	+	31.25	-	-	-	-	-	+	15.62
S$_5$	-	-	+	+	+	+	125	-	-	-	+	+	+	62.5
S$_6$	-	-	-	+	+	+	62.5	-	-	-	-	+	+	31.25
S$_7$	-	+	+	+	+	+	250	-	+	+	+	+	+	250
S$_8$	-	-	-	+	+	+	62.5	-	-	-	+	+	+	62.5
S$_9$	-	-	-	-	+	+	31.25	-	-	-	-	+	+	31.25
S$_{10}$	-	-	-	-	-	+	15.62	-	-	-	-	-	+	15.62

Standard drug Ampiciline showed MIC at 6.25 µg/ml and Ciprofloxacin showed MIC at 6.25 µg/ml.

"-" growth of the organism in test tube not observed, "+" growth of the organism in test tube observed

Table 6. Antifungal activity data of 1-[5-(substituted aryl)-1H-pyrazol-3-yl]-3,5-diphenyl-1H-1,2,4-triazole derivatives.

Comp	Concentration in µg/ml against C. albicans						MIC µg/ml	Concentration in µg/ml against A. niger						MIC µg/ml
	250	125	62.5	31.25	15.62	7.81		250	125	62.5	31.25	15.62	7.81	
S$_1$	-	-	-	-	+	+	31.25	-	-	-	-	+	+	31.25
S$_2$	-	-	-	-	-	+	15.62	-	-	-	-	+	+	31.25
S$_3$	-	-	-	+	+	+	62.5	-	-	+	+	+	+	125
S$_4$	-	-	-	-	+	+	31.25	-	-	-	-	-	+	15.62
S$_5$	-	-	+	+	+	+	125	-	-	+	+	+	+	125
S$_6$	-	-	-	-	-	+	15.62	-	-	-	-	-	+	15.25
S$_7$	-	-	+	+	+	+	125	-	-	-	+	+	+	62.5
S$_8$	-	-	-	-	+	+	31.25	-	-	-	-	-	+	15.25
S$_9$	-	-	-	+	+	+	62.5	-	-	-	+	+	+	62.5
S$_{10}$	-	-	-	-	+	+	31.25	-	-	-	-	+	+	31.25

Standard drug Fluconazole showed MIC at 6.25 µg/ml

"-" growth of the organism in test tube not observed, "+" growth of the organism in test tube observed

Results and Discussion

The synthesis of 1-[5-(substituted aryl)-1H-pyrazol-3-yl]-3,5-diphenyl-1H-1,2,4-triazole derivatives (S_1-S_{10}) depicted in Figure 2. The previously synthesized chalcones were cyclized with hydrazine hydrate in acidic medium to get various pyrazoles clubbed with 1,2,4-triazole. Infra-red spectrum of compounds S_1-S_{10} showed a sharp absorption at 1557, 779-785, 1157, 3149, 696, 3359 and 3068-3081 cm^{-1} which is accredited to -NO_2, -Cl, -OCH_3, -N-(CH_3)$_2$, Br, OH and aromatic region. Synthesized compounds showed appropriate ^{1}H-NMR signals aromatic protons showed multiplets in the range of δ 6.45-8.59, the anticipated signals with proper multiplicities for different types of protons were observed for the compounds. Mass spectra of the compounds showed molecular ion peaks with high abundance at m/z in concurrence with their molecular formula.

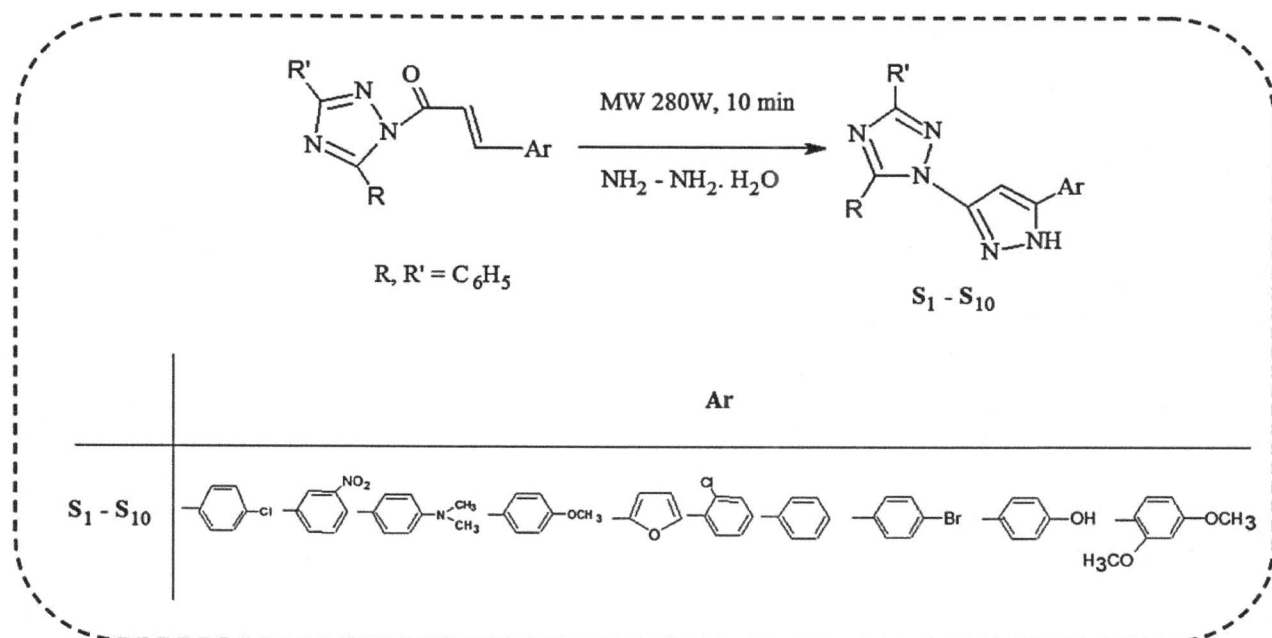

Figure 2. Microwave assisted synthesis of compounds S_1-S_{10}

All compounds are tested for their central and peripheral antinociceptive activity, in acetic acid induced writhing method compounds S_1, S_2, S_4, S_6 and S_{10} were found to be excellent analgesic agents with 66, 61, 67, 62 and 63 percentage of protection respectively. SAR study for peripherally acting analgesics stated that electron withdrawing groups (EWG) such as chloro and nitro on para, meta and ortho positions and electron releasing group (ERG) like methoxy on ortho and para position of phenyl ring present on pyrazole nucleus exhibited potential activity. Bromo, hydroxy and dimethylamino substituted analogues showed moderate antinociceptive activity. The ortho, meta and para positions of phenyl ring substituted on 5th position of pyrazole ring are found to be crucial and important site for lead modification.

Hot plate method was studied to perceive the centrally acting analgesic effect of newly synthesized compounds, Pentazocine 5 mg/kg significantly increased the hot plate latency producing a highest %MPE at 69.02. Compounds S_1, S_2, S_3, S_4 and S_6 significantly increased the hot plate latency when compared to the control group. Compounds S_8, S_9 and S_{10} showed moderate activity. The highest antinociception induced by compounds S_3, S_6 and S_1 at dose of 100 mg/kg were observed with 68.92, 68.21 and 67.79% MPE respectively. Compounds substituted with 3-nitro, phenyl, 4-chloro, 2-chloro, 4-methoxy, 4-bromo, 4-hydroxy and 2,4-dimethoxy groups demonstrated dynamic analgesic activity. Dimethyl aminophenyl and 2-furyl substituted analogues found to be weak analgesic agents from the tested series.

Newly synthesized compounds were furthermore tested for their *in vitro* antimicrobial activity against various NCIM reference bacterial strains of *B. subtillis*, *E. coli* and fungal strains of *C. albicans* and *A. niger*. The MIC values were calculated using liquid broth method of two fold serial dilution technique. All compounds showed a reasonable level of antibacterial and antifungal activity at the µg/ml level, antibacterial activity ranging from the lowest MIC value of 15.62 µg/ml for compound S_{10} against *B. subtillis* and *E. coli*, compound S_4 against *E. coli* to the highest of 250 µg/ml for compound S_7 against *B. subtillis* and *E. coli*. The MIC values of antifungal activity ranging from the lowest MIC value of 15.62 µg/ml for compound S_2 and S_6 against *C. albicans*, compounds S_4, S_6 and S_8 against *A. niger* to the highest of 125 µg/ml for compound S_5 against *C. albicans* and *A. niger*. The order of the antimicrobial activity in tested compounds seems to depend on the nature of the EWG in position 2, 3 and 4 of phenyl ring of pyrazole nucleus varies in the order 2-

chloro > 3-nitro > 4-chloro > 4-bromo, moreover the ERG like methoxy in position 2 and 4 of phenyl ring of pyrazole nucleus. The screening results also suggested that 3, 5 disubstituted triazole ring might be performing vital role in the antimicrobial activity.

Conclusion
A new class of pyrazole containing 3,5-disubstituted triazole was synthesized and evaluated as antimicrobial, centrally and peripherally acting analgesic agents and found to be potential therapeutic agent. The increase in biological activity is attributed to the presence of 3-nitro, 2-chloro, 4-chloro and 4-methoxy groups on phenyl ring of pyrazole ring. These results suggest that novel series of pyrazoles clubbed with triazole moiety are interesting lead molecules for further synthetic and biological evaluation.

Acknowledgments
Authors are highly thankful to *BCUD, University of Pune*, Pune, India for providing financial assistance for entire course of investigation. Authors are also grateful to Principal M.E.S. College Pharmacy, Sonai and *Prashant Patil Gadakh*, Secreatary, Mula Education Society for providing excellent research facilities for this work.

Conflict of interest
All the authors report no conflicts of interest.

References
1. Al-Soud YA, Al-Masoudi NA, Ferwanah Ael R. Synthesis and properties of new substituted 1,2,4-triazoles: potential antitumor agents. *Bioorg Med Chem* 2003;11(8):1701-8.
2. Khanage SG, Mohite PB, Raju SA. Synthesis, anticancer and antibacterial activity of some novel 1,2,4-triazole derivatives containing pyrazole and tetrazole rings. *Asian J Res Chem* 2011;4(4):567-73.
3. Lingappa B, Girisha KS, Kalluraya BN, Rai S, Kumari NS. Regioselective reaction: Novel Mannich bases derived from 3-(4,6-disubstituted-2-thiomethyl)3-amino-5-mercapto-1,2,4-triazoles and their antimicrobial properties. *Indian J Chem* 2008;47B:1858-64.
4. Rao G, Rajasekran S, Attimarad M. Synthesis and Antimicrobial activity of Some 5-phenyl-4-substituted amino-3-mercapto (4*H*) 1,2,4-triazoles. *Indian J Pharm Sci* 2000;62(6):475-7.
5. Jalilian AR, Sattari S, Bineshmarvasti M, Shafiee A, Daneshtalab M. Synthesis and in vitro antifungal and cytotoxicity evaluation of thiazolo-4H-1,2,4-triazoles and 1,2,3-thiadiazolo-4H-1,2,4-triazoles. *Arch Pharm (Weinheim)* 2000;333(10):347-54.
6. Lazarevic M, Dimova V, Molnar GD, Kakurinov V, Colanceska RK. Synthesis of some N1-aryl/heteroarylaminomethyl/ethyl-1,2,4-triazoles and their antibacterial and antifungal activities. *Heterocycl Commun* 2001;7(6):577-82.
7. Chimirri A, Bevacqua F, Gitto R, Quartarone S, Zappala MD, Sarro A, et al. Synthesis and anticonvulsant activity of new 1-*H*-triazolo[4,5-c][2,3]benzodiaze-pines. *Med Chem Res* 1999;9:203-12.
8. Hunashal RD, Ronad PM, Maddi VS, Satyanarayana D, Kamadod MA. Synthesis, anti-inflammatory and analgesic activity of 2-[4-(substituted benzylideneamino)-5-(substitutedphenoxymethyl)-4*H*-1,2,4-triazol-3-yl-thio] acetic acid derivatives. *Arab J Chem* 2011;1-9.
9. Khanage SG, Mohite PB, Pandhare RB, Raju SA. Study of analgesic activity of novel 1,2,4-triazole derivatives bearing pyrazole and tetrazole moiety. *J Pharm Res* 2011; 4(10):3609-11.
10. Kane JM, Dudley MW, Sorensen SM, Miller FP. Synthesis of 1,2,4-Dihydro-3*H*-1,2,4-triazole-3-thiones as potential antidepressant agents. *J Med Chem* 1988;31(6):1253-8.
11. Husain MI, Amir M, Singh E. Synthesis and antitubercular activities of [5-(2furyl)-1,2,4-triazoles-3yl thio] acehydrazide derivatives. *Indian J Chem* 1987;26B:2512-54.
12. Khanage SG, Mohite PB, Pandhare RB, Raju SA. Investigation of pyrazole and tetrazole derivatives containing 3,5 disubstituted-4*H* 1,2,4-triazole as a potential antitubercular and antifungal agent. *Bioint Res Appl Chem* 2012; 2(2):277-83.
13. Xiao Z, Waters NC, Woodard CL, Li Z, Li PK. Design and synthesis of Pfmrk inhibitors as potential antimalarial agents. *Bioorg Med Chem Lett* 2001;11(21):2875-8.
14. Mhasalkar MY, Shah MH, Pilankar PD, Nikam ST, Anantanarayanan KG, Deliwala CV. Synthesis and hypoglycaemic activity of 3-aryl(or pyridyl)-5-alkyl amino-1,3,4, Thiadiazole and some sulfonyl ureas derivatives of 4*H*-1,2,4 triazoles. *J Med Chem* 1971;14(10):1000-3.
15. Badawey E, El-Ashmawey IM. Anti-inflammatory, analgesic and antipyretic activity of some new 1-(pyrimidin-2-yl)-3-pyrazoline-5-ones and 2-(pyrimidin-2- yl)-1,2,4,5, 6,7-hexahydro-3H-indazol-3-ones. *Eur J Med Chem* 1998;33:349-61.
16. Tanitame A, Oyamada Y, Ofuji K, Terauchi H, Kawasaki M, Wachi M, et al. Synthesis and antibacterial activity of a novel series of DNA gyrase inhibitors: 5-[(E)-2-arylvinyl]pyrazoles. *Bioorg Med Chem Lett* 2005;15(19):4299-303.
17. Sahu SK, Banerjee M, Samantray A, Behera C, Azam MA. Synthesis, analgesic, anti-inflammatory and antimicrobial activities of some novel pyrazoline derivatives. *Trop J Pharm Res* 2008;7(2):961-8.
18. Bouabdallah I, M'barek LA, Zyad A, Ramdani A, Zidane I, Melhaoui A. Anticancer effect of three pyrazole derivatives. *Nat Prod Res* 2006;20(11):1024-30.

19. Lv PC, Li HQ, Sun J, Zhou Y, Zhu HL. Synthesis and biological evaluation of pyrazole derivatives containing thiourea skeleton as anticancer agents. *Bioorg Med Chem* 2010;18(13):4606-14.

20. Castagnolo D, De Logu A, Radi M, Bechi B, Manetti F, Magnani M, et al. Synthesis, biological evaluation and SAR study of novel pyrazole analogues as inhibitors of Mycobacterium tuberculosis. *Bioorg Med Chem* 2008;16(18):8587-91.

21. Sanjay K, Gyanendra K, Mili K, Avadhesha S, Namita S. Synthesis and evaluation of substituted pyrazoles: potential antimalarials targeting the enoyl-acp reductase of plasmodium falciparum. *Synth Commun* 2006;36(2):215-26.

22. Khanage SG, Mohite PB, Pandhare RB, Raju SA. Synthesis, characterization and antimicrobial evaluation of 3,5 diphenyl-1*H*-1,2,4-triazole containing pyrazole function. *Bioint Res Appl Chem* 2012;2(3):313-9.

23. Khanage SG, Raju SA, Mohite PB, Pandhare RB. Analgesic Activity of Some 1,2,4-Triazole Heterocycles Clubbed with Pyrazole, Tetrazole, Isoxazole and Pyrimidine. *Adv Pharm Bull* 2013;3(1):13-8.

24. Miller LC, Tainter ML. Estimation of LD_{50} and its error by means of log-probit graph paper. *Proc Soc Exp Bio Med* 1944;57:261-4.

25. Siegmund E, Cadmus R, Lu G. A method for evaluating both non-narcotic and narcotic analgesics. *Proc Soc Exp Biol Med* 1957;95(4):729-31.

26. Eddy NB, Leimbach D. Synthetic analgesics. II. Dithienylbutenyl- and dithienylbutylamines. *J Pharmacol Exp Ther* 1953;107(3):385-93.

27. Gibbons S, Ohlendorf B, Johnsen I. The genus Hypericum--a valuable resource of anti-Staphylococcal leads. *Fitoterapia* 2002;73(4):300-4.

22

Thin Layer Chromatographic Analysis of Beta-Lactam Antibiotics

Gabriel Hancu[1]*, Brigitta Simon[1], Hajnal Kelemen[1], Aura Rusu[1], Eleonora Mircia[2], Árpád Gyéresi[1]

[1] *Department of Pharmaceutical Chemistry, Faculty of Pharmacy, University of Medicine and Pharmacy, Târgu Mureş, Romania.*

[2] *Department of Organic Chemistry, Faculty of Pharmacy, University of Medicine and Pharmacy, Târgu Mureş, Romania.*

A R T I C L E I N F O

Keywords:
Thin layer chromatography
Beta-lactam antibiotics
Penicillins
Cephalosporins
Separation

A B S T R A C T

Purpose: The paper describes some thin layer chromatographic procedures that allow simple and rapid separation and identification of penicillins and cephalosporins from complex mixtures. *Methods:* Using silicagel GF254 as stationary phase and selecting different mobile phases we succeeded in the separation of the studied beta-lactamins. Our aim was not only to develop a simple, rapid and efficient method for their separation but also the optimization of the analytical conditions. *Results:* No system will separate all the beta-lactams, but they could be identified when supplementary information is used from color reactions and/or by using additional chromatographic systems. *Conclusions:* The right combination of solvent system and detection method allows the identification of the studied penicillins and cephalosporins and can be successfully used in the preliminary analysis beta-lactam antibiotics.

Introduction

Among all the antibiotics, the group of beta-lactams ranks first regarding both the number of compounds on the market and also in terms of their use in the treatment of infectious disease. The most frequently used beta-lactams are the group of penicillins and cephalosporins respectively.[1]

The most popular analytical methods for the determination of beta-lactams are the chromatographic ones, including high performance liquid-chromatography (HPLC) and thin layer chromatography (TLC). HPLC offers high sensitivity and separation efficiency, establishing itself as the first choice method for the analysis of beta-lactams; however it is expensive and requires sophisticated equipment. TLC is a less expensive and less complicated chromatographic procedure, which can be successfully used, in the preliminary screening of pharmaceutical substances. In modern analysis, TLC is usually used as a separation method, which establishes the presence or absence of beta-lactam antibiotics above a defined level of concentration.[2,3]

TLC is used in 7th edition of the European Pharmacopoeia (Ph.Eur. 7) for separations of a particular beta-lactam antibiotic from its specific impurities, but the methods described refers to only one antibiotic and to its structure-related impurities and are less suitable for identification purposes from complex mixtures.[4]

A number of publications regarding the identification and separation of beta-lactams by TLC have appeared in literature, but few of them discuss the simultaneous separation from complex mixtures of structurally related derivatives.[5-8]

Structurally, penicillins are based on a heterocyclic skeleton, penam, formed by condensation of a beta-lactam ring with a thiazolidine one. In this study we analyzed four of the most frequently used penicillin derivatives with different structural characteristics: benzylpenicillin (PEN) – the first natural penicillin introduced in therapy; ampicillin (AMP) and amoxicillin (AMO) – two semisynthetic aminopenicillins; oxacillin (OXA) – a semisynthetic izoxazolilpenicillin. Penicillins differ from one another in the substituent R attached to the 6-aminopenicillanic acid residues. The chemical structures of the studied penicillins are presented in Figure 1.

The skeleton of the cephalosporins consits in a heterocycle, cefem, formed by condensation of a beta-lactam ring with a dihydrothiazine one. In this study we analyzed six frequently used cephalosporin derivatives: cefalexin (CEL), cefadroxil (CFD), cefaclor (CFC) – first generation oral cephalosporins, cefuroxim (CFR) – second generation parenteral cephalosporin, ceftazidim (CZI), ceftriaxon (CTR) – third generation parenteral cephalosporins. Substitution of the various R and R' groups results in cephalosporins with different pharmacological and pharmacokinetic properties. The chemical structures of the studied cephalosporins are presented in Figure 2.

*Corresponding author: Gabriel Hancu, Faculty of Pharmacy, University of Medicine and Pharmacy Târgu Mureş, GhMarinescu 38, 540000 Târgu Mureş, Romania. E-mail: g_hancu@yahoo.com

Figure 1. The chemical structure of the studied penicillins[4,9]

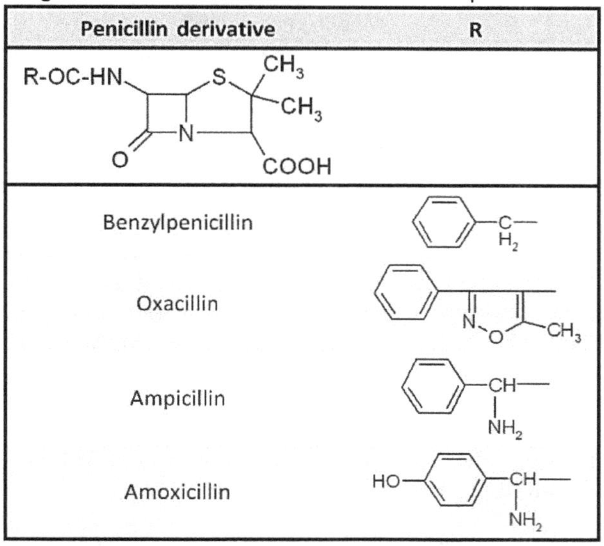

Our aim was the separation of beta-lactams from complex mixtures and also the „optimization" of the generic chromatographic process, in order to enhance the quality of the separation.

Materials and Methods
Instrumentation
The TLC system consisted of a Camag Nanomat III automatic sampler, a Camag Linomat IV semiautomatic sampler (Camag, Switzerland), a 2-µl Hamilton microsyringe (Hamilton, USA), a Camag Normal Development Chamber and a Camag fluorescence inspection lamp (Camag, Switzerland). As stationary phase we used 10x20 and 20x20 cm pre-coated silicagel GF254 HPTLC glass plates (Merck, Germany).

Figure 2. The chemical structure of the studied cephalosporins[4,9]

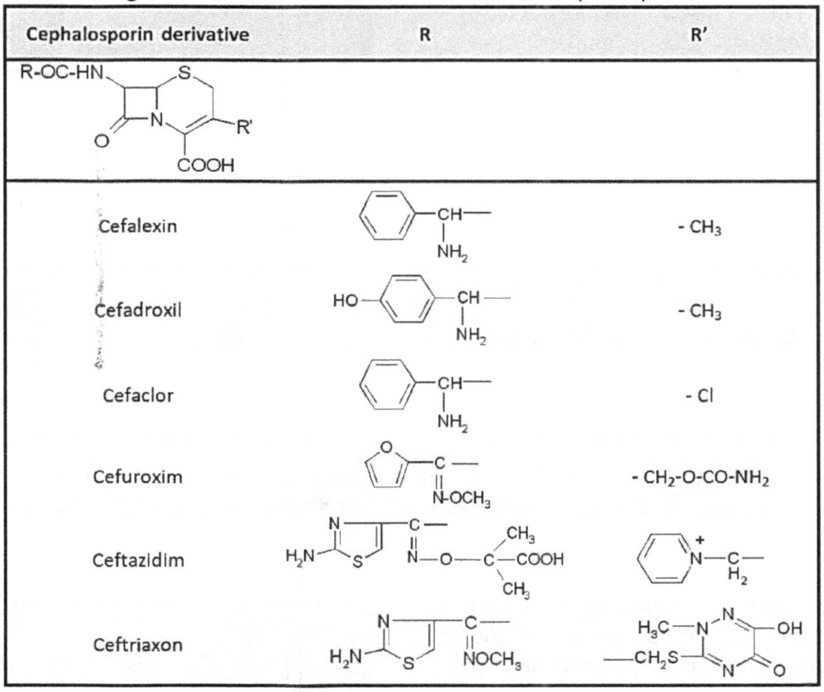

Reagents
Penicillins: amoxicillin trihydrate, ampicillin trihydrate, benzylpenicillin sodium, oxacillin sodium (Antibiotice Iaşi, Romania). Cephalosporins: cefalexin monohydrate, cefadroxil monohydrate, cefaclor monohydrate (Sandoz, Romania), cefuroxim sodium (Medochemie, Cyprus), ceftazidim pentahydrate, ceftriaxon sodium (Antibiotice Iaşi, Romania). All the studied beta-lactams were of pharmaceutical grade.
Reagents: acetone, acetic acid, benzene, butanol, ethanol, ethyl acetate, formaldehyde, methanol, sulphuric acid (Reactivul Bucureşti, Romania). All reagents were of analytical grade.

Samples
PEN and OXA, were used as sodium salts, consequently samples were prepared in water at a concentration of 0.2%. AMP and AMO, used as trihydrates, exhibit poor solubility in water; consequently samples of 0.2% were prepared in a 2% sodium bicarbonate solution. Cephalosporin samples were prepared by dissolving the substances in methanol and then diluting with water (1:1). Amounts of 0.5 µl were applied on the chromatoplates using a Hamilton syringe.

Method

The chromatographic chambers were saturated with the mobile phase for 30 minutes. The plates were developed over a distance of 15 cm in filter-paper-lined chromatographic chambers, dried in a stream of hot air, and examined under UV radiation at wavelengths of 254 and 366 nm. The spots were then visualized by placing the plates in a chromatographic chamber saturated with iodine vapors. Some specific in situ color reactions were used in order to increase specificity of the method. All experiments were carried out at room temperature. Photographs of the chromatoplates were taken with a Nikon D-3100 camera, equipped with a UV filter.

Chromatographic detection procedure

Three detection procedures were used; first with iodine vapors and then using in situ plate color reactions with iodine and ninhydrine, after an alkaline hydrolysis.

A few iodine crystals were placed on the base of tightly sealed chromatographic chamber, stored in a fume cupboard. After a few hours during which violet iodine vaporizes and distributes itself homogenously throughout the interior of the chamber, the chromatographic plates were introduced in the chamber. After 30 minutes the plates were sprayed with a 1% starch solution.

Chromatograms were first sprayed with a 1N sodium hydroxide solution, in order to hydrolyze the beta-lactam ring, and after 15 minutes with a solution containing 0.2 g potassium iodine, 0.4 g iodine dissolved in 20 ml ethanol and 5 ml 10% hydrochloric acid.

Chromatoplates were first sprayed with a 1N sodium hydroxide solution, in order to hydrolyze the beta-lactam ring, and after 15 minutes with a 0.1% ninhydrine solution in ethanol, and heated in an oven at 120 °C for 10 minutes.

Results and Discussion

The purpose of the method (simultaneous separation of a multicomponent mixture), and the information about the samples (structure, polarity, solubility, stability) were important as initial hints for the choice of the chromatographic system, using the rule of the Stahl's triangle.[2,10,11]

The most widely used stationary phase for the analysis of beta-lactam is silicagel, but if we consult the literature reversed-phase or cellulose plates have also been used. Silicagel surface bears Si-OH groups capable of hydrogen bonding with polar substances. Mobile phases for the separation of both penicillins and cephalosporins are polar, usually containing variable quantities of water.[5-7,12]

An acid (acetic acid) was added to the mobile phase in order to avoid decomposition of the beta-lactam ring on silicagel.

Around twenty solvents were tested and six mobile phases were selected (Table 1).

Table 1. The selected mobile phases

No	Mobile phases (V/V)
I	butanol – water – ethanol – acetic acid 50:20:15:15
II	butanol – water –acetic acid 60:20:20
III	ethyl acetate – water – acetic acid 60:20:20
IV	ethyl acetate – methanol – acetic acid 45:50:5
V	acetone – acetic acid 95:5
VI	acetone – benzene – water – acetic acid 65:14:14:7

All beta-lactams can be detected in UV light at 254 nm (green fluorescence) and 366 nm (blue fluorescence). Applying reagents such as ninhydrin or exposing the chromatoplate to iodine vapor can diminish the detection limit.

Figure 3 and 4 show photographs of the chromatograms obtained with mobile phase III in UV light at 254 and 366 nm respectively.

Figure 3. Chromatogram obtained at the separation of penicillins using mobile phase III (ethyl acetate – water – acetic acid 60:20:20), detection in UV light at 254 nm(A) and 366 nm(B) (1 - AMP, 2 - AMO, 3 – PEN, 4 - OXA)

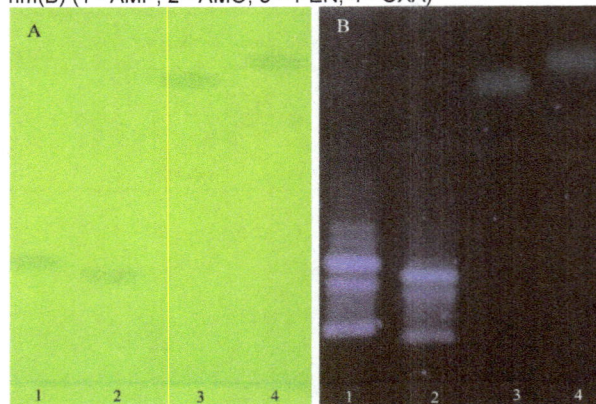

Figure 4. Chromatogram obtained at the separation of cephalosporins using mobile phase III (ethyl acetate – water – acetic acid 60:20:20), detection in UV light at 254 nm (A) and 366 nm (B) (1 - CFD, 2 - CEL, 3 – CFC, 4 – CFR, 5 – CZI, 6 - CTR)

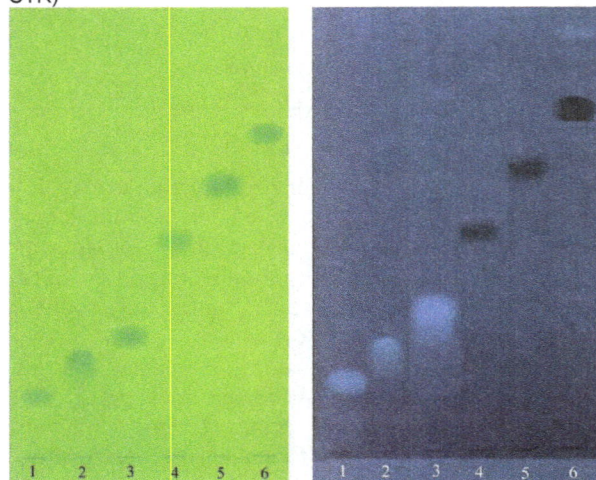

The Rf values, colors and fluorescence of the spots are mentioned in Table 2 and 3 respectively.

Table 2. Rf values of the studied beta-lactams in the six-development system

Beta-lactam derivative	Rf values					
	I	II	III	IV	V	VI
AMP	0.43	0.45	0.48	0.36	0.40	0.45
AMO	0.38	0.41	0.42	0.34	0.38	0.39
PEN	0.79	0.82	0.87	0.66	0.75	0.80
OXA	0.84	0.85	0.92	0.71	0.77	0.84
CFD	0.15	0.17	0.19	0.14	0.15	0.18
CEL	0.20	0.20	0.22	0.18	0.21	0.24
CFC	0.23	0.23	0.26	0.18	0.19	0.21
CFR	0.42	0.45	0.48	0.36	0.40	0.46
CZI	0.58	0.60	0.61	0.46	0.51	0.57
CTR	0.67	0.69	0.72	0.55	0.60	0.64

Difficulties appear at the separation of the two aminopenicillins (AMP, AMO) and of the three first generation oral cephalosporins (CEL, CFD, CFC)

respectively; substances with similar structural and physico-chemical characteristics.

It is often advantageous in TLC to be able to obtain preliminary impression of a substance separation by exposing the plate to a rapidly carried out, economically priced universal reaction before passing on to final characterization using group-specific specific reactions.[2,3,12] Detection by iodine is usually based on physical concentration of iodine molecule in the lipophilic chromatogram zones, without the occurrence of any chemical reaction. Iodine is more strongly enriched in the substance zones than in the neighboring polar substance-free silicagel layer.[2] The result was the appearance of brown chromatogram zones on a yellow background. The chromatogram zones can be stabilized by spraying them with 1 % starch solution; when the well-known blue clathrates are formed (starch-iodine inclusion compounds), which remain stable for months. The presence of different beta-lactams is demonstrated by the appearance of pale spots on a blue-purple background.

Table 3. Colours and fluorescence of beta-lactams developed by the six TLC systems

Beta-lactam derivative	-	Detection	in (with)	-
-	UV 254	UV 366 nm	Iodine vapors	Ninhydrine reaction
AMP	brown	fluorescent blue	yellow-brown	reddish
AMO	brown	fluorescent blue	yellow-brown	reddish
PEN	brown	fluorescent green	yellow	pale red
OXA	brown	fluorescent green	yellow	pale red
CFD	brown	fluorescent blue	yellow-orange	pale red
CEL	brown	fluorescent blue	yellow-orange	pale red
CFC	brown	fluorescent blue	yellow-orange	pale red
CFR	brown	fluorescent dark blue	yellow-orange	negative
CZI	brown	fluorescent dark blue	yellow-orange	negative
CTR	brown	pale dark blue	yellow-orange	negative

When detection takes place by spraying the chromatoplate with an iodine-potassium iodide solution, the iodine contained in the reagent reacts chemically with the penicilloic acid, as the beta-lactam ring is initially opened by alkaline hydrolysis. The subsequent treatment with starch solution employed after the iodine treatment for the stabilization and enhancement of the "iodine" chromatogram zones cannot be employed here since the layers - even after evaporation of the excess iodine - still contain so much iodine that the whole background is colored blue.

Aminopenicillins (AMP, AMO) proved to be more sensitive to ninhydrin reaction after an alkaline hydrolysis than PEN or OXA, which were scarcely visible. Cephalosporins couldn't be detected clearly with ninhydrine, as ninhydrine reacts actually with a degradation product of penicillins in alkaline environment, D-penicillamine. In general, amino - acid related compounds could be visualized using the ninhydrin reagent.

Penicillins can be also detected by spraying the plates with sulphuric acid – formaldehyde reagent (37% formaldehyde solution in conc. sulphuric acid 1:10), dark yellow spots were detected for the two aminopenicillins (AMP, AMO), PEN gave a brown spot while OXA a yellow one. All the cephalosporins gave pale yellow spots with this reagent. Heating was not necessary.

Dragendorff reagent (solution of potassium bismuth iodide) was also applied for detection, but beta-lactams proved to be less sensitive to this commonly used chromatographic reagent, as all the penicillins gave a very pale orange spot.

Although the stability of beta-lactam antibiotics in solid state is generally satisfying, beta-lactams dissolved in water or other solvents gradually convert to different degradation products through hydrolysis. After dissolution of each antibiotic the sample solutions were analyzed using mobile phase III, several times over duration of a week. The extent of the hydrolysis of beta-lactams is highly dependant on the time and temperature. Some degradation products detectable by TLC were found in the case of PEN after 48 hours storage. Possible degradation was noticeable on the chromatoplate for OXA, CEL, CFD and CFC after samples were stored in a refrigerator for a week, as they produced more than one spot on the TLC plate. Therefore the concentration value of beta-lactams determined in a certain sample solution is valid just for the application time on the chromatoplate, but does not provide valid information about the amount of beta-lactam at the time of the sampling step. It is highly advisable for sample solutions to be stored under refrigeration, especially if the sample cannot be analyzed shortly after dissolution of the antibiotic. This is especially important if the TLC method is applied for direct determination from biological samples.

With the unstable nature of these antibiotics in mind, degradation of the drugs may occur during the run and shadow spots and tailing may result from interactions between the sample and the developing solvent; however in our case these disadvantages were insignificant with the selected chromatographic systems.

Conclusion

All the studied beta-lactam derivatives may be separated using silicagel as stationary phase with an appropriate mobile phase. The use of a mobile phase, or a combination of two mobile phases, or a combination of a mobile phase and a color reaction enables the identification of the studied substances from complex mixtures. No system will separate all the beta-lactams, but they could be identified when supplementary information is obtained from color reactions and/or by using additional TLC systems. This identification technique is easy to perform and can be applied in preliminary analytical screening.

With some restriction regarding stability of beta-lactam antibiotics, the solvents and detection system mentioned above allow a rapid and convenient separation and detection of a large number of penicillins and cephalosporins and can find useful applications in the purity and stability control of beta-lactams in solution and dosage forms.

Conflict of Interest

The authors report no conflicts of interest.

References

1. Cristea A. Tratat de Farmacologie. Bucureşti: Editura Medicală; 2011.
2. Fried B, Sherma J. Thin-layer Chromatography. 4th ed. New York: Marcel Dekker Inc; 1999.
3. Wall P. Thin-layer chromatography – A modern practical approach, RSC Chromatography Monographs. London: Royal Society of Chemistry; 2005.
4. European Pharmacopoeia. 7th ed. Strasbourg: Council of Europe; 2010.
5. Hendrickx S, Roets E, Hoogmartens J, Vanderhaeghe H. Identification of penicillins by thin-layer chromatography. *J Chromatogr A* 1984;291:211-8.
6. Quintens I, Eykens J, Roets E, Hoogmartens J. Identification of cephalosporins by thin layer chromatography and color reactions. *J Plan Chromatogr* 1993;6:181-6.
7. Nabi SA, Laiq E, Islam A. Selective separation and determination of cephalosporins by TLC on stannic oxide layers. *Acta Chromatogr* 2004;14:92-101.
8. Choma IM. TLC Separation of cephalosporins: searching for better selectivity. *J Liq Chromatogr Relat Technol* 2007;30(15):2231-40.
9. Block JH, Beale JM. Wilson and Gisvold's textbook of Organic Medicinal and Pharmaceutical Chemistry. 11th ed. Philadelphia: Lippincott Williams and Wilkins; 2004.
10. Sadek PC. Ilustrated Pocket Dictionary of Chromatography. New Jersey: Wiley and Sons Inc; 2004.
11. Cazes J. Encyclopedia of Chromatography. 3rd ed. New York: Marcel Dekker Inc; 2009.
12. Pachaly P. DC-Atlas – Dünnschicht Chromatographie in der Apotheke. Stuttgart: Wissenschaftliche mbH; 2010.

23

Application of Liquisolid Technology for Enhancing Solubility and Dissolution of Rosuvastatin

Pavan Ram Kamble[1], Karimunnisa Sameer Shaikh[1]*, Pravin Digambar Chaudhari[1]

Department of Pharmaceutics, Modern College of Pharmacy, Nigdi, Pune, Maharashtra, India-411044.

ARTICLE INFO

Keywords:
Rosuvastatin calcium
Liquisolid compacts
Liquid load factor
Excipient ratio
Tablets
Dissolution rate

ABSTRACT

Purpose: Rosuvastatin is a poorly water soluble drug and the rate of its oral absorption is often controlled by the dissolution rate in the gastrointestinal tract. Hence it is necessary to increase the solubility of the Rosuvastatin.

Methods: Several liquisolid tablets formulations containing various drug concentrations in liquid medication (ranging from 15% to 25% w/w) were prepared. The ratio of Avicel PH 102 (carrier) to Aerosil 200 (coating powder material) was kept 10, 20, 30. The prepared liquisolid systems were evaluated for their flow properties and possible drug-excipient interactions by Infrared spectra (IR) analysis, differential scanning calorimetry (DSC) and X- ray powder diffraction (XRPD).

Results: The liquisolid system showed acceptable flow properties. The IR and DSC studies demonstrated that there is no significant interaction between the drug and excipients. The XRPD analysis confirmed formation of a solid solution inside the compact matrix. The tabletting properties of the liquisolid compacts were within the acceptable limits. Liquisolid compacts demonstrated significantly higher drug release rates than those of conventional and marketed tablet due to increasing wetting properties and surface area of the drug.

Conclusion: This study shows that liquisolid technique is a promising alternative for improvement of the dissolution rate of water insoluble drug.

Introduction

Solubility is one of the important parameters to achieve desired concentration of drug in systemic circulation for achieving required pharmacological response. Poorly water soluble drugs often require high doses in order to reach therapeutic plasma concentrations after oral administration. Low aqueous solubility is the major problem with formulation development of new chemical entities. Water is the solvent of choice for liquid pharmaceutical formulations. Most of the drugs are either weakly acidic or weakly basic having poor aqueous solubility. A great number of new and possibly beneficial chemical entities do not have suitable pharmaceutical dosage form because of their poor solubility and poor dissolution rate. The oral absorption of drugs is most often controlled by dissolution in the gastrointestinal tract.[1]

Rosuvastatin calcium is a BCS class II drug used as a lipid lowering agent by acting as HMG CoA reductase inhibitor.[2] Different methods are employed to improve the dissolution characteristics of poorly water soluble drugs like solubilization, pH adjustment, cosolvents, microemulsion, self emulsification, polymeric modification, drug complexation, particle size reduction, use of a surfactant as a solubilizing agent,

the pro-drug approach and solid solutions.[3] Amongst these, the most promising method for promoting dissolution is the use of the liquisolid system (LS).[4-13] Liquisolid systems are acceptably flowing and compressible powdered forms of liquid medications. The term 'liquid medication' involves oily liquid drugs and solutions or suspensions of water insoluble solid drugs carried in suitable nonvolatile solvent systems termed liquid vehicles. Employing this liquisolid technique, a liquid medication may be converted into a dry-looking, non-adherent, free flowing and readily compressible powder by simple blending with selected powder excipients referred to as carrier and coating materials.

To attain the flowability and compressibility of liquisolid compacts, the ''mathematical model for liquisolid systems'' was employed as follows to calculate the appropriate quantities of excipients required to produce liquisolid systems of acceptable flowability and compressibility. Various grades of cellulose, starch and lactose may be used as the carriers, whereas very fine particle size silica powders may be used as the coating (or covering) materials.[14]

*Corresponding author: Karimunnisa Sameer Shaikh, Department of Pharmaceutics, Modern College of Pharmacy, Sector No.21, Yamunanagar, Nigdi, Pune- 411044. Email: karima78@rediffmail.com

Due to low solubility, Rosuvastatin shows low bioavailability. Various approaches to enhance dissolution properties of Rosuvastatin are complexation with β-cyclodextrin, solid dispersion, hydrotropy, micellar solibilisation and microemulsion.[2,3]

Therefore, the present work is aimed towards enhancing the solubility, dissolution and thereby the bioavailability of Rosuvastatin by using liquisolid compact technology.

Materials and Methods
Materials
The following gift samples were received: Rosuvastatin (Biocon Pvt Ltd. Benglore, India); Avicel PH 102 and Sodium starch glycolate (Maple biotech Pvt. Ltd. Pune, India); Aerosil 200(Research lab Pune India) propylene glycol (PG), polyethylene glycol 400 (PEG400), polyethylene glycol (PEG200) and Acetonitrile (Research lab, Pune, India). All reagents used were of analytical grade.

Saturation solubility studies
Solubility studies of Rosuvastatin were carried out in distilled water, propylene glycol, PEG 400 and PEG 200. Saturated solutions prepared in above vehicles were kept in an orbital shaker (Remi motors Pvt. Ltd Mumbai, India.) for 72 h at 25 °C. The solutions were filtered and their concentration was determined by UV-spectrophotometry (Shimadzu Corporation Pvt. Ltd. Nishinokyo-Kuwabara-cho, Nakagyo-ku, Kyoto 604-8511, Japan) at 241 nm. The results were determined as the percent w/w of Rosuvastatin in its saturated solution with the solvent under investigation.

Application of a mathematical model for liquisolid system
To attain the flowability and compressibility of liquisolid compacts, the "new formulation mathematical model of liquisolid systems" was employed as follows to calculate the appropriate quantities of excipients required to produce liquisolid systems of acceptable flowability and compressibility. This mathematical model was based on new fundamental powder properties (constants for each powder material with the liquid vehicle) called the flowable liquid retention potential (Φ-value) and compressible liquid retention potential (Ψ-number) of the constituent powders (carrier and coating materials) according to Spireas et al (Spireas. 2002; Spireas et al. 1999). According to the new theories, the carrier and coating powder materials can retain only certain amounts of liquid while maintaining acceptable flow and compression properties. Depending on the excipients ratio (R) or the carrier: coating ratio of the powder system used, where

$$R = Q/q \dots (1)$$

As R represents the ratio between the weights of carrier (Q) and coating (q) materials present in the formulation. An acceptably flowing and compressible liquisolid system can be prepared only if a maximum liquid on the carrier material is not exceeded; such a characteristic amount of liquid is termed the liquid load factor (Lf) and defined as the ratio of the weight of liquid medication (W) over the weight of the carrier powder (Q) in the system, which should be possessed by an acceptably flowing and compressible liquisolid system. i.e.

$$Lf = W/Q \dots (2)$$

Spireas et al. used the flowable liquid retention potentials (Φ -values) of powder excipients to calculate the required ingredient quantities. Hence the powder excipients ratios R and liquid load factors Lf of the formulations are related as follows:

$$Lf = \Phi + \Phi (1/R) \dots (3)$$

So, in order to calculate the required weights of the excipients used, first, from equation (3), Φ and Φ are constants. Therefore, according to the ratio of the carrier/ coat materials (R), Lf was calculated from the linear relationship of Lf versus 1/R. Next, according to the used liquid vehicle concentration, different weights of the liquid drug solution (W) will be used. So, by knowing both Lf and W, the appropriate quantities of carrier (Q) and coating (q) powder materials required to convert a given amount of liquid medication (W) into an acceptably flowing and compressible liquisolid system, could be calculated from equations (1) and (2).[15]

Preparation of conventional tablet and liquisolid compacts
A conventional formulation of micronized Rosuvastatin calcium (denoted as DC) was directly compressed into cylindrical tablets, each containing 5 mg drug. In addition, each DC tablet contained the following powder excipients: 140 mg Avicel PH 102, 70 mg lactose monohydrate, 10 mg Aerosil 200, and 20 mg sodium starch glycolate. A 10 tablet batch was mixed in a mortar for 10 min. and the final admixture was compressed using a manual compression machine (Cip Machinaries.Pvt. Ltd. Ahrmadabad, Gujarat). Various liquisolid compacts containing 5 mg Rosuvastatin were prepared by dispersing in nonvolatile vehicles such as PEG 200. Then a binary mixture of carrier (Avicel PH 102) and coating material (Aerosil-200) was prepared at a ratio of 20:1,10:1 and 30:1. This binary mixture was added to the admixture of drug and vehicle. From the calculated Φ-value, the liquid load factor (Lf) was calculated.[16] Depending upon the drug concentration in liquid medication, different liquid load factors were employed in liquisolid preparations. Different concentrations of Avicel and silica were used to prepare different liquisolid formulations. Finally, sodium starch glycolate as a disintegrant was added to the above powder blend and mixed. The final powder blend was subjected to compression by using manual compression machine (Cip Machinaries. Pvt. Ltd. Ahemadabad, Gujarat.). The composition of the liquisolid compacts are shown in Table 1.

Table 1. Composition of the liquisolid compacts

Drug in conc of PEG 200	Batch	R value	Drug (mg)	Liquid load (Lf)	Avicel PH 102 (mg)	Aerosil (mg)	SSG (mg)	PEG 200 (mg)	Unit dose (mg)
15%	F1	10	5	0.326	102.24	10.22	7.28	28.33	153.07
	F2	20	5	0.163	204	10.20	12.37	28.33	259.9
	F3	30	5	0.109	305.77	10.19	17.46	28.33	366.75
20%	F4	10	5	0.326	76.68	7.66	5.44	20	114.78
	F5	20	5	0.163	218.57	10.92	12.72	20	367.21
	F6	30	5	0.109	229.35	7.645	13.09	20	275.08
25%	F7	10	5	0.326	61.34	6.13	4.37	15	191.84
	F8	20	5	0.163	122.69	6.13	7.44	15	156.231
	F9	30	5	0.109	183.48	6.11	10.47	15	220.06

Pre-compression studies of the liquisolid system

Flow properties of the liquisolid system

The flow properties of the liquisolid systems were estimated by determining the angle of repose, Carr's index and Hausner's ratio. The angle of repose was measured by the fixed funnel method. The bulk density and tap density were determined for the calculation of Hausner's ratio and Carr's index.[17]

Infra red spectra analysis

IR spectrum of optimized formulation was recorded by KBr method using Jasco M4100 Fourier Transform InfraRed spectrophotometer. A baseline correction was made by using dried potassium bromide and then the spectrum of powder with potassium bromide was recorded. Sample was scanned from 4000 to 400 cm^{-1}. The compatibility of drug and other excipients in formulation was confirmed by comparing drug and formulation spectra.

X-ray powder diffraction

Crystallinity study was carried out by comparing XRD spectrum of drug with formulation to check peak of drug in individual state and in formulation. Study was carried out on Elementer Vario E L III XRD Sophisticated Analytical Instrument Facility, at Cochin. The data was recorded at 2θ range of 10 to 60 °C at time of 0.5 sec. the relative intensity I/I0 and inter-planar distance (d) corresponding to 2θ value were reported and compared.

Differential scanning calorimetry (DSC)

Thermograms of the rosuvastatin and its liquisolid formulations were recorded on Mettler STAR SW 9.01 instruments. The analysis was carried out by heating 2 to 3 mg of sample on an aluminum crimp pan at rate of 10 °C/min in nitrogen atmosphere.

In vitro evaluation of liquisolid compacts

Content uniformity of rosuvastatin liquisolid tablets

Ten tablets from each batch were taken randomly to examine its content uniformity. Each tablet was weighed and crushed individually. The crushed tablet powders were dissolved in acetonitrile water system.

The solution was filtered using Whatman filter paper.The drug content was measured using UV spectrophotometer (Shimadzu corporation Pvt. Ltd Nishinokyo-Kuwabara-cho, Nakagyo-ku, Kyoto 604-8511, Japan) at 241 nm.

Weight variation test

Weight variation test was performed as per USP.[18]

Hardness and friability

The hardness of formulated liquisolid tablets was assessed using a Monsanto hardness tester and the mean hardness of three tablets was determined. The friability of the prepared liquisolid tablets was measured in a Roche type apparatus (Electrolab Pvt. Ltd Mumbai, India.) and the percentage loss in weight was calculated and used as a measure of friability.

Disintegration test

The disintegration test was carried out using disintegration test apparatus as specified in the Indian Pharmacopoeia.

In vitro dissolution studies

The in-vitro release profiles of rosuvastatin from liquisolid compacts and directly compressed tablets were obtained using a dissolution test apparatus USP-II (Electrolab Electrolab Pvt. Ltd Mumbai, India.)The dissolution study was carried out in 900 ml phosphate buffer pH 6.8 as the dissolution medium at 37 °C ± 2 °C and 50 rpm. Then 5 ml samples were collected for up to 60 min at 5-min intervals . The dissolution medium was replaced with 5 ml fresh dissolution fluid to maintain sink conditions. The withdrawn samples were filtered and analyzed spectrophotometrically at 241 nm. The mean of three determinations was used to calculate the drug release from each of the formulations.[18]

Estimation of fraction of molecularly dispersed drug

The fraction (FM) of the dissolved or molecularly dispersed drug in the liquid medication is the ratio the drug's saturation solubility (CL) in the liquid vehicle over the drug concentration (Cd) in the liquid medication.

$$FM = CL / Cd \quad (1)$$
$$(\text{Where } FM = 1 \text{ when } CL / Cd > 1)$$

The fractions of the molecularly dispersed drug in any system cannot exceed unity.

Effect of aging on tabletting properties

The study was performed under accelerated stability conditions at 40 °C ± 2 °C/75% RH ± 5% RH for three months.

Results and Discussion
UV analysis and solubility study

Rosuvastatin in acetonitrile-water solution obeyed Beer's law and displayed linearity over the concentration range tested from 2–20 µg/ml. The solubility of the drug was studied in different solvents like propylene glycol, polyethylene glycol 200, polyethelene glycol 400, distilled water, Phosphate Buffer pH 6.8. Saturation solubility of rosuvastatin in various solvent is given in Table 2.

Table 2. Saturated solubility of rosuvastatin in various solvent.

Solvent	Solubility (%w/w)
Distilled water	0.00000043±0.037
Buffer ph 6.8	0.0025±0.075
PEG400	4.55±0.115
Propylene glycol	9.96 ±0.180
PEG200	11.57 ±0.205

Selection of non volatile solvent

Rosuvastatin has highest solubility in PEG 200. Since the aim of this study was to enhance the dissolution rate of drug, PEG 200 was chosen as the non volatile liquid vehicle for formulation of liquisolid compacts of Rosuvastatin.

Application of a mathematical model for liquisolid system

To determine the quantities of the ingredients of the compacts,, the flowable liquid-retention potentials (Φ-values) and liquid load factor(Lf value) and the carrier to coating ratio (R value).

Determination of flowable liquid-retention potential (Φ-values)

"Angle of slide" measurement was used to evaluate the flow property of powder excipients (Avicel PH102 and Aerosil20 with PEG200). Several uniform liquid vehicle/powder admixtures which contain 10 g of the carrier or coating materials with increasing amounts of liquid vehicle (PEG200) were prepared. To measure the angle of slide, the prepared liquid/powder admixtures were placed on polished metal plates, the plate was then tilted gradually until the liquid/powder admixture was about to slide. The angle formed between the plate and the horizontal surface was defined as the angle of slide (h). The flow properties of excipients will be change due to adsorption of the liquid vehicle. The flowable liquid-retention potential (Φ values) of each liquid/powder admixture was calculated using the following equation.

Φ value=weight of liquid/weight of solid

The Φ -values for Avicel PH102 and Aerosil with PEG 200 were 0.007 and 3.26 respectively.

Determination of liquid load factor

Using the Φ –values the liquid load factor, Lf, was calculated according to equation

$$Lf = \Phi + \Phi \, (1/R)$$

The Lf values were used to calculate the required quantities of excipients.

Pre-compression studies of the liquisolid system
Flow properties of the Rosuvastatin liquisolid system

The flow properties of the liquisolid powder system are influenced by physical, mechanical as well as environmental factors. Therefore, different flow parameters were employed and results are depicted in Table 3. Batch F3 showed good flow properties with a θ value of 30.02 and was considered as the liquisolid system with acceptable flowability. Carr's index up to 16 was considered acceptable as a flow property. Hausner's ratio was related to the inter particle friction; powders with a low interparticle friction had a ratio of approximately 1.25 indicating a good flow. Batch F3 with a Carr's index of 12.10 and a Hausner's ratio of 1.17 was considered for further study for preparing batches of rosuvastatin liquisolid compacts.

Table 3. Flow properties of rosuvastatin liquisolid system

Batch	Tap density (gm/cm3)	Bulk density (gm/cm3)	Angle Of repose (θ)	Cars index	Hausner's ratio
F1	0.502±0.04	0.421±0.04	28.14±1.46	16.14±2.78	1.18±0.03
F2	0.472±0.01	0.410±0.009	29.14±1.03	14.12±1.59	1.16±0.02
F3	0.503±0.17	0.442±0.01	30.02±1.88	12.10±0.30	1.13±0.005
F4	0.456±0.02	0.390±0.042	30.10±2.30	16.25±0.791	1.16±0.05
F5	0.497±0.009	0.437±0.007	29.66±1.15	11.98±0.18	1.13±0.00
F6	0.417±0.009	0.379±0.007	30.94±0.554	11.29±1.55	1.12±0.023
F7	0.465±0.01	0.386±0.01	31.77±1.74	16.33±2.20	1.2±0.04
F8	0.620±0.03	0.516±0.02	32.85±0.39	16.33±0.62	1.19±0.01
F9	0.497±0.01	0.406±0.01	25.49±1.53	18.33±0.433	1.22±0.001

IR spectra analysis

The IR spectrum showing percentage transmission (T%) versus wave number of Rosuvastatin is shown in Figure 1 with characteristic peaks of aromatic N-H stretching and C=O stretching at 3316 cm-1 and 1600 cm-1, respectively. From the figure it was observed that functional group of rosuvastatin was retained in liquisolid compact, suggesting absence of chemical interaction with any of the excipients used in the preparation of liquisolid compacts.[10]

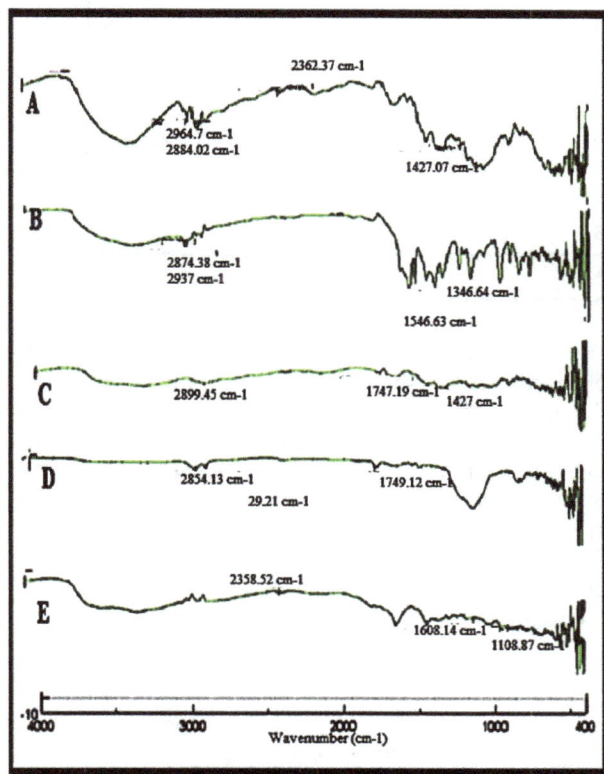

Figure 1. FTIR spectra A) Liquisolid formulation, F3 B) Rosuvastatin C) Avicel D) Aerosil E) Sodium starch glycolate.

X-ray powder diffraction (XRPD)

Powder X-RD is used to determine the crystallinity of compounds. Polymorphic changes of drug are important factor which might affect the dissolution rate and in turn bioavailability. Crystallinity of the drug and the liquisolid compacts samples was determined. The X-Ray Diffraction pattern (Figure 2) of pure drug (Rosuvastatin) showed sharp diffraction peaks at 2θ values of 16.04, 22.45, and 34.3 while liquisolid powder showed sharp peak at 2θ values of 19.87. The absence of characteristics peak in formulation indicated that drug had probably converted from crystalline to amorphous form.[10]

Differential scanning calorimetry (DSC)

The possible interactions between a drug entity and excipients in liquisolid compacts were determined by DSC. Figure 3 shows the thermal behavior of the pure components as well as of the final liquisolid system

prepared. The rosuvastatin peaks appeared clear, demonstrating a sharp characteristic endothermic peak at 125.38 °C (Figure 3A) corresponding to its melting temperature (Tm); such a sharp endothermic peak shows that the rosuvastatin used was in a pure crystalline state. On the other hand, the liquisolid system (Figure 3B) showed that the characteristic peaks of rosuvastatin had disappeared; this agrees with the formation of a solid solution in the liquisolid powdered system, *i.e.*, the drug was molecularly dispersed within the liquisolid matrix. That was accompanied by the formation of a new endothermic peak at 93.5.°C indicating the melting and decomposition of whole liquisolid system. This disappearance of drug peaks upon formulation into a liquisolid system was in agreement with McCauley and Brittain who declared that the complete suppression of all drug thermal features undoubtedly indicates the formation of an amorphous solid solution. In addition, Mura et al. found that the total disappearance of the drug melting peak indicates that drug amorphization had taken place.[10]

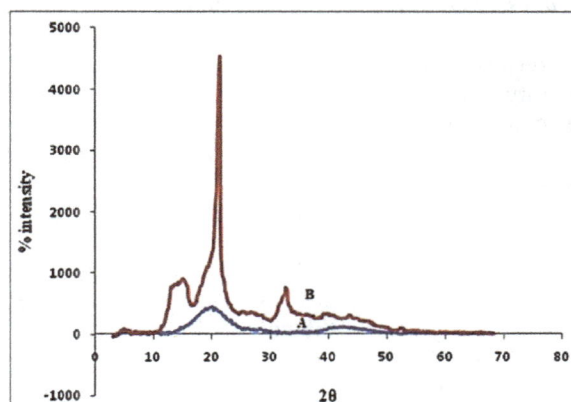

Figure 2. X-ray diffractograms of A) Liquisolid powder system (F3) and B) Pure drug, Rosuvastatin.

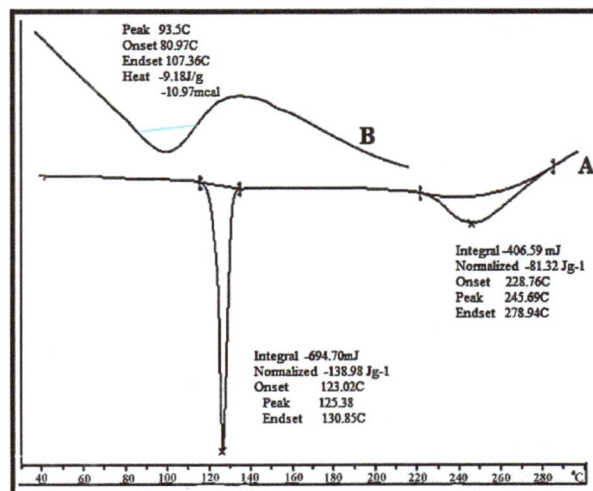

Figure 3. DSC thermogram of (A) Pure drug Rosuvastatin, (B) Liquisolid powder system (F3).

In vitro evaluation of liquisolid compacts

Rosuvastatin liquisolid compact content uniformity

A fundamental quality attribute for all pharmaceutical preparations is the requirement for a constant dose of drug between individual tablets. The percent drug content as shown in Table 4 varied from 90 to 97% w/w.

Table 4. Post compression evaluation of Rosuvastatin liquisolid tablets

Batch	Thickness (mm)	Hardness (kg/cm^2)	Weight variation (mg)	Friability	Disintegration time (sec)	Drug content (%)	FM
F1	3.02±0.01	4.20±0.24	151.45±0.95	0.095	175.00±0.63	96.66±1.31	0.771
F2	3.53±0.01	4.08±0.25	256.51±0.95	0.126	210.00±0.89	92.83±1.32	0.771
F3	3.45±0.01	4.00±0.15	363.64±0.85	0.274	143.33±0.81	96.66±1.31	0.771
F4	2.06±0.01	3.33±0.51	110.96±1.10	0.089	253.5±1.37	92.85±1.28	0.578
F5	3.42±0.01	4.00±0.44	363.62±0.91	0.072	307.0±0.89	96.66±1.31	0.578
F6	3.63±0.00	3.66±0.51	272.27±0.95	0.099	226.83±1.16	90.58±1.36	0.578
F7	3.00±0.02	3.5±0.44	187.25±1.19	0.094	354.66±0.81	90.58±1.36	0.462
F8	2.84±0.00	3.58±0.58	151.8±0.92	0.199	182.83±0.75	92.11±1.28	0.462
F9	2.65±0.01	4.00±0.31	216.20±0.44	0.168	254.66±1.03	95.13±1.32	0.462

*All readings are average ± SD (n=3)

Hardness, Friability, Weight variation, Disintegration test

The results of thickness, hardness, weight variation, friability, disintegration test and fraction of molecularly dispersed drug (FM)of liquisolid tablet are mentioned in Table 4. All the selected Rosuvastatin tablets had acceptable friability as none of the tested formulae had percentage loss in tablet weights that exceed 0.5%. Also none of the tablets was cracked, split or broken. The liquisolid tablet disintegrated in less than 5 minutes which is as per specifications given for the uncoated tablets in the IP. Uniform drug content was observed for all the formulation (90 to 100).

In vitro dissolution studies

The drug dissolution profile of the liquisolid compact, the directly compressed compacts and marketed tablet of rosuvastatin at different dissolution volume and medium was studied. Phosphate buffer pH 6.8, 900 ml, was used as the dissolution medium. As seen in Figure 4, liquisolid compacts (F3) showed better in-vitro release than those of the directly compressed tablet and marketed tablet. The liquisolid compacts contain a solution of the drug in PEG 200 which facilitates the wetting of drug particle by decreasing the interfacial tension between tablet and dissolution medium. The drug surface available for dissolution is tremendously increased. After disintegration, the liquisolid primary particles suspended in the dissolving medium contain the drug in a molecularly dispersed state, whereas the directly compressed compacts are merely exposed micronized drug particles. Therefore, in the case of liquisolid compacts, the surface area of drug available for dissolution is much greater than that of the directly compressed compacts. According to Noyes and Whitney, the drug dissolution rate (DR) is directly proportional to the concentration gradient (Cs-C) of the drug in the stagnant diffusion layer and its surface area (S) available for dissolution. The significantly increased surface area of the molecularly dispersed rosuvastatin in the liquisolid compacts may be principally responsible for their observed higher dissolution rates. The consistent and higher dissolution rate displayed by liquisolid compacts will improve the absorption of drug from the GI tract.

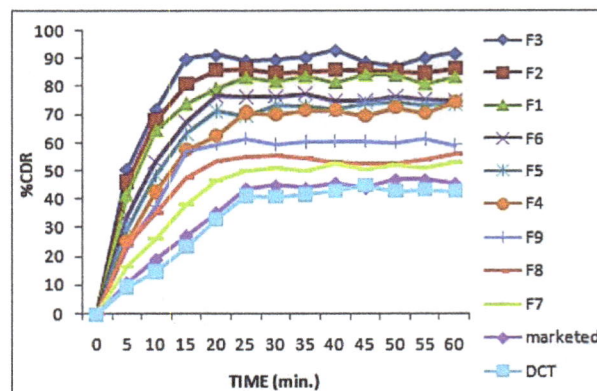

Figure 4. Dissolution profile of liquisolid, marketed and directly compressed tablet.

Effect of R Value on drug release from Rosuvastatin Liquisolid compacts: Spireas et al in their patent have stated that R value ranging from 10 to 30 gives optimal result. In the present study different drug concentrations in liquid medication were used between 15-25%. Further for each drug to non volatile solvent R value was varied from 10 to 30 and its *in vitro* drug release patterns were studied. The drug release followed the following pattern: $R_{30} > R_{20} > R_{10}$

Liquisolid compacts with lower R-values contain relatively smaller amounts of carrier powder and larger quantities of fine drug loaded silica particles. Also, the ratios of the amounts of their liquid medication per powder substrate are relatively higher. On the other hand, liquisolid compacts with higher R-values contain low liquid/powder ratios, high presence of cellulose and low presence of silica. This could be directly associated with enhanced wicking, disintegration and deaggregation properties. Therefore, the liquisolid tablets with low R-values showed relatively poor dissolution.

Effect of different drug concentrations in liquid medication on drug release: PEG 200 was selected as nonvolatile vehicle as the drug rosuvastatin showed maximum solubility in it. Concentrations of drug in liquid medication were varied from 15 to 25%. The drug release when compared suggested that 15% showed highest dissolution profile followed by 20 and there on . The drug release was high as higher fraction of drug was in solubilized or molecular state as compared to other concentrations.

Thus, formulations with smaller drug concentration (15%w/w) have a higher dissolution than higher drug concentration (25%w/w) in liquisolid tablets formulated with PEG 200. This can be explained by the dissolved drug in the liquid medication. The drug release follows the following pattern: F3 > F6 > F9

$$F_M = C_l / C_d \text{----------------------} (4)$$

Where FM is the fraction of molecularly dispersed or dissolved drug in liquid medication of the prepared liquisolid formulation, C_l is the saturation solubility of Rosuvastatin in the liquid vehicle and C_d is the concentration of the liquid. According to Spireas et al. F_M value cannot exceed unity. The saturation solubility of rosuvastatin in PEG 200 is 11.57 % w/w. By applying Equation 4, it was again seen that F_M value is not greater than 1 .

Effect of aging on tabletting properties
The optimized formulation was subjected to stability studies to evaluate any change in the formulation. Stability study of optimized formulation was performed under accelerated stability conditions at 40 °C ± 2 °C/75% RH ± 5% RH for three months. The hardness, drug content and dissolution rate were measured for the aged tablets. The results showed that there was no significant different between hardness of fresh (4Kg/Cm^2) and aged (4Kg/Cm^2) of the liquisolid tablets. Figure 5. too shows similar dissolution profiles between the fresh and aged formulation. This means that aging had no significant effect on drug release profile of rosuvastatin liquisolid tablets. The study concluded that the tested formulations are found to be stable.

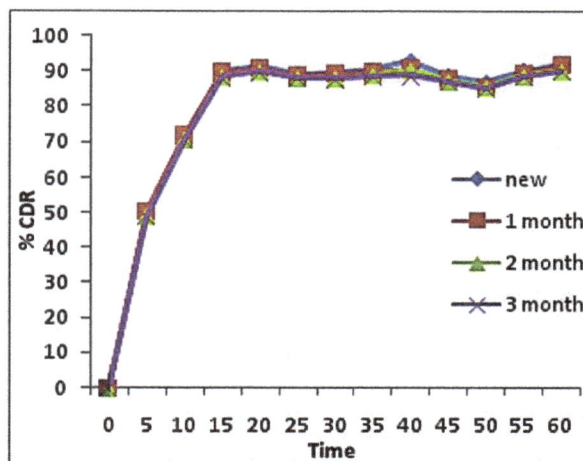

Figure 5. Disolution profile of F3 during Stability studies.

Conclusion
Rosuvastatin exhibits high permeability through biological membranes, but its absorption after oral administration is limited by its low dissolution rate due to its very low aqueous solubility. Hence, the use of the liquisolid technique was chosen to enhance the dissolution properties of rosuvastatin. The rosuvastatin liquisolid compacts were prepared using Avicel PH 102 and Aerosil 200 as the carrier and coating material, respectively. The P-XRD studies showed complete inhibition of crystallinity in the rosuvastatin liquisolid compacts. The DSC study confirmed the absence of any interaction between the drug and excipients used in the preparation of Rosuvastatin liquisolid compacts. The hardness, friability, weight variation and disintegration tests were within acceptable limits. The in vitro dissolution study confirmed enhanced drug release from liquisolid compacts compared with directly compressed tablet and marketed tablet. It was observed that aging had no significant effect on the hardness, disintegration time and dissolution profile of the liquisolid compacts.

Acknowledgements
The authors are thankful to Maple Biotech Pvt. Ltd. Bhosari Pune for providing gift samples of the polymers and Biocon Pharma Bangalore for providing gift sample of the rosuvastatin.

Conflict of Interest
The authors declare that they have no conflict of interest.

References
1. Vemula VR, Lagishetty V, Lingala S. Solubility enhancement techniques. *Int J Pharm Sci Rev Res* 2010;5(1):41-51.
2. Akbari BV, Valaki BP, Mardiya VH, Akbari AK, Vidyasagar G. Enhancement of solubility and dissolution rate of rosuvastatin calcium by complexation with β cyclodextrin. *Int J Pharm Biol Arch* 2011;2(1):511-20.

3. Nainwal P, Sinha P, Singh A, Nanda D, Jain DA, Bhoomi D. A comparative solubility enhancement study of rosuvastatin using solubilization technique. *Int J Appl Biol Pharm Technol* 2011;2(4):14-8

4. Fahmy RH, Kassem MA. Enhancement of Loratidine dissolution rate through liquisolid tablets formulation: in vitro and in vivo evaluation. *Eur J Pharm Biopharm* 2008;69(3):993-1003.

5. Spireas S, Sadu S. Enhancement of prednisolone dissolution properties using liquisolid compacts. *Int J Pharm* 1998;166(2):177-88.

6. Spireas S, Wang T, Grover R. Effect of powder substrate on the dissolution properties of methyclothiazide liquisolid compacts. *Drug Dev Ind Pharm* 1999;25(2):163-8.

7. Karmarkar AB, Gonjari ID, Hosmani AH, Dhabale PN, Bhise SB. Dissolution rate enhancement of fenofibrate using liquisolid tablet technique. Part II: Evaluation of in vitro dissolution profile comparison methods. *Lat Am J Pharm* 2009;28(4):538-43.

8. Nokhodchi A, Javadzadeh Y, Siahi-Shadbad MR, Barzegar-Jalali M. The effect of type and concentration of vehicles on the dissolution rate of a poorly soluble drug (indomethacin) from liquisolid compacts. *J Pharm Pharm Sci* 2005;8(1):18-25.

9. Khaled KA. Formulation and evaluation of hydrochlorothiazide liquisolid tablets. *Saudi Pharm J* 1998;6(1):39-46.

10. Gubbi SR, Jarag R. Formulation and characterization of atorvastatin calcium liquisolid compacts. *Asian J Pharm Sci* 2010;5(2):50-60.

11. Burra S, Kudikala S, Reddy GJ. Formulation and evaluation of Simvastatin liquisolid tablets. *Der Pharmacia Lettre* 2011;3(2):419-26.

12. Javadzadeh Y, Navimipour B, Nokhodchi A. Liquisolid technique for dissolution rate of piroxicam using liquisolid compact. *Int J Pharm* 2005;(60):361-5.

13. Singh SK, Srinivasan KK, Gowthamarajan K, Prakash D, Gaikwad NB, Singare DS. Influence of formulation parameters on dissolution rate enhancement of glyburide using liquisolid technique. *Drug Dev Ind Pharm* 2012;38(8):961-70.

14. Gavali SM, Pacharane SS, Sankpal SV, Jadhav KR, Kadam VJ. Liquisolid compact: A new technique for enhancement of drug dissolution. *Int J Res Pharm Chem* 2011;1(3):705-13.

15. Vaskula S, Vemula SK, Bontha VK, Garrepally P. Liquisolid Compacts: An Approach to Enhance the Dissolution Rate of Nimesulide. *J Appl Pharm Sci* 2012;2(5):115-21.

16. Tiong N, Elkordy AA. Effects of liquisolid formulations on dissolution of naproxen. *Eur J Pharm Biopharm* 2009;73(3):373-84.

17. Ansel HC, Allen LV, Popovich NG. Pharmaceutical dosage forms and drug delivery systems. Philadelphia: Lippincott williams and wilkins; 1999.

18. United States Pharmacopeia and National Formulary. 29th ed. Rockville, MD, USA: United States Pharmacopeial Convention; 2006.

24

Synthesis, Characterization and Antioxidant Property of Quercetin-Tb(III) Complex

Jafar Ezzati Nazhad Dolatabadi[1], Ahad Mokhtarzadeh[2], Seyed Morteza Ghareghoran[1], Gholamreza Dehghan[3]*

[1] *Research Center for Pharmaceutical Nanotechnology, Tabriz University of Medical Sciences, Tabriz, Iran.*

[2] *Faculty of Pharmacy, Mashhad University of Medical Sciences, Mashhad, Iran.*

[3] *Department of Plant Biology, Faculty of Natural Science, University of Tabriz, Tabriz, Iran.*

ARTICLE INFO

Keywords:
Flavonoid
Antioxidant
Quercetin–Tb(III) complex
DPPH
FRAP
ABTS

ABSTRACT

Purpose: Nearly all of flavonoids are good metal chelators and can chelate many metal ions to form different complexes. This article describes a synthesis of Quercetin–Tb(III) in methanol, characterized by using elemental analysis, UV–visible and evaluation of its antioxidant properties.

Methods: The formation of complexes is realized from the UV–visible spectra which shows that the successive formation of Quercetin–Tb(III) occurs. To find out the antioxidant activity variation and the role of Tb(III) ion on the antioxidant activity of the complexes different radical scavenging methods such as: 1,1-diphenyl-2-picrylhydrazyl (DPPH), ferric reducing antioxidant power (FRAP) and 2,2′-azinobis 3-ethylbenzothiazoline-6-sulphonic acid (ABTS) were used.

Results: The results from DPPH, ABTS and FRAP methods showed that Quercetin and Quercetin–Tb(III) complex are capable of donating electron or hydrogen atom, and consequently could react with free radicals or terminate chain reactions in a time- and dose-dependent manner.

Conclusion: This study showed that the chelation of metal ions by Quercetin decrease the redox potential of Quercetin-metal complex.

Introduction

Flavonoids are antioxidants, which are recognized to affect bio-availability of the metal in the body. They have a basic structure of 2-phenyl-benzo-γ-pyrones, frequently polyphenolic in nature. A large number of substitution patterns in the two benzene rings (A and B) of the basic structure occur in nature. Variations in their heterocyclic rings give rise to flavonols, flavones, catechins, flavanones, anthocyanidins and isoflavones.[1-4] Flavonoids, and particularly quercetin derivatives, have received more attention as dietary constituents during the last few years. Experimental studies showed that they have frequent beneficial effects on human health, including cardiovascular protection, anticancer activity, antiulcer effects, and antiallergic, antiviral, and anti-inflammatory properties. These health-promoting activities seem to be related to the natural antioxidant (free-radical scavenging) activity of flavonoids.[2]

Reactive oxygen species (ROS) induce oxidative damage to biomolecules and organelles, and then lead to many diseases like Parkinson's disease, heart disease, and cancer. Researches demonstrated that exogenous antioxidants or free radical scavengers can scavenge the excess free radicals and be benefic to those diseases effectively. Thus, evaluating and developing novel antioxidant is becoming one of the noteworthy topics recently.[2,5] Most of flavonoids are strong metal chelators which can chelate many metal ions to form different complexes. Those complexes are reported to have various important biological activities, and most of them exhibit higher antioxidant abilities than the ligand flavonoids. However, the antioxidant mechanism of the complexes has not been exactly elucidated so far.[5,6] The aim of this study, was to compare the efficiency of DPPH, FRAP and ABTS assays to estimate antioxidant activities of Quercetin–Tb(III) complex and to find the role of Tb(III) ion on the antioxidant activity of Quercetin.

Materials and Methods
Chemical and Materials
All reagents used for experiments were analytical reagent grade. Extra pure methanol was purchased from Scharlau chemical company. Quercetin and DPPH (2,2-diphenyl-1-picrylhydrazyl) was purchased from Sigma. The standard solutions at 1.0×10^{-3} M concentration of antioxidant compounds were all prepared in 100% MeOH. All working solutions of antioxidant compounds were freshly prepared.

Corresponding author: Gholamreza Dehghan, Department of Plant Biology, Faculty of Natural Science, University of Tabriz, Tabriz, Iran. Email: gdehghan@tabrizu.ac.ir

Instrumentation

Spectroscopic study of Quercetin and its metal complex was performed using analytic jena UV-visible spectrophotometer specord 40 for obtaining UV spectra.

Synthesis of the complex

The synthesis of the Quercetin–Tb(III) complex had been carried out according to our previous work.[6] Briefly, in a 50-cm^3 two-necked round-bottomed flask equipped with an electromagnetic stirrer and thermometer, quercetin·2H$_2$O (0.05 g, 0.008 mol) dissolved in MeOH (20 ml) within 15 min, the color of the solution was light yellow. Consequently, TbCl$_3$.6H$_2$O (0.12 g, 0.016mol) was added quickly in the reaction mixture, now the color of the solution was brownish yellow and the solution was stirred at room temp for 4 h. After stirring the reaction mixture was filtered, and the filtrate was evaporated slowly at room temperature. The resulting dark brownish yellow product was washed with t-butanol and dried in a vacuum desiccator. A brownish yellow product, Quercetin–Tb(III) complex, was obtained in 82% yield.[2,6-8]

Antioxidant activity of the complex by DPPH method

Free radical scavenging capacity of the complex was determined by previously reported procedure using the stable 2,2-diphenyl-1-picrylhydrazylradical (DPPH•).[1,9] Methanol solution (0.1 ml) containing different concentrations of standards (0, 5, 10, 15, 20, 25 μmol) was added to 1.95 ml of freshly prepared (57.65μmol) DPPH in methanol. The reduction of the DPPH was followed by monitoring the decrease in absorbance at 517 nm in each 5 min for about 25 min (A_S). As a control, the absorbance of blank solution of DPPH (2 ml) was also determined at 515 nm (A_C). The following equation has been used for the calculation of the percentage of radical scavenging activity (RSA%):[1,9]

$$RSA \% = \frac{100\ (AC - AS)}{AC}$$

FRAP assay of total antioxidant capacity

FRAP assay was carried out by the method of Benzie and Strain with minor modifications. The method is based on the reduction of a ferric 2,4,6-tripyridyl-s triazine complex (Fe^{3+}-TPTZ) by antioxidants to the ferrous form (Fe^{2+}-TPTZ). FRAP reagent was prepared freshly by mixing 2.5 ml of solutions TPTZ (10 mM, dissolved in 40 mM HCl) and FeCl$_3$ (20 mM) in 25 ml of acetate buffer (300 mM concentration and pH 3.6), the light blue reagent contains Fe^{3+}–TPTZ that changes to dark blue after interaction with antioxidants, which is clarified by the presence of Fe^{2+}–TPTZ in the reagent. These changes were due to the absorbance increase as monitored at a wavelength of 593 nm for different concentrations (5, 10, 15, 20 and 25 mM) of the Quercetin and Quercetin–Tb(III) complex in FRAP reagent. The standard calibration curve obtained by using different concentrations of FeSO$_4$·7H$_2$O as standard for calculation of the FRAP values for both Quercetin and complex.[9]

ABTS radical scavenging activity of Quercetin and Quercetin–Tb(III) complex

ABTS radical scavenging activity was based on the method of Dehghan et al. Briefly, 54.2 mg of ABTS powder was dissolved in 10 ml of phosphate buffer (5 mM, pH 7.0) and then mixed with 1 g of MnO$_2$ and incubated in room temperature within 30 min for generation of green colored ABTS$^+$. After that the prepared solution was centrifuged for 5 min and after filtration; the filtrate was diluted with phosphate buffer until the absorbance of solution equals with 0.70 ± 0.01 in 734 nm. Different concentrations (0–12.5 μM) of Quercetin and its Quercetin–Tb(III) complex were mixed with 2 ml of ABTS solution and incubated for 10 min at room temperature. The decrease of absorbance was monitored at 734 nm after 10 min.[9]

Results

Interaction of quercetin with Tb(III)

The changes in UV–vis absorption of Quercetin in the presence of Tb(III) were examined in the methanol solution. The UV–vis spectra of Quercetin showed an intense absorbance at 280 and 372 nm. When the solution of Tb(III) was added, decrease in absorption observed. The results indicated formation of a complex between Quercetin and Tb(III) (Figure 1).[1,6,10]

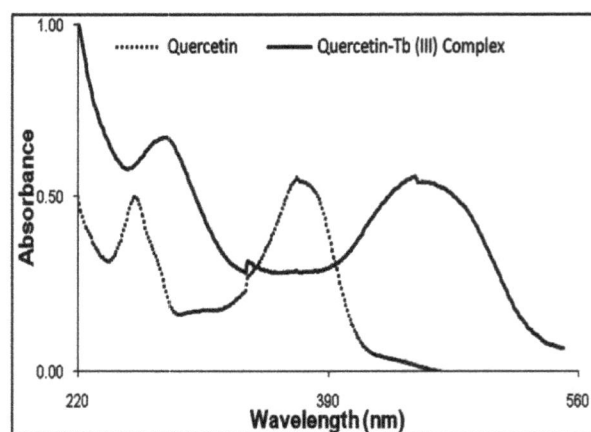

Figure 1. UV-vis spectrum of Quercetin and Quercetin-Tb (III) complex in methanol.

DPPH radical scavenging analysis

The results of DPPH radical scavenging analysis can be seen in Figure 2. Quercetin and Quercetin–Tb(III) complex can scavenge DPPH radical effectively. The scavenging activity of Quercetin–Tb(III) complex is obviously less than that of Quercetin, indicating that this complex is a much weaker free radical scavenger and antioxidant than Quercetin.[1,10] Radical scavenging activity of Quercetin was increased in a dose- and time-dependent manner, at the same time, antioxidant ability of Quercetin decreased after chelation of stannous cation (Figure 3). The antioxidant activity of flavonoids was owing to their molecular structure. The higher antioxidant activity of Quercetin may be because of the highly contribution of the 3', 4' hydroxyl groups on the B-ring. Besides, it may be supposed that 3', 4' hydroxyl groups are mainly involved in H-atom transfer reactions to DPPH.

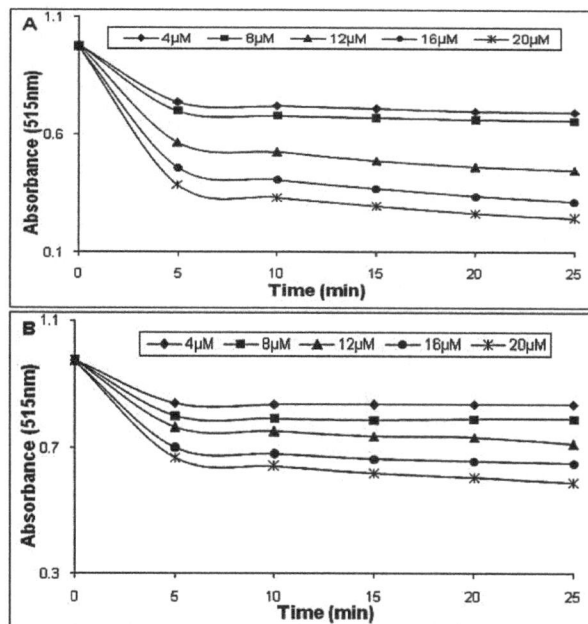

Figure 2. Decrease in absorbance at (λ=517 nm) of DPPH methanol solution in the presence of different concentrations of (A) Quercetin and (B) Quercetin-Tb (III) complex (0–20μM).

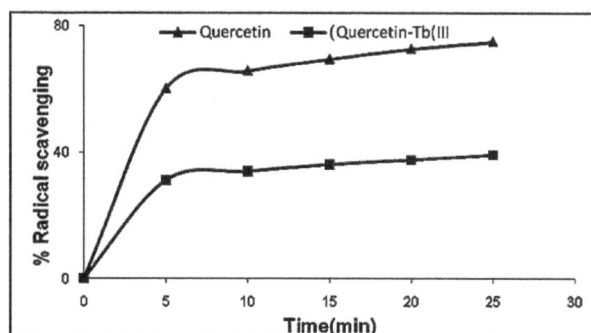

Figure 3. Dependence of the ligand Quercetin and Quercetin-Tb(III) complex concentration in the DPPH, scavenging activities evaluated through the absorbance decrease at 517 nm caused by the addition of Quercetin and Quercetin-Tb (III) complex.

Ferric reducing antioxidant power of Quercetin and Quercetin–Tb(III) complex

Antioxidants may exert their protective effects by reduction of metal ions and therefore influencing the oxidative stress caused by these metal ions. This reduced ability can be assessed for antioxidants such as flavonoids according to the FRAP method. The ability of antioxidants to reduce Fe^{3+} to Fe^{2+} in the presence of TPTZ and forming an intense blue Fe^{2+}–TPTZ complex

with an absorption maximum at 593 nm is the basic theory of the FRAP assay. The absorbance increase is proportional to the antioxidant content. Herein, the FRAP results for the Quercetin and Quercetin–Tb(III) complex were measured via absorbance variations during 10 min of interaction of subjected compounds with FRAP reagent and the relevant data are shown in Figure 3, which again confirm the decline of antioxidant power of the resultant complex in comparison with free Quercetin. These findings propose that Quercetin and Quercetin–Tb(III) complex are capable of donating electrons, and could therefore react with free radicals or terminate chain reactions, whereas metal chelation reduces electron transfer from Quercetin after complex formation. It is reasonable that the chelation of metal ions by Quercetin decreases the redox potential of metal-Quercetin complex.[9]

ABTS radical scavenger activity of Quercetin and Quercetin–Tb(III) complex

For confirming the anti-radical potential of the synthesized complex, we used the ABTS assay as well. The effect of Quercetin and Quercetin–Tb(III) complex on ABTS radical is shown in Figure 4. Absorption of active ABTS solution at 734 nm obviously decreased in the presence of different concentrations of both Quercetin and Quercetin–Tb(III) complex (Figure 5). While, similar to previous methods, radical scavenging activity of free Quercetin was better than Quercetin–Tb(III) complex.

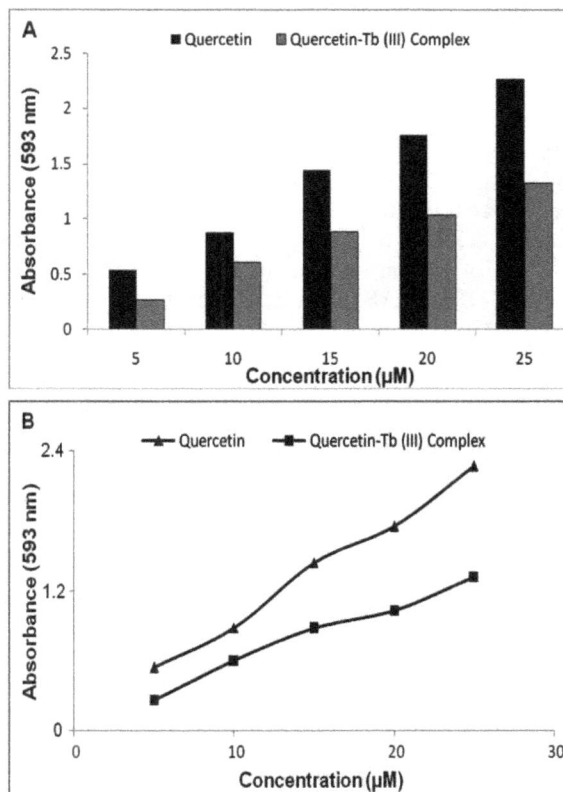

Figure 4. Time dependent ferric reducing antioxidant power (mmolFe^{2+}/L) of Quercetin and the Quercetin-Tb (III) complex.

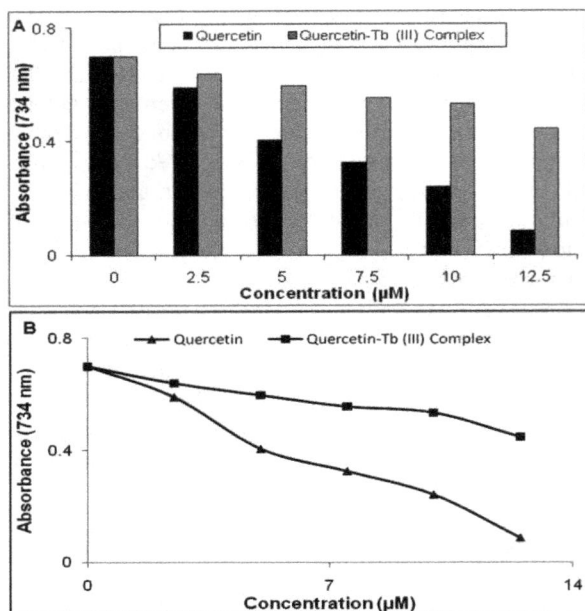

Figure 5. Decrease in absorbance at (λ=734 nm) of ABTS at different concentrations of Quercetin and the Quercetin-Tb (III) complex.

Discussion

Antioxidant property of various flavonoids is more considerably related to their molecular structure. Hydrogen atom transferring and electron donation are two major mechanisms through which phenolic compounds can exert their antioxidative functions. Pure Quercetin showed more antioxidant activity in comparison with the Quercetin–Tb(III) complex. The higher antioxidant activity of the Quercetin may be due to the considerable contribution of the hydroxyl groups that their hydrogens are replaced by Tb (III), therefore decreasing their ability for hydrogen donation or radical scavenging of Quercetin.

It can be concluded that a radical inhibitory and metal reducing activity of Quercetin was decreased after chelation of cation, taking into consideration three methods: DPPH, ABTS radical scavenging activities and FRAPS assays. Therefore, this study proposed that metal ions significantly alter the chemical properties of Quercetin and influence its antioxidant activity. Also the results arisen from DPPH, FRAP and ABTS assays showed that Quercetin and Quercetin–Tb(III) complex can scavenge free radicals or reduce Fe^{3+} in a concentration- and time- dependent manner.

Conclusion

The complex of Tb(III) with Quercetin was prepared and characterised by several spectroscopic techniques. Using UV–vis the coordination to the carbonyl group of the ligand and one of the adjacent hydroxyl groups is assumed. Spectroscopic data suggest that Quercetin molecule can chelate lanthanide cations such as Tb from both 3-hydroxy-carbonyl and the 3', 4'-dihydroxyl (catechol) chelation sites. The results from DPPH, ABTS and FRAP methods demonstrated that Quercetin

and Quercetin–Tb(III) complex are capable of donating electron or hydrogen atom, and consequently could react with free radicals or terminate chain reactions in a time- and dose-dependent manner. The results of this study showed that the chelation of metal ions by Quercetin decrease the redox potential of Quercetin-metal complex and the metal ions Tb(III) considerably change the chemical properties of the Quercetin.

Acknowledgments
The Authors are grateful for financial support from the Research Center for Pharmaceutical Nanotechnology, Tabriz University of Medical Sciences and University of Tabriz.

Conflict of Interest
The authors report no conflicts of interest.

References
1. Bukhari SB, Memon S, Mahroof-Tahir M, Bhanger MI. Synthesis, characterization and antioxidant activity copper-quercetin complex. *Spectrochim Acta A Mol Biomol Spectrosc* 2009;71(5):1901-6.
2. Ahmadi SM, Dehghan G, Hosseinpourfeizi MA, Dolatabadi JE, Kashanian S. Preparation, characterization, and DNA binding studies of water-soluble quercetin--molybdenum(VI) complex. *DNA Cell Biol* 2011;30(7):517-23.
3. Jamali A, Tavakoli A, Ezzati Nazhad Dolatabadi J. Analytical overview of DNA interaction with Morin and its metal complexes. *Eur Food Res Technol* 2012;235:367-73.
4. Hu YJ, Yue HL, Li XL, Zhang SS, Tang E, Zhang LP. Molecular spectroscopic studies on the interaction of morin with bovine serum albumin. *J Photochem Photobiol B* 2012;112:16-22.
5. Chen WJ, Sun SF, Cao W, Liang Y, Song JR. Antioxidant property of quercetin-Cr(III) complex: The role of Cr(III) ion. *J Mol Struct* 2009;918:194-7.
6. Dehghan G, Dolatabadi JE, Jouyban A, Zeynali KA, Ahmadi SM, Kashanian S. Spectroscopic studies on the interaction of quercetin-terbium(III) complex with calf thymus DNA. *DNA Cell Biol* 2011;30(3):195-201.
7. Xie WL, Yang PH, Cai JY. Synthesis, Characterization and Antioxidation Activity of Germanim(IV)-Quercetin Complex. *Chinese J Anal Chem* 2010;38:1809-12.
8. Cornard JP, Merlin JC. Spectroscopic and structural study of complexes of quercetin with Al(III). *J Inorg Biochem* 2002;92(1):19-27.
9. Dehghan G, Khoshkam Z. Tin(II)-quercetin complex: Synthesis, spectral characterisation and antioxidant activity. *Food Chem* 2012;131:422-6.
10. Zhang GW, Guo JB, Pan JH, Chen XX, Wang JJ. Spectroscopic studies on the interaction of morin-Eu(III) complex with calf thymus DNA. *J Mol Struct* 2009;923(1-3):114-9.

Modifications to the Conventional Nanoprecipitation Technique: an Approach to Fabricate Narrow Sized Polymeric Nanoparticles

Moorthi Chidambaram*, Kathiresan Krishnasamy

Department of Pharmacy, Annamalai University, Chidambaram, Tamil Nadu, India.

ARTICLE INFO

Keywords:
Nanoparticles
Polymeric Nanoparticles
Nanoprecipitation Method
Eudragit E 100

ABSTRACT

Purpose: Nanoprecipitation is the convenient and commonly used method for the preparation of polymeric nanoparticles around 170 nm but yield particles with broad distribution, which require filtration step to produce particles with narrow distribution. Hence, the primary aim of the present study was to implement few modifications to the conventional nanoprecipitation method to reduce the mean particle size less than 150 nm and to produce particles with narrow distribution without filtration step.

Methods: Eudragit E 100 nanoparticles were prepared using modified nanoprecipitation method 1 and 2. Prepared nanoparticles were characterized for the mean particle size, surface area and uniformity.

Results: Eudragit E 100 nanoparticles prepared using modified nanoprecipitation method 1 has shown a mean particle size of 196 nm with surface area of 50.9 m^2g^{-1} and uniformity of 0.852 whereas, Eudragit E 100 nanoparticles prepared using modified nanoprecipitation method 2 has shown a mean particle size of 114 nm with surface area of 57.9 m^2g^{-1} and uniformity of 0.259.

Conclusion: Modification to the conventional nanoprecipitation method (method 2) has produced mean particle size less than 150 nm and produced nanoparticles with narrow distribution without filtration step.

Introduction

Nanotechnology is a branch of science that deals with engineering particles on a near atomic scale with at least one dimension between 1-100 nanometer (nm). Manipulation of particle size below 100 nm significantly increases the particle surface area and alters the physicochemical properties of the size reduced compound, which offers significant improvement in various fields including automotive, construction, electronics, textiles, sports, military, energy, and medicine. Nanotherapeutics is a rapidly progressing area in the field of nanomedicine, which is being utilized to overcome several limitations of conventional drug including poor aqueous solubility, lack of site specific targeting, rapid systemic clearance, intestinal metabolism and systemic toxicities. Nanotherapeutics includes but not limited to solid-lipid nanoparticles, gold nanoparticles, silver nanoparticles, mesoporous silica nanoparticles, nanocrystals, magnetic nanoparticles, carbon nanotubes, nanosponges, albumin nanoparticles, fullerene nanoparticles and polymeric nanoparticles.[1-4] However, polymeric nanoparticles offer potential advantages such as enhancement of solubility, protection of encapsulated drug, improvement in the bio-distribution, offer sustain release of the drug, reduces the number of required dose, reduces the systemic toxicities,

targets the drug to specific site, increases the intercellular concentration of drug by enhanced permeability and retention effect.[5-7] Polymeric nanoparticles can be prepared using solvent evaporation method, salting-out method, nanoprecipitation method, emulsion diffusion method, dialysis method, double emulsification method, nano spray drying method, layer by layer method, desolvation method, supercritical fluid technology and ionic gelation method.[8,9] Particle size of the prepared polymeric nanoparticles decides the performance such as solubility, dissolution, drug release, cellular uptake, circulation half-life, and bio-distribution. Similarly, uniformity of the prepared polymeric nanoparticles is the most significant parameter that decides the consistency of performance. Particles with broad distribution leads to difficulty in establishing the conclusion on which sized particles are responsible for the biological effects.[6] Based on these two parameters, nanoprecipitation is the most convenient and widely used method to prepare polymeric nanoparticles around 170 nm but yield particles with broad distribution and requires additional filtration step to yield particles with narrow distribution.[10] Hence, we intend to implement few modifications to the conventional nanoprecipitation method to reduce the mean particle size less than 150 nm

*Corresponding author: Moorthi Chidambaram, Department of Pharmacy, Annamalai University, Chidambaram, Tamil Nadu, India. Email: cmoorthitgodu@gmail.com

and to produce particles with narrow distribution without filtration step.

Materials and Methods

Cationic copolymer Eudragit E 100 was obtained from Degussa (India). Poloxamer 188 was procured from Sigma Aldrich (India). Analytical grade ethanol was purchased from Brampton (Canada).

Fabrication of Eudragit E 100 nanoparticles using modified nanoprecipitation method

In conventional nanoprecipitation method, polymer was dissolved in acetone, which was poured in to distilled water containing poloxamer 188 with moderate stirring and the prepared nanosuspension was subjected to filtration to yield narrow sized particle.[10] However, Eudragit E 100 nanoparticles were prepared using modified nanoprecipitation method 1 and modified nanoprecipitation method 2, which were described in subsequent section.

Modified nanoprecipitation method 1

Briefly, about 250 mg of cationic copolymer Eudragit E 100 was dissolved in 6 mL of ethanol, which was diluted with 4 mL of distilled water under the influence of sonication (40 kHz, Lark, India). Prepared organic phase was loaded in to a syringe equipped with needle (with inner diameter of 0.30 x 8 mm). The loaded organic phase was injected at the rate of 2 mL per minute by inserting the needle (submerged position) in to 20 mL of aqueous phase containing 250 mg of poloxamer 188 under the influence of sonication (40 kHz, Lark, India). Subsequently, nanoparticles were formed and turned the aqueous phase slightly milky with bluish opalescence. However, sonication process was continued up to 60 minutes to aid size reduction and to evaporate residual solvent present in the nanoformulation.

Modified nanoprecipitation method 2

Briefly, about 250 mg of cationic copolymer Eudragit E 100 was dissolved in 6 mL of ethanol, which was diluted with 4 mL of distilled water under the influence of sonication (40 kHz, Lark, India). Prepared organic phase was added at once in to 20 mL of aqueous phase containing 250 mg of poloxamer 188 under sonication (40 kHz, Lark, India). Subsequently, nanoparticles were formed and turned the aqueous phase slightly milky with bluish opalescence. However, sonication process was continued up to 60 minutes to aid size reduction and to evaporate residual solvent present in the nanoformulation.

Characterization of prepared Eudragit E 100 nanoparticles

Prepared Eudragit E 100 nanoparticles were characterized for mean particle size, surface area and uniformity using Mastersizer (Malvern Instruments, UK), which function based on Mie and Fraunhofer laser light scattering principle.

Statistical analysis

Student t test (GraphPad Prism V5.04) was used to evaluate the significance of difference between modified nanoprecipitation method 1 and 2. Any difference between method 1 and 2 were evaluated at confidence levels 90%, 95% and 99%.

Results and Discussion

In nanoprecipitation method, addition of organic phase containing cationic copolymer Eudragit E 100 in to the aqueous phase containing poloxamer 188 results in rapid miscibility of ethanol in the distilled water leading to increase in the polarity of ethanol, which decreases the solubility of Eudragit E 100 and initiate the nucleation. Concurrently, sonication process produce bubble which oscillate non-linearly and finally collapse resulting in production of high temperature, pressure and shock waves, which not only inhibit the nucleation of Eudragit E 100 at the initial stage but also helps in evaporation of residual organic solvent present in nanosuspension. Cationic nature of Eudragit E 100 provides higher positive zeta potential to the prepared nanoparticles, which generates an electrostatic force and maintains the nanoparticles in Brownian motion. Additionally, particles in Brownian motion can effectively overcomes the Van der Waals force of attraction and gravitational force, which in turn prevent the aggregation and sedimentation of Eudragit E 100 nanoparticles.[6,11,12]

In conventional nanoprecipitation method, Poly(lactic-co-glycolic acid) (PLGA) nanoparticles were prepared as follows. 15 mg of PLGA was dissolved in 5 ml of acetone, which was poured in to 15 mL of distilled water containing 75 mg of poloxamer 188 with moderate stirring. Prepared PLGA nanosuspension was filtered using 1.0 μm cellulose nitrate membrane filter to yield narrow sized particle. Prepared PLGA nanoparticles were in the size range of 160 nm to 170 nm and uniformity were around 0.2 after filtration.[10]

However, we have implemented few modifications to the conventional nanoprecipitation method (which has been described in modified nanoprecipitation method 1 and 2) and prepared Eudragit E 100 nanoparticles were characterized for particle size, surface area and uniformity (Table 1, Figure 1 and 2).

Out of two modified nanoprecipitation methods, Eudragit E 100 nanoparticles prepared using modified nanoprecipitation method 2 has shown significantly much lesser mean particle size (114 nm) and uniformity (0.259) than the modified nanoprecipitation method 1. Moreover, modified nanoprecipitation method 2 has produced much lesser mean particle size and comparable uniformity than the conventional nanoprecipitation method without filtration step.

Conclusion

Modification to the conventional nanoprecipitation method (method 2) has produced mean particle size less than 150 nm and produced nanoparticles with narrow distribution without filtration step. Hence, the proposed modification (method 2) to the conventional nanoprecipitation method can be utilized to fabricate least mean particle size and highly narrow sized polymeric nanoparticles.

Table 1. Characterization of Eudragit E 100 nanoparticles prepared using modified nanoprecipitation methods

Method	Distribution Width (nm)			Mean Particle Size (nm)	Surface Area (m²g⁻¹)	Uniformity
	d 10	d 50	d 90			
Method 1	74±1.0	123±2.0*	226±3.0*	196±2.0*	50.9±0.7*	0.852±0.011*
Method 2	73±0.0	108±0.0	162±0.0	114±0.0	57.7±0.0	0.259±0.000

* P<0.10, P<0.05, P<0.01 as compared to Method 2

Concentration: 0.2147 %Vol   Span: 1.235   Uniformity: 0.852   Result units: Volume
Specific Surface Area: 50.9 m²/g   Surface Weighted Mean D[3,2]: 0.118 um   Vol. Weighted Mean D[4,3]: 0.196 um
d(0.1): 0.074 um   d(0.5): 0.123 um   d(0.9): 0.226 um

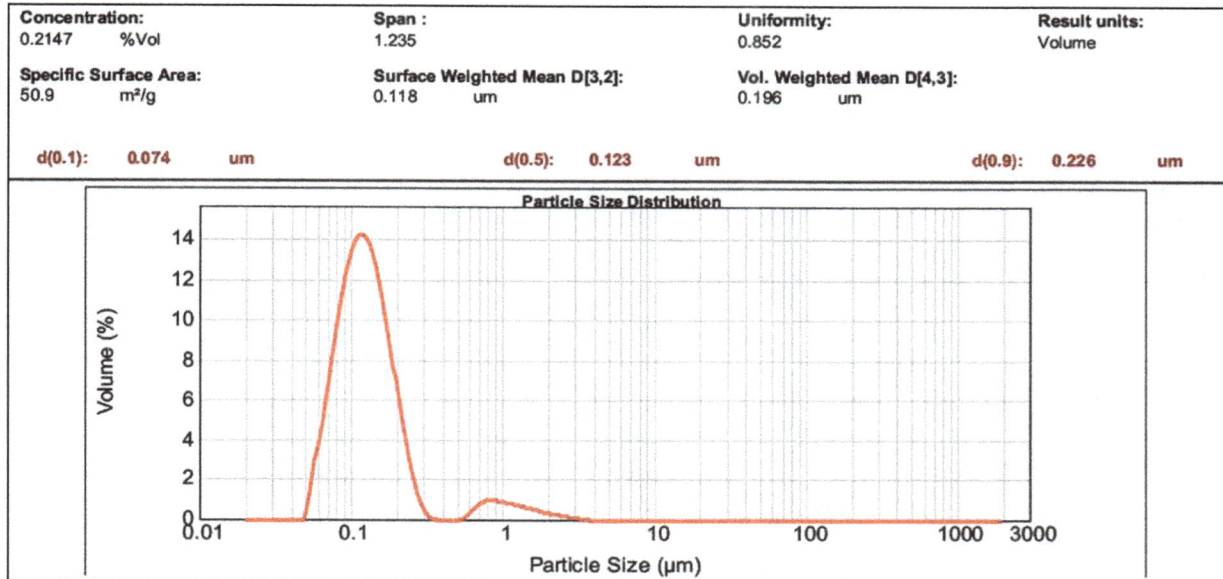

Figure 1. Characterization of Eudragit E 100 nanoparticles prepared using modified nanoprecipitation method 1.

Concentration: 0.6980 %Vol   Span: 0.821   Uniformity: 0.259   Result units: Volume
Specific Surface Area: 57.7 m²/g   Surface Weighted Mean D[3,2]: 0.104 um   Vol. Weighted Mean D[4,3]: 0.114 um
d(0.1): 0.073 um   d(0.5): 0.108 um   d(0.9): 0.162 um

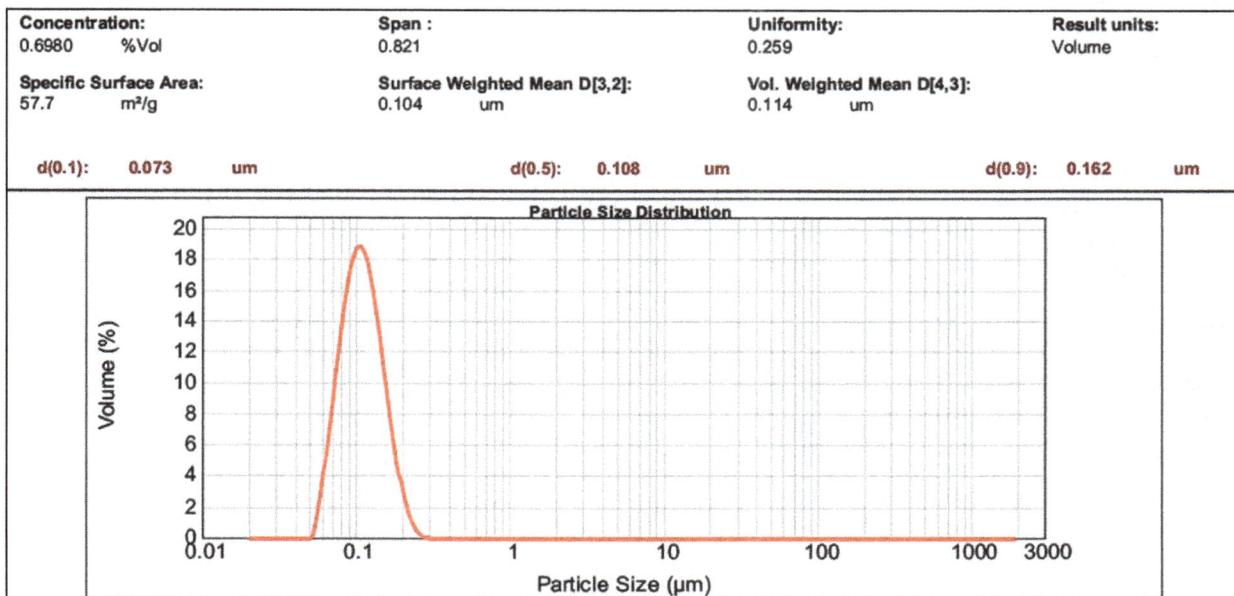

Figure 2. Characterization of Eudragit E 100 nanoparticles prepared using modified nanoprecipitation method 2.

Conflict of Interest
The authors declare that they have no conflict of interest.

References
1. Chidambaram M, Manavalan R, Kathiresan K. Nanotherapeutics to overcome conventional cancer

chemotherapy limitations. *J Pharm Pharm Sci* 2011;14(1):67-77.

2. Moorthi C, Kathiresan K. Nanotoxicology: Toxicity of engineered nanoparticles and approaches to produce safer nanotherapeutics. *Int J Pharm Sci* 2012;2(4):117-24.

3. Kesisoglou F, Panmai S, Wu Y. Nanosizing--oral formulation development and biopharmaceutical evaluation. *Adv Drug Deliv Rev* 2007;59(7):631-44.

4. Moorthi C, Kathiresan K. Curcumin–Piperine/Curcumin–Quercetin/Curcumin–Silibinin dual drug-loaded nanoparticulate combination therapy: A novel approach to target and treat multidrug-resistant cancers. *J Med Hypotheses Ideas* 2013;7(1):15-20.

5. Gelperina S, Kisich K, Iseman MD, Heifets L. The potential advantages of nanoparticle drug delivery systems in chemotherapy of tuberculosis. *Am J Respir Crit Care Med* 2005;172(12):1487-90.

6. Moorthi C, Kathiresan K. Application of Plackett-Burman factorial design in the development of curcumin loaded Eudragit E 100 nanoparticles. *Nano Biomed Eng* 2013;5(1):28-33.

7. De Jong WH, Borm PJ. Drug delivery and nanoparticles:applications and hazards. *Int J Nanomedicine* 2008;3(2):133-49.

8. Moorthi C, Kathiresan K. Fabrication of dual drug loaded polymeric nanosuspension: Incorporating analytical hierarchy process and data envelopment analysis in the selection of a suitable method. *Int J Pharm Pharm Sci* 2013;5(2):499-504.

9. Mora-Huertas CE, Fessi H, Elaissari A. Polymer-based nanocapsules for drug delivery. *Int J Pharm* 2010;385(1-2):113-42.

10. Barichello JM, Morishita M, Takayama K, Nagai T. Encapsulation of hydrophilic and lipophilic drugs in PLGA nanoparticles by the nanoprecipitation method. *Drug Dev Ind Pharm* 1999;25(4):471-6.

11. Moorthi C, Kathiresan K. Fabrication of highly stable sonication assisted curcumin nanocrystals by nanoprecipitation method. *Drug Invention Today* 2013;5(1):66-9.

12. Moorthi C, Krishnan K, Manavalan R, Kathiresan K. Preparation and characterization of curcumin-piperine dual drug loaded nanoparticles. *Asian Pac J Trop Biomed* 2012;2(11):841-8.

26

Preparation, Physicochemical Characterization and Performance Evaluation of Gold Nanoparticles in Radiotherapy

Ali Kamiar[1], Reza Ghotaslou[2], Hadi Valizadeh[3]*

[1] Faculty of Pharmacy, Student Research Committee, Tabriz University of Medical Sciences, Tabriz, Iran.

[2] Department of Microbiology, School of Medicine, Tabriz University of Medical Sciences, Tabriz, Iran.

[3] Research Center for Pharmaceutical Nanotechnology and Faculty of Pharmacy, Tabriz University of Medical Sciences, Tabriz, Iran.

ARTICLE INFO

Keywords:
Gold Nano particle
Dose enhancement
Radiation therapy
Gel dosimetry
Anti-bacterial

ABSTRACT

Purpose: The aim of the present study was preparation, physicochemical characterization and performance evaluation of gold nanoparticles (GNPs) in radiotherapy. Another objective was the investigation of anti-bacterial efficacy of gold nanoparticle against E. coli clinical strains. ***Methods***: Gold nanoparticles prepared by controlled reduction of an aqueous $HAuCl_4$ solution using Tri sodium citrate. Particle size analysis and Transmission electron microscopy were used for physicochemical characterization. Polymer gel dosimetry was used for evaluation of the enhancement of absorbed dose. Diffusion method in agar media was used for investigation of anti-bacterial effect. ***Results***: Gold nanoparticles synthesized in size range from 57 nm to 346 nm by planning different formulation. Gold nanoparticle in 57 nm size increased radiation dose effectiveness with the magnitude of about 21 %. At the concentration of 400 ppm, Nano gold exhibited significant anti-bacterial effect against E. coli clinical strains. ***Conclusion***: It is concluded that gold nanoparticles can be applied as dose enhancer in radiotherapy. The Investigation of anti-bacterial efficacy showed that gold nanoparticle had significant effect against E. coli clinical strains.

Introduction

Nanotechnology is beginning to show its impact on the way the health care is administered. These include new interventions in disease detection, treatment and prevention, which are collectively termed as nanomedicine.[1] The most well-studied nanoparticles include quantum dots, carbon nanotubes, paramagnetic nanoparticles, liposomes, gold nanoparticles (GNPs), and many others.[2] In recent years, gold nanoparticles have attracted much attention. They are agents with numerous applications in biomedicine like cancer research, diagnostic assay,[3-5] thermal ablation, gene and drug delivery,[6-8] etc. Nano gold have several unique properties, For example they are inert and nontoxic[9] and have good anti-bacterial,[10] anti-angiogenesis properties,[11] etc. GNPs have been prepared by both "physical" and "chemical" methods. For the "physical" preparation method, Au bulk is broken down by a strong attack force, for example, ion irradiation in air or arc discharge in water, to generate GNPs. Chemical method including chemical reduction of Au salts, electrochemical pathways and decomposition of organometallic compounds. Among them, the chemical reduction method is simple and controllable to prepare various sizes and shapes of GNPs.[12,13]

Today Cancer is the third leading cause of death in developed countries and the second leading cause of death in the United States.[2] Treatment of Cancer includes chemotherapy, surgery and radiotherapy. Although radiation therapy is one of the most preferred cure and has been practiced for about 100 years in cancer treatment, but this treatment has a lot of side effects. So scientists are looking for new ways to enhance effect of radiotherapy and lower damage to the normal cell.[14] The concept of using high-*Z* materials as dose enhancement in cancer radiotherapy has long been investigated. Several studies have focused on the potential application of GNPs in conjunction with radiation therapy.[15] The aim of this project was preparation, characterization of GNPs with the intention of absorbed dose enhancement in tumor cells. Anti-bacterial effect of prepared GNPs against clinical strains of E. coli was also investigated.

Materials and Methods
Materials
$HAuCl_4$ was purchased from Alfa Aesar (Great Britain). Tri sodium citrate was obtained from Scharlau (Spania). N,N'-methylenebis-acrylamide (bis) acrylamide (AA), Tetrakis (Hydroxymethyl)

Corresponding author: Hadi Valizadeh, Department of Pharmaceutics, Faculty of Pharmacy, Tabriz University of Medical Sciences, Tabriz, Iran.
Email: valizadeh@tbzmed.ac.ir

Phosphonium Chloride and Gelatin were obtained from Sigma chemical company. Mueller Hinton agar was purchased from Liofilchem. De-ionized water was used to prepare aqueous solutions.

Gold nanoparticles preparation
Gold nanoparticles were prepared by the classical citrate reduction (frens method). Briefly, 20ml of $HAuCl_4$ water solution (1 mM) was kept boiling. Various volume of 1% sodium citrate water solution was then added to the solution and stirred for about 10 min, until the formation of a colored gold nanoparticle suspension. Table 1 shows different citrate volume that use for preparation of GNPs.

Table 1. Different formulation for preparation of gold nanoparticle and their particle size and polydispersity index

Formulation No.	Volume of $HAuCl_4$ 1mM(ml)	Volume of citrate 1% (ml)	Particle size(nm)	Polydispersity Index
F_1	20	1.9	-	-
F_2	20	1.8	-	-
F_3	20	1.7	57	1.21
F_4	20	1.6	74	1.85
F_5	20	1.5	136	1.20
F_6	20	1.3	259	1.11
F_7	20	1.2	346	1.08

Characterization of GNPs
The mean particle-size values of GNPs were measured by using a laser diffraction particle-size analyzer (Sald 2101, Shimadzu, Japan) equipped with Wing software (version 1.20). The morphology of the nanoparticles was investigated by Transmission electron microscopy (TEM) (LEO906, Germany). Drops of the gold suspension (formulation F_6) were deposited and dried onto a Formvar-coated copper grid. The UV–visible absorption spectra of the one of the prepared colloidal solutions recorded using a spectrophotometer (Shimadzu, Japan), from 400 to 900 nm.

Gel dosimetry
Gel fabrication
The gel solution consists of water (89 % of total mass), acrylamide (3 %), N,N-methylene-bisacrylamide (3 %) and gelatin (5 %). The gel components were mixed together at 35-40 °C in a 500 ml beaker. An oxygen scavenger, Tetrakis (hydroxyl methyl) phosphonium chloride (THPC), was added to the gel mixture at a concentration of 10 mM as anti-oxidant. Nano gold (formulation F_3) was used as a part of water in gel preparation to fabricate gel with GNPs batch. The GNPs were observed to mix homogeneously in the gel. Another batch of gel without GNPs served as a control. The gel was then quickly poured into separate tubes.

Irradiation
The tubes of the both batches were irradiated with CT scanner after put them in a head and neck phantom.

The gel samples were exposed to radiation doses of 40, 80 and 120 Gy. Irradiation of the gel samples was carried out at Day CT scanner center with following parameters: slice thickness=1 cm, t=0.8 s/turn, mA=200, kVp =140.

Magnetic Resonance Imaging (MRI)
Irradiated and non-irradiated gel samples were scanned using a 1.5 T MRI scanner (GE Sigma, Milwaukee, USA), to measure spin–spin relaxation time of the free protons using a head coil. A fast-spin echo sequence was used with following parameters: field of view $=105 \times 120$ mm^2, slice thickness = 5 mm (kV X-ray beams), effective echo time TE = 22 ms, turbo factor = 14, repetition time (TR) = 5,710 ms, the field of view = 128×128 matrix, total imaging time = 20 min. At least 24 h elapsed after irradiation prior to imaging to allow for polymerization. All the samples were scanned at room temperature.

Data analysis
Analysis of the image was performed using MATLAB software (version 3.5.7) (The Math Works Inc, Natick, Massachusetts, USA). The program examined the data before analyzing it to determine the region of interest. T_2 values were calculated and formed T_2 maps on a pixel-by-pixel basis. The levels of the polymerization of the irradiated gels with and without GNPs were compared by calculating the R_2 ($1/T_2$).

Anti-bacterial test
Antibacterial activity was studied by the agar-well-diffusion method, wherein 100 µl bacterial suspension was added to 20-mL sterile nutrient Mueller Hinton agar at 45 °C and the mixture was solidified on a Petri dish. After the medium had solidified, 7-mm-diameter wells were made in the agar (three wells per dish) that were equidistant from one another and from the dish edge. The wells received 150 µL of different concentration of GNPs from formulation F_2 (400 ppm, 200 ppm, 100 ppm). The petri dishes were incubated in a thermostat at 37 °C for 24 h. After incubation, the diameter of the zone of bacterial-growth inhibition was measured. All experiments were done for five clinical strains of E. coli and repeated thrice.

Results and Discussion
Physicochemical properties of GNPs
The influence of citrate volume in particle size is shown in Table 1. This data indicated that as citrate volume increase, the particle size of gold nanoparticle get smaller. TEM image show that synthesized GNPs are spherical in shape (Figure1). Narrow range of sizes was achieved using reduction method (Figure 2). The formation of GNPs was confirmed from an absorption maximum at 532 nm. The absence of absorbance at wavelengths greater than 600 nm confirmed their well dispersed state in solution[16] (Figure 3).

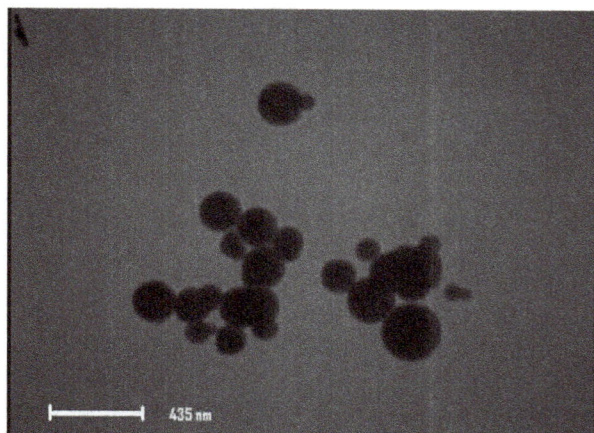

Figure 1. TEM image of gold nanoparticle (formulation F_6)

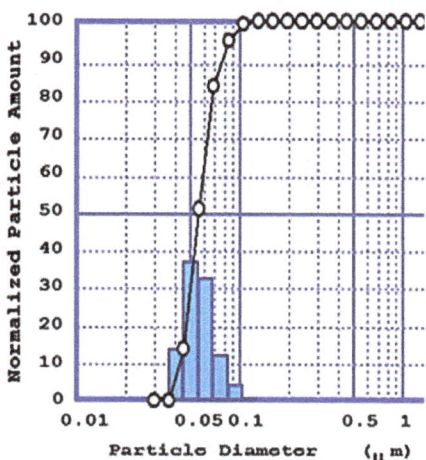

Figure 2. Particle size distribution of gold nanoparticles (formulation F_1)

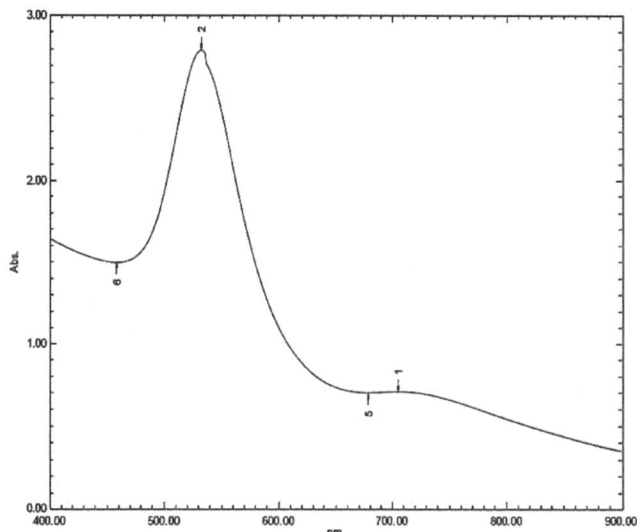

Figure 3. UV–Vis spectra of 250 nM gold nanoparticles (formulation F_3)

Gel dosimetry

The relationship between the delivered X-ray dose and the R_2 (spin–spin relaxation rate) was investigated to characterize the effect of GNPs using polymer gel. R_2 is equal to $1/T_2$ (spin–spin relaxation time) and is a function of dose (dose delivered to water). A linear relationship is found between delivered dose and R_2 (Figure 4). The dose–response slopes for R_2 versus delivered X-ray dose for gel–GNP and pure gel were calculated. The ratio of these slopes was taken as the dose enhancement factor (DEF). The DEF of 1.21 was obtained for the dose–response relationship. Dose enhancement by high Z material is believed to be caused predominantly by enhancing the likelihood of the photoelectric interaction. When GNPs are added to the gel prior to irradiation and bombarded with kilovoltage X-rays, the photoelectric interaction cross section will increase. This can be clearly inferred from the interaction probability of these X-ray photons with gold atoms compared to their interaction with the tissue equivalent medium such as water.

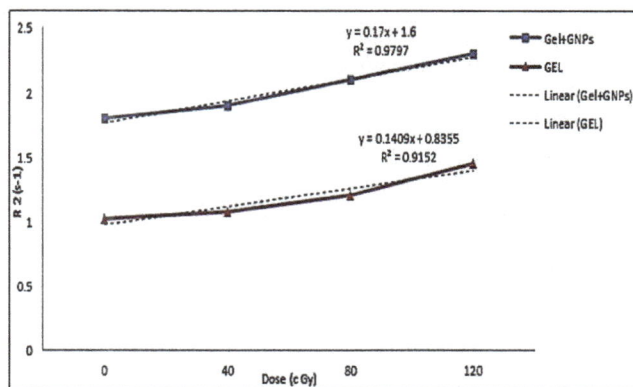

Figure 4. dose–response curve for pure gel and gel–GNPs

Antimicrobial activity of GNPs against E. coli clinical strains

Table 2 indicates Mean inhibitory diameters related to different concentrations of GNPs (formulation F_2). At the concentration of 400 ppm GNPs exhibited good effect against E. coli clinical strains. The concentration 200 ppm had a little effect and 100 ppm almost had no effect. GNPs exert their antibacterial action mainly by two ways: one is to change membrane potential and inhibit ATP synthase activities to decrease the ATP level, indicating a general decline in metabolism. The other mechanism is to inhibit the subunit of ribosome for tRNA binding, indicating a collapse of biological process.[17] Nishat et al. reported a simple one step microwave irradiation method for the synthesis of GNPs using citric acid as reducing agent and cetyl trimethyl ammonium bromide (CTAB) as binding agent. They investigated antibacterial efficacy of the nano gold against E. coli standard strain and reported high antibacterial activity with zone of inhibition of about 22 mm against E. coli.[18] This result showed more anti-bacterial effectiveness of nano gold against E. coli.

CTAB is a potent anti-microbial agent, so this difference may be related to use of this material.

Table 2. Inhibition zone diameter (mm) of different concentration of nano gold loaded in plates with *E. coli* clinical strains inoculums

Strain	100 ppm	200 ppm	400 ppm
1	0	8.33	10
2	5.5	9	11
3	0	8.66	11.33
4	0	5.33	11.33
5	0	2.66	8.16

Conclusion

We reported here the measurement of radiation dose enhancement generated by GNPs using polymer gel dosimeters as a phantom. This study has found a significant dose enhancement from the inclusion of the GNPs within polymer gels irradiated with kilovoltage X-rays beams from a therapy machine. Besides, GNPs exhibited a good anti-microbial effect against E. coli clinical strains at 400 ppm concentration.

Acknowledgements

The authors would like to thank the authority of student research committee, Tabriz university medical sciences for their support.

Conflict of Interest

The authors report no conflicts of interest.

References

1. Rees M, Moghimi SM. Nanotechnology: From fundamental concepts to clinical applications for healthy aging. *Nanomed Nanotechnol Biol Med* 2012;8(Suppl 1):S1-4.
2. Cai W, Gao T, Hong H, Sun J. Applications of gold nanoparticles in cancer nanotechnology. *Nanotechnol Sci Appl* 2008;1(1):17-32.
3. Sun IC, Eun DK, Na JH, Lee S, Kim IJ, Youn IC, et al. Heparin-coated gold nanoparticles for liver-specific CT imaging. *Chemistry* 2009;15(48):13341-7.
4. Fournelle M, Bost W, Tarner IH, Lehmberg T, WeiB E, Lemor R, et al. Antitumor necrosis factor-α antibody-coupled gold nanorods as nanoprobes for molecular optoacoustic imaging in arthritis. *Nanomed* 2012;8(3):346-54.
5. Lee H, Lee K, Kim IK, Park TG. Synthesis, characterization, and in vivo diagnostic applications of hyaluronic acid immobilized gold nanoprobes. *Biomaterials* 2008;29(35):4709-18.
6. Lee SH, Bae KH, Kim SH, Lee KR, Park TG. Amine-functionalized gold nanoparticles as non-

cytotoxic and efficient intracellular siRNA delivery carriers. *Int J Pharm* 2008;364(1):94-101.
7. Ryou SM, Kim S, Jang HH, Kim JH, Yeom JH, Eom MS, et al. Delivery of shRNA using gold nanoparticle-DNA oligonucleotide conjugates as a universal carrier. *Biochem Biophys Res Commun* 2010;398(3):542-6.
8. Rivera Gil P, Huhn D, Del Mercato LL, Sasse D, Parak WJ. Nanopharmacy: Inorganic nanoscale devices as vectors and active compounds. *Pharmacol Res* 2010;62(2):115-25.
9. Patra CR, Bhattacharya R, Mukhopadhyay D, Mukherjee P. Fabrication of gold nanoparticles for targeted therapy in pancreatic cancer. *Adv Drug Deliv Rev* 2010;62(3):346-61.
10. Dastjerdi R, Montazer M. A review on the application of inorganic nano-structured materials in the modification of textiles: focus on anti-microbial properties. *Colloids Surf B Biointerfaces* 2010;79(1):5-18.
11. Mukherjee P, Bhattacharya R, Wang P, Wang L, Basu S, Nagy JA, et al. Antiangiogenic properties of gold nanoparticles. *Clin Cancer Res* 2005;11(9):3530-4.
12. Schmid G, Corain B. Nanoparticulated gold: Syntheses, structures, electronics, and reactivities. *Eur J Inorg Chem* 2003;2003(17):3081-98.
13. Nguyen DT, Kim DJ, Kim KS. Controlled synthesis and biomolecular probe application of gold nanoparticles. *Micron* 2011;42(3):207-27.
14. Cho SH, Jones BL, Krishnan S. The dosimetric feasibility of gold nanoparticle-aided radiation therapy (gnrt) via brachytherapy using low-energy gamma-/x-ray sources. *Phys Med Biol* 2009;54(16):4889-905.
15. Chang MY, Shiau AL, Chen YH, Chang CJ, Chen HH, Wu CL. Increased apoptotic potential and dose-enhancing effect of gold nanoparticles in combination with single-dose clinical electron beams on tumor-bearing mice. *Cancer Sci* 2008;99(7):1479-84.
16. Lasagna-Reeves C, Gonzalez-Romero D, Barria MA, Olmedo I, Clos A, Sadagopa Ramanujam VM, et al. Bioaccumulation and toxicity of gold nanoparticles after repeated administration in mice. *Biochem Biophys Res Commun* 2010;393(4):649-55.
17. Cui Y, Zhao Y, Tian Y, Zhang W, Lu X, Jiang X. The molecular mechanism of action of bactericidal gold nanoparticles on Escherichia coli. *Biomaterials* 2012;33(7):2327-33.
18. Arshi N, Ahmed F, Kumar S, Anwar MS, Lu J, Koo BH, et al. Microwave assisted synthesis of gold nanoparticles and their antibacterial activity against escherichia coli (E. Coli). *Curr Appl Phys* 2011;11(1 Supplement):S360-3.

27

Electrochemical Studies for the Determination of Quetiapine Fumarate and Olanzapine Antipsychotic Drugs

Manal A. El-Shal

National Organization for Drug Control and Research (NODCAR), Pyramid Ave., P. O. B 29 Cairo, Egypt.

ARTICLE INFO

Keywords:
Olanzapine
Quetiapine fumarate
Voltammetry
Pharmaceuticals
Urine

ABSTRACT

Purpose: Cyclic voltammetry and differential pulse voltammetry were used to explore the diffusion behavior of two antipsychotic drugs at a glassy carbon electrode. A well-defined oxidation peak was obtained in Britton-Robinson (BR) buffer (pH 2.0). The response was evaluated as a function of some variables such as the scan rate, and pH. ***Methods:*** A simple, precise, inexpensive and sensitive voltammetric method has been developed for the determination of the cited drugs Olanzapine (OLZ) and Quetiapine fumarate (QUT). ***Results:*** A linear calibration was obtained from 3×10^{-8} M to 4×10^{-6} M and 2×10^{-8} M to 5×10^{-6} M, with R. S. D. were 1.6 % and 1.2 % for OLZ and QUT, respectively. The limit of detection (LOD) was 1×10^{-8} M, while the limit of quantification (LOQ) was 3×10^{-8} M. ***Conclusion:*** The method was applied to the determination of investigated drugs in urine and serum samples and dosage forms.

Introduction

Olanzapine (OLZ) **I**, and Quetiapine fumarate (QUT) **II** are psychotropic agents that belongs to the thienobenzodiazepine class, a relatively new benzodiazepine, which has been found useful in the treatment of, among other psychosis, schizophrenia.[1-3] The cited drugs are the antipsychotic that has the highest serotonin/dopamine binding ratio,[4] being the serotonin type 2 (5-HT2)-receptor blocking effect about twice as strong as the dopamine D2-receptor blocking effect.[5] The chemical formula of olanzapine is 2-methyl-4-(4-methyl-1-piperazinyl)-10 H –thieno [2,3- b] [1,5] benzodiazepine and Quetiapine fumarate (bis [2-(2-[4-(dibenzo[b,f][1,4]thiazepin-11-yl)] ethoxy) ethanol]. The molecular formula is $C_{17}H_{20}N_4S$ and $C_{42}H_{50}N_6O_4S_2 \cdot C_4H_4O$, which corresponds to a molecular weight of 312.44 and 883.11 (fumarate salt) for OLZ and QUT, respectively. The chemical structures are shown in Figure 1:

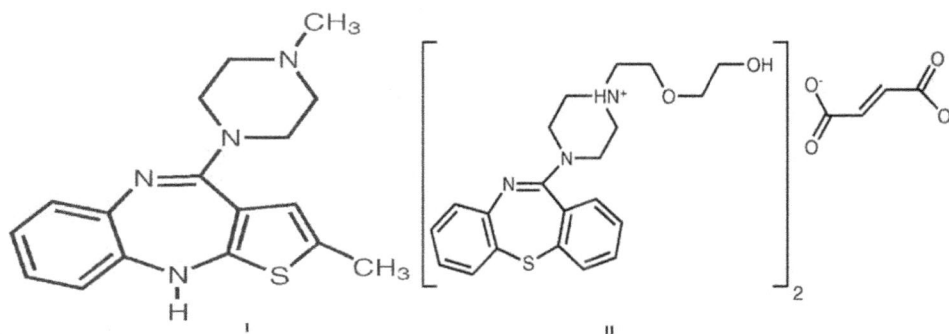

Figure 1. Chemical structures of Olanzapine (OLZ) I and Quetiapine fumarate (QUT) II.

A literature search showed that until now, high-performance liquid chromatography (HPLC) has been the major technique used for the quality control of pharmaceutical formulations containing these drugs. Therefore, the aim of the present work was to design easy electrochemical method for determination of the cited drugs in pure, in the pharmaceutical formulations and in biological fluids.

Several methods have been reported for analysis of investigated drugs in pharmaceutical formulations including biological fluids and flow injection titration,[6] voltammetry,[7] gas chromatography,[8-10] high

Corresponding author: Manal A. El-Shal, National Organization for Drug Control and Research (NODCAR), Pyramid Ave., P. O. B 29 Cairo, Egypt. Email: manalelshal@hotmail.com

performance liquid chromatograpgy,[11-16] capillary zone electrophoresis,[17] HPTLC,[18] X-ray powder diffraction,[19] and Spectrophotometry.[20-22] However, these methods require multi-step extraction procedures and selective detectors. Therefore, it was felt useful to develop electrochemical method for its determination. The problem in the reported assay is the precise, specific and easy measurement of this potent drugs in dosage forms especially they only possess a very low absorption in the UV region. This weak absorption means that a conventional UV spectrophotometric assay is susceptible to interference from excipients. This work reported an example of using electrochemical method in drug analysis. The possibility of performing more in this field is still opened for further trials. I have tried to contribute to the field of drug analysis as much as possible and according to available facilities. The research is in progress with a direction to apply the analytical techniques in clinical studies and to solve problems facing the local pharmaceutical industry. Hence, the proposed electrochemical method to analysis our cited drugs are simple, accurate and inexpensive. They can adapt for quality control testing and drug stability monitoring (antidepressant, vitamins, antibiotic, etc).

Good electrical conductivity of the electrodes is an important factor. Carbon-based electrodes usually have a wider potential range than the other solid electrodes because of their broad potential window, low background current, rich surface chemistry, chemical inertness, low cost and suitability for various sensing and detection applications.

Glassy carbon electrode (GCE) is a class of nongraphitizing carbon that is widely used as an electrode material in electrochemistry. It is also known as vitreous carbon. Glassy carbon electrode is used very commonly because of its excellent mechanical and electrical properties, impermeability to gases and extremely low porosity. Electro analytical application[23,24] of carbon based electrodes to determine pharmaceutical compounds in their dosage forms and in biological samples using modern electrochemical techniques were published.

Materials and Methods
Materials
Olanzapine and quetiapine were provided from Lilly (Brussels, Belgium) and AstraZeneca (Mölndal, Sweden) respectively. Pharmaceutical preparations, Zyprexa (olanzapine, Lilly), and Seroquel (quetiapine fumarate, AstraZeneca) were used for quantitative determinations. Stock solutions of 1×10^{-3} M of OLZ, and QUT were prepared by dissolving a calculated weight of the active ingredient drugs in deionized water and stored in dark bottles at 4°C. More dilute solutions were prepared daily just before use. Britton–Robinson (B–R) buffer solutions (pH 2 – 6) were used as supporting electrolytes. All solutions were prepared from Analar-grade reagents (Merck and Sigma) in doubly distilled water.

Instrumentation
The cyclic and DPV experiments at a stationary electrode were performed using 797VA Computrace software (1.0) from Metrohm, Switzerland, electrochemical analyzer. A three electrode cell system incorporating the glassy carbon disc electrode as working electrode: an Ag/AgCl (3M KCl) reference electrode and a platinum-wire auxiliary electrode were also used. Before each measurements the glassy carbon electrode was polished manually with alumina (φ = 0.01_m) in the presence of bi-distilled water on a smooth polishing cloth. The data were treated with Microcal Origin (Ver. 5) software to transform the initial signal. A Mettler balance (Toledo-AB104) was used for weighing the solid materials. A cyberscan 500 digital (EUTECH Instruments, USA) pH-meter with a glass combination electrode was served to carry out pH measurements. A micropipette (Eppendorf-multipette® Plus) was used throughout the present experimental work. Deionized water used throughout the present study was supplied from a Purite still plus deionized connected to a Hamilton-Aqua-Matic deionized water system.

Test solution
Ten tablets of Zyprexa and Seroquel, were weighed, and the average mass per tablet was determined. A weighed portion of a finely grounded powder equivalent to the calculated weight of pharmaceutical preparations was dissolved to produce a 1×10^{-3} M solution. The solution was then filtered through a 0.45 µm Millipore filter, in order to separate out the insoluble excipients, and reject the first portion of the filtrate. The solution was directly analyzed, according to the general analytical procedures without the necessity for sample pretreatment or any extraction step.

Biological sampling
Accurately measured aliquots of OLZ, and QUT solutions were pipetted into centrifugation tubes containing 500 µl human urine or plasma, then vortex was done for 5 min. Into each tube, 0.5 ml of methanol, 0.1 ml NaOH (0.1 M), 0.5 ml $ZnSO_4.7H_2O$ (5% w/v),[25] were added, then centrifuged for 8 min at 4000 rpm. The clear supernatant layer was filtered through 0.45 µm Milli-pore filter. A 0.1 ml of the supernatant liquor was transferred into the voltammetric cell then completed to 10 ml with a pH 2.0 BR buffer. Then, OLZ, and QUT were quantified by means of the proposed voltammetric procedure.

Voltammetric analyses
Voltammetric analyses were performed in 25 ml of BR buffer. The solution was continuously stirred at 1200 rpm when accumulation was applied for a certain time

and potential to the working electrode. At the end of accumulation, the stirring was stopped and a 5 sec rest period was allowed for the solution to become quiescent. The used drug was determined by using Cyclic CV and differential pulse voltammetry DPV methods. Aliquots of the drug solution were introduced into the electrolytic cell and the procedures were repeated. The voltammograms were recorded. The peak current was evaluated as the difference between each voltammogram and the background electrolyte voltammogram. All data were obtained were carried out at room temperature.

Results and Discussion
Influence of the Type and pH of the Supporting Electrolyte
The effect of different supporting buffers (B-R, acetate, borate, citrate and phosphate) on the current response of OLZ, and QUT were studied in order to assess their impact on the monitored electroanalytical signal. The best results with respect to sensitivity accompanied with sharper response were obtained with B-R.

Anodic cyclic voltammogram peaks for the oxidation of 1×10^{-5} M of OLZ and QUT in B–R buffer of pH 2-6 at GCE was studied. The pH of the electrolyte medium is one of the variables that commonly and strongly influence the shape of the voltammogram, and therefore it was important to investigate the effect of the pH on the electrochemical behavior of the drugs. Definite anodic peaks, corresponding to oxidation of the used drugs, were observed at +0.60 and +0.65 V for OLZ and QUT, Figure 2. In a forward scan, a single anodic peak was observed with no cathodic peak in the reverse sweep, which indicates that the oxidation process of OLZ and QUT is irreversible. The graph of Ip vs. pH (Figure 2) revealed that the peak current decreases from pH 2.0 to 5.0. The decreasing in magnitude is related to interaction between the electrode surface and the positive charge of nitrogen atom. After the pKa value, there is no charge and the intensity is almost the same from pH 5 to 12.

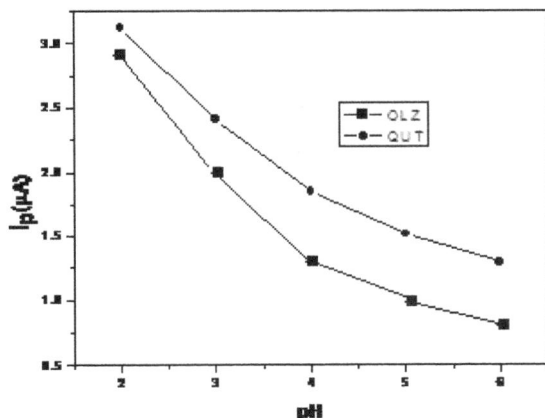

Figure 2. The effect of pH on the peak current in a B-R buffer.

Effect of the Scan Rate
The influence of the scan rate on the peak current (Ip) was studied Figure 3 within the range $10 - 200$ mV s^{-1} for OLZ and QUT. The peak potential moves to a more positive potential with increasing the scan rate, which confirms the irreversibility of the process. A plot of the peak current versus scan rate for OLZ and QUT gave a straight line. linear relationship between log Ip and log υ over the scan range 10-200 mV s-1 with slope values of 0.51 , 0.47 is close to the theoretically expected value of 0.50 for a diffusion controlled process.[26]

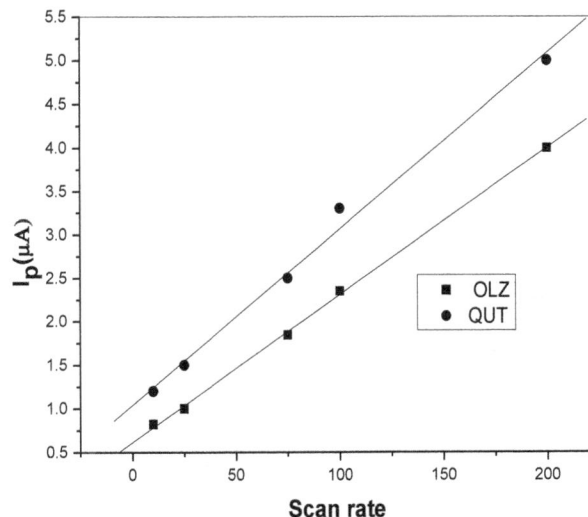

Figure 3. Anodic peak current response of (1×10^{-6} M) OLZ and QUT as a function of the scan rate (mV/S) at a GCE.

Effect of Instrumental Parameters
It was found that the peak current was increased with the increasing pulse amplitude and scan rate, while it decreased with the increasing pulse width. To obtain relatively high and narrow peaks the values of 50 mV, 30 ms, and 10 mV s^{-1} were finally chosen for pulse amplitude, pulse width and scan rate, respectively.

Interferences
The tolerance limit was defined as the maximum concentration of the interfering substances that caused an error less than ±2%. Under optimized experimental conditions, the effects of potential interferents on the voltammetric response of 3.4 g/mL OLZ and QUT as a standard at GCE were evaluated. The experimental results show that 200-fold concentration of glucose, starch, lactic acid, dextrose, talk, gum acacia, magnesium stearate and ascorbic acid did not interfere. In brief proposed method has good selectivity for determination of OLZ and QUT.

Analytical Applications
Validation of the Proposed Method
In order to develop a voltammetric methodology for determining the drugs, we selected the DPV mode, since the peaks were sharper and better-defined at lower concentration of OLZ and QUT than those

obtained by cyclic voltammetry, with a lower background current, resulting in improved resolution. The peak potential versus pH plots were similar to that obtained by cyclic voltammetry for DPV. According to the obtained results, it was possible to apply these techniques to the quantitative analysis of OLZ and QUT. The precision of the method was evaluated by repeating six experiments on the same day and in the same standard solution (repeatability) and over 6 days from the different standard solutions (reproducibility).[27] For these studies, 1×10^{-7} M OLZ and QUT standard solutions were used. The results were given as shown in Table 1.

Table 1. Characteristics of OLZ and QUT calibration plots

Parameters	OLZ	QUT
Linearity range (M)	3×10^{-8} M to 4×10^{-6}	2×10^{-8} - 5×10^{-6}
Correlation Coefficient	0.9970	0.9956
(R.S.D., %)	1.4	1.1
LOD (M)	1×10^{-8}	1×10^{-8}
LOQ (M)	3×10^{-8}	3×10^{-8}
Repeatability (%)	98.5	99.1

In order to provide the DPV quantitative procedure, the dependence of the peak current on the drugs concentration was investigated. Using the optimum conditions described linear calibration curves was obtained in Figure 4.

The characteristics of these graphs were as shown in Table 1. Related statistical data of the calibration curves were obtained from three different calibration curves. The limit of detection (LOD) and quantification (LOQ) were also as shown in Table 1. The LOD and LOQ were calculated on the peak current using the following equations:

$$LOD = 3s/m \qquad\qquad LOQ = 10s/m$$

Where s is the standard deviation and m is the slope of the calibration curve.[27] Sample solutions recorded after 48 h did not show any appreciable change in the assay values.

The F- and student t-test were carried out on the data and statistically examined the validity of the obtained results. At the 95% of the confidence level, the values of t- and F-tests (calculated from the experiments) were less than that of theoretical t- and F-tests values showing that there is no significative difference between the proposed DPV method and reference HPLC method.

The reproducibility was evaluated in terms of repeatability and between-day reproducibility. The coefficient of variation (cv) of ten consecutive measurements of the peak current corresponding to an OLZ and QUT concentration of 1×10^{-7} mol/L was calculated as 0.5 and 0.7%, for three times in four successive days which demonstrates the good repeatability of the voltammetric method.

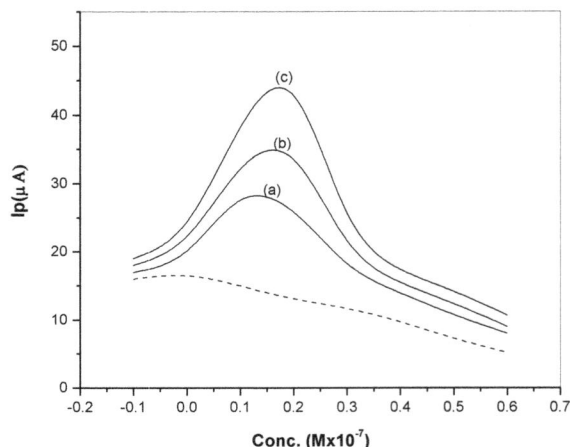

Figure 4. Anodic differential voltammogrames of OLZ at scan rate 10 mV s^{-1} with concentrations (a) 0.4 (b) 0.8 (c) 1.2×10^{-7} M , The (---) line represents the blank BR.

The robustness[28] of the results of the procedure is the ability to remain unaffected by small changes in its operational parameters, such as the pH. In the present work, this was examined by studying the effect of a variation of pH (2.0 –2.7). The recovery values were not significantly affected by these variations and consequently the optimized procedure was reliable for the assay of drugs. It could be robust. The ruggedness is the degree of reproducibility of the results obtained by analysis of the same sample under a variety of normal test conditions, such as different laboratories, different analysts, and different lots of reagents, Table 2. This was examined by applying the proposed procedures to an assay under experimental conditions using two different analysts. The result obtained due to lab. (1) to lab. (2) and even day to day were found to be reproducible, since there is no significant difference between the recovery and the SD values.

Table 2. The robustness and ruggedness of the conditions of the proposed procedure for determination of OLZ and QUT.

Variables	Drug	Recovery % ±RSD
Robustness results at pH =2.5	OLZ	98.0 ± 0.60
	QUT	98.7 ± 0.70
Ruggedness Analyst 1	OLZ	98.4 ± 0.60
	QUT	98.9 ± 0.50
Ruggedness Analyst 2	OLZ	98.1 ± 0.60
	QUT	99.0 ± 0.70

Determination of OLZ and QUT in Tablets

The proposed analysis procedure was successfully applied for the assay of OLZ and QUT in their pharmaceutical formulations. For this reason the HPLC methods[8,12] were used for comparison and for the reliability of the developed procedures. The results obtained for the formulation are listed in Table 3 and compared with the HPLC method which has been described in the literature.

Table 3. Statistical evaluation for Assay of OLZ and QUT in pharmaceutical dosage forms by the proposed and official methods.

Sample	% Found	Proposed method (%±RSD, n = 5)	Reported method (%± RSD)	F – test[a]	t– test[a]
OLZ(Zyprexa) 5 mg\tab	98.8	98.8 ± 0.50	98.7 ± 0.42	1.60	0.60
QUT (Seroquel) 25 mg\tab	98.1	99.0 ± 0.40	98.7 ± 0.55	1.30	0.80
(a) Theoretical values of F and t - test at 95% confidence limit (n = 5) are 6.39 and 2.61, respectively.					

Determination of Spiked Biological Samples

The modified DPV method could be successfully applied to the determination of the investigated drugs in spiked urine and serum. Calibration curves were constructed by using the standard addition method of the prepared spiked samples. The percent recoveries in spiked urine were 98.2 ±0.42, and 98.0 ±0.65, while in spiked serum were 96.7 ±0.75 and 97.0 ± 0.58 for OLZ and QUT, respectively (Table 4).

Table 4. Statistical evaluation for Assay of OLZ and QUT in biological fluids.

	Proposed method with GCE in spiked urine	Proposed method with GCE in spiked serum
OLZ	98.2 ±0.42	96.7 ±0.75
QUT	98.0 ±0.65	97.0 ± 0.58

Conclusion

This paper on the electrochemical behavior of OLZ and QUT at glassy carbon electrode has described how the compound is irreversibly oxidized at positive potentials. voltammetric technique has been developed for the determination of OLZ and QUT in pharmaceutical dosage forms and biological samples. Application of the DPV technique to pharmaceuticals is possible after a simple dilution step. The principal advantage of the proposed methods, over the published HPLC procedures, is that the excipients do not interfere and the separation procedure is not necessary. The methods are rapid, requiring <5 min to run sample and involves no sample preparation other than dissolving and transferring an aliquot to the supporting electrolyte.

Conflict of Interest

The authors report no conflicts of interest.

References

1. Dossenbach MR, Folnegovic-Smalc V, Hotujac L, Uglesic B, Tollefson GD, Grundy SL, et al. Double-blind, randomized comparison of olanzapine versus fluphenazine in the long-term treatment of schizophrenia. *Prog Neuropsychopharmacol Biol Psychiatry* 2004;28(2):311-8.
2. Heresco-Levy U, Ermilov M, Lichtenberg P, Bar G, Javitt DC. High-dose glycine added to olanzapine and risperidone for the treatment of schizophrenia. *Biol Psychiatry* 2004;55(2):165-71.
3. Sclar DA, Skaer TL, Robison LM, Dickson WM, Markowitz JS, DeVane CL. Use and cost patterns of risperidone versus olanzapine for the treatment of schizophrenia: An assessment of medicaid children and adolescents age 5-18 years. *Eur Neuropsychopharmacol* 2003;13:S281-S2.
4. Worrel JA, Marken PA, Beckman SE, Ruehter VL. Atypical antipsychotic agents: a critical review. *Am J Health Syst Pharm* 2000;57(3):238-55.
5. Gefvert O, Bergstrom M, Langstrom B, Lundberg T, Lindstrom L, Yates R. Time course of central nervous dopamine-D2 and 5-HT2 receptor blockade and plasma drug concentrations after discontinuation of quetiapine (Seroquel) in patients with schizophrenia. *Psychopharmacology (Berl)* 1998;135(2):119-26.
6. Jasinska A, Nalewajko E. Batch and flow-injection methods for the spectrophotometric determination of olanzapine. *Anal Chim Acta* 2004;508(2):165-70.
7. Raggi MA, Casamenti G, Mandrioli R, Izzo G, Kenndler E. Quantitation of olanzapine in tablets by HPLC, CZE, derivative spectrometry and linear voltammetry. *J Pharm Biomed Anal* 2000;23(6):973-81.
8. Pujadas M, Pichini S, Civit E, Santamarina E, Perez K, De La Torre R. A simple and reliable procedure for the determination of psychoactive drugs in oral fluid by gas chromatography-mass spectrometry. *J Pharm Biomed Anal* 2007;44(2):594-601.
9. Sanchez TC, Martinez MA, Almarza EA. Determination of several psychiatric drugs in whole blood using capillary gas–liquid chromatography with nitrogen phosphorus detection: comparison of two solid phase extraction procedures. *Forensic Sci Int* 2005;155(2-3):193-204.
10. Mandrioli R, Fanali S, Ferranti A, Raggi MA. HPLC analysis of the novel antipsychotic drug quetiapine in human plasma. *J Pharm Biomed Anal* 2002;30(4):969-77.
11. Yuan SL, Li XF, Jiang XM, Zhang HX, Zheng SK. Simultaneous Determination of 13 Psychiatric Pharmaceuticals in Sewage by Automated Solid Phase Extraction and Liquid Chromatography-Mass Spectrometry. *Chinese J Anal Chem* 2013;41(1):49-56.
12. Bellomarino SA, Brown AJ, Conlan XA, Barnett NW. Preliminary evaluation of monolithic column high-performance liquid chromatography with tris(2,2'-bipyridyl)ruthenium(II) chemiluminescence detection for the determination of quetiapine in human body fluids. *Talanta* 2009;77(5):1873-6.
13. Zhang G, Terry AV Jr., Bartlett MG. Sensitive liquid chromatography/tandem mass spectrometry

method for the simultaneous determination of olanzapine, risperidone, 9-hydroxyrisperidone, clozapine, haloperidol and ziprasidone in rat brain tissue. *J Chromatogr B Analyt Technol Biomed Life Sci* 2007;858(1-2):276-81.

14. D'arrigo C, Migliardi G, Santoro V, Spina E. Determination of olanzapine in human plasma by reversed-phase high-performance liquid chromatography with ultraviolet detection. *Ther Drug Monit* 2006;28(3):388-93.

15. Nirogi RV, Kandikere VN, Shukla M, Mudigonda K, Maurya S, Boosi R, et al. Development and validation of a sensitive liquid chromatography/electrospray tandem mass spectrometry assay for the quantification of olanzapine in human plasma. *J Pharm Biomed Anal* 2006;41(3):935-42.

16. Kirchherr H, Kuhn-Velten WN. Quantitative determination of forty-eight antidepressants and antipsychotics in human serum by HPLC tandem mass spectrometry: a multi-level, single-sample approach. *J Chromatogr B Analyt Technol Biomed Life Sci* 2006;843(1):100-13.

17. Izzo G, Raggi MA, Maichel B, Kenndler E. Separation of olanzapine, carbamazepine and their main metabolites by capillary electrophoresis with pseudo-stationary phases. *J Chromatogr B Biomed Sci Appl* 2001;752(1):47-53.

18. Spangenberg B, Selgel A, Kempf J, Weinmann W. Forensic drug analysis by means of diode-array HPTLC using R F and UV library search. *J Planar Chromat Mod TLC* 2005;18(5):336-43.

19. Polla GI, Vega DR, Lanza H, Tombari DG, Baggio R, Ayala AP, et al. Thermal behaviour and stability in Olanzapine. *Int J Pharm* 2005;301(1-2):33-40.

20. Sudha Lakshmi PB, Rambabu C. Use of Ion-Association Reactions for the Spectrophotometric Determination of Quetiapine. *Asian J Chem* 2012;24(8):3521-3.

21. Vinay KB, Revanasiddappa HD. Spectrophotometric determination of quetiapine fumarate through ion-pair complexation reaction with tropaeolin ooo. *Indian J Chem Technol* 2012;19(3):205-12.

22. Rajendraprasad N, Basavaiah K, Vinay KB. Extractive Spectrophotometric Determination of Quetiapine Fumarate in Pharmaceuticals and Spiked Human Urine. *Croat Chem Acta* 2012;85(1):9-17.

23. El-Shal MA, Attia AK. Adsorptive Stripping Voltammetric Behavior and Determination of Zolmitriptan Using Differential Pulse and Square Wave Voltammetry. *Anal Bioanal Electrochem* 2013;5(1):32-45.

24. Uslu B, Özkan SA, Sentürk Z. Electrooxidation of the antiviral drug valacyclovir and its square-wave and differential pulse voltammetric determination in pharmaceuticals and human biological fluids. *Anal Chim Acta* 2006;555(2):341-7

25. Al-Ghamdi AH, Al-Ghamdi AF, Al-Omar MA. Electrochemical studies and square-wave adsorptive stripping voltammetry of spironolactone drug. *Anal Lett* 2008;41(1):90-103.

26. Gosser DK. Cyclic Voltammetry Simulation and Analysis of Reaction mechanism. New York: VSH; 1994.

27. Swartz E, Krull IS. Analytical Method Development and Validation. New York: Marcel Dekker; 1997.

28. USP 26, The United States Pharmacopoeia. The National Formularly, Rockville, MD, 2003; 2442.

Chiral Separation of Indapamide Enantiomers by Capillary Electrophoresis

Amelia Tero-Vescan[1], Gabriel Hancu[2]*, Mihaela Oroian[2], Anca Cârje[3]

[1] *Department of Biochemistry, Faculty of Pharmacy, University of Medicine and Pharmacy, Târgu Mureș, Romania.*

[2] *Department of Pharmaceutical Chemistry, Faculty of Pharmacy, University of Medicine and Pharmacy, Târgu Mureș, Romania.*

[3] *Department of Drug Analysis and Analytical Chemistry, Faculty of Pharmacy, University of Medicine and Pharmacy, Târgu Mureș, Romania.*

ARTICLE INFO

Keywords:
Indapamide
Capillary electrophoresis
Chiral separation
Cyclodextrines

ABSTRACT

Purpose: Indapamide is probably the most frequently prescribed diuretic drug, generally being used for the treatment of hypertension. It contains a chiral center in its molecule; is marketed as a racemic mixture; but there are rather few studies regarding the pharmacokinetic and the pharmacological effect differences of the two enantiomers. Our aim was the development of a simple, rapid and precise analytical procedure for the chiral separation of indapamide enantiomers.

Methods: In this study capillary zone electrophoresis was used for the enantiomeric separation of indapamide using a systematic screening approach involving different native and derivatized; neutral and charged cyclodextrines as chiral selectors. The effects of pH value and composition of the background electrolyte, capillary temperature, running voltage and injection parameters have been investigated.

Results: After preliminary analysis a charged derivatized CD, sulfobuthyl ether- β-CD, proved to be the optimum chiral selector for the enantioseparation. Using a buffer solution containing 25 mM disodium hydrogenophosphate – 25 mM sodium didydrogenophosphate and 5 mM sulfobuthyl ether- β-CD as chiral selector at a pH - 7, a voltage of + 25 kV, temperature 15°C and UV detection at 242 nm, we succeeded in the separation of the two enantiomers in approximately 6 minutes, with a resolution of 4.30 and a separation factor of 1.08.

Conclusion: Capillary zone electrophoresis using cyclodextrines as chiral selectors proved to be a suitable method for the enantioseparation of indapamide. Our method is rapid, specific, reliable, and cost-effective and can be proposed for laboratories performing indapamide routine analysis.

Introduction

Indapamide is a "thiazide-like" diuretic drug, generally used for the treatment of hypertension, alone or in combination with other antihypertensive drugs, as well as for the treatment of salt and fluid retention associated with congestive heart failure or edema.[1]

The benzamide-sulfonamide-indole chemical structure of indapamide (4-chloro-N-(2-methylindolin-1-yl)-3-sulphamoylbenzamide) is presented in Figure 1.[2]

Its molecule contains both a polar sulfamoyl chlorobenzamide moiety and a lipid-soluble methylindoline moiety. It differs chemically from the thiazides in that it does not possess the thiazide ring system and contains only one sulfonamide group.

Indapamide appears to cause vasodilation, probably by inhibiting the passage of calcium and other ions (sodium, potassium) across membranes. Overall, indapamide has an extra-renal antihypertensive action resulting in a decrease in vascular hyperreactivity and a reduction in total peripheral and arteriolar resistance.[1]

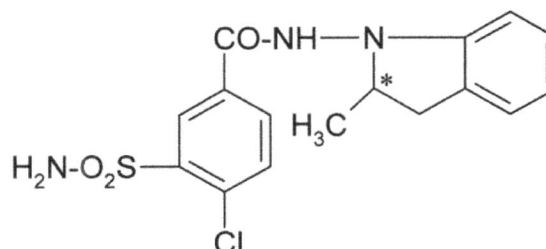

Figure 1. Indapamide chemical structure. The asterix denote the chiral center

---

*Corresponding author: Gabriel Hancu, Faculty of Pharmacy, University of Medicine and Pharmacy Târgu Mureș, GhMarinescu 38, 540000 Târgu Mureș, Romania. Email: g_hancu@yahoo.com

Indapamide posses an asymmetric carbon atom adjacent to an amino group in its molecule, resulting in the existence of a S- and R-enatiomer, but is marketed as a racemic mixture. Despite the great prevalence of indapamide in modern therapy, studies' regarding the pharmacokinetics and the pharmacological effect differences of the two enantiomers are few and the results are inconclussive.[3]

Several chiral separation methods for the indapamide have been reported in recent years using especially high performance liquid chromatographiy (HPLC) methods.[3-5] Capillary electrochromatography (CEC) was also used as an alternative to HPLC methods for the separation of indapamide enantiomers.[6-8] But these methods require derivatization or the use of expensive chiral columns or chiral capillary packings.

Capillary electrophoresis (CE) has been found to be a powerful alternative to HPLC techniques as several chiral separation principles successfully applied in HPLC have been transferred also to CE. The main advantage of using CE in chiral separations is the small amounts of sample, chiral selector and solvents required. This permits the use of a large variety of chiral selectors and also makes it easy to change rapidly the chiral selector and the buffer electrolyte when screening for the suitable selector and electrophoretic conditions.[9,10]

The most frequently used technique in chiral separations by CE is the capillary zone electrophoresis (CZE), with the direct addition of the chiral selector in the background electrolyte (BGE). Interaction between analytes and the chiral selector will depend on the stability of the formed diastereomeric complex. When a chiral selector is added to the BGE, the mobility of the complex will differ in most cases from the mobility of the free analyte. As a consequence, a difference in complex stability between two enantiomers, will result in a difference in the average velocity of these compounds.[9,10]

Cyclodextrins (CD's) are by far the most popular chiral selectors used in CE. CD's are cyclic D-glucooligosaccharides, having a relatively hydrophobic interior cavity, while the outside of the rim is more hydrophilic. The inclusion mechanism is sterically selective because analytes must fit the size of the cavity, the diameter of which depends on the number of glucose units in the CD structure. Because of the chirality of the hydroxyls in the glucose molecules, which form the rim of the CD cavity, the inclusion complex formation will be chirally selective.[11,12]

Our aim was the development of an alternative simple, rapid and cost-effective method for the chiral separation of indapamide enantiomers using a systematic screening of different native and derivatized CDs as chiral screening approach and the optimization of electrophoretic conditions in order to obtain a good chiral resolution in a short analysis time.

Materials and Methods

R,S–indapamide of pharmaceutical grade was purchased from Moehs Productos Quimicos (Barcelona, Spain). For the determination of carvedilol from commercial products we used Indapamid (Labormed, Romania) tablets containing 2.5 mg indapamide. The following reagents of analytical grade were used: phosphoric acid, sodium tetraborate, disodium hydrogenophosphate, sodium didydrogenophosphate (Merck, Germany), methanol, sodium hydroxide (Lach Ner, Czech Republic). Purified water was provided by a Milli-Q Plus water purification system (Millipore, USA).

As chiral selectors we used the following cyclodextrine (CD) derivatives of research grade: native neutral CD (α-CD, β-CD, γ-CD), derivatized neutral CD (hydroxypropyl-β-CD - HP-β-CD, randomly methylated β-CD – RAMEB), anionic substituted charged CD (sulfobuthyl ether- β-CD – SBE-β-CD). All CDs were obtained from Cyclolab (Budapest, Hungary) with the exception of SBE-β-CD - Capsitol (Cydex, USA).

The experiments were made on an Agilent 6100 CE system (Agilent, Germany) equipped with a diode array UV detector. Separations were performed on a 48 cm length (40 cm effective length) x 50 μm I.D uncoated fused silica-capillaries (Agilent, Germany). The electropherograms were recorded and processed by Chemstation 7.01 (Agilent, Germany). The pH of the buffer solutions was determined with the Terminal 740 pH–meter (Inolab). The UV spectrum of indapamide was recorded with Specord 210 spectrophotometer (Analytik Jena, Germany).

Indapamide sample stock solutions were prepared by dissolving the substance in methanol in a concentration of 100 μg/ml and later diluted with the same solvent to the appropriate concentration. The samples were introduced in the system at the anodic end of the capillary by hydrodynamic injection. All samples and buffers were filtered through a 0.45 μm syringe filter and degassed by ultrasound for 5 minutes before use.

Ten Indapamid tablets (each containing 2.5 mg indapamide) were weighed, and the net weight of each tablet was calculated. The tablets were powdered in a mortar, and an amount of powder equivalent to the average weight was accurately weighed, methanol was added to dissolve the active substance, and the solution was sonicated for 10 minutes. A sample of the tablet solution was then centrifuged at 3500 rpm for 10 minutes. The supernatant was diluted following the same procedure as for the preparation of the standard solution, before the CE analysis.

The capillaries were conditioned before use with 0.1 M sodium hydroxide for 15 minutes and with the background electrolyte used in the analysis for 15 minutes. The capillary was rinsed for 1 minute with 0.1M sodium hydroxide and buffer solutions before each electrophoretic separation.

The separation factors (α) were calculated as the ratio of the migration times of the optical isomers, and the resolution (R) was obtained by the $R = 2(t_2 - t_1)/(w_1 + w_2)$ equation, where the migration times (t_1 and t_2) and the peak-widths at half height (w_1 and w_2) were marked for the slow and fast migrating enantiomers, respectively.

Results and Discussion
Preliminary analysis
In the initial experiments the indapamide sample solution was injected in the absence of CDs and its effective electrophoretic mobility was calculated. Then we performed the measurements using the same BGE, containing a relatively low amount of chiral selector in order to verify the decrease in the effective mobility of the analyte.

We recorded previously the UV spectra of indapamide and found its absorption maximum at 242 nm, which was elected as detection wavelength in the CE separations. We applied some "standard" electrophoretic conditions for a CZE analysis: temperature 20 °C, applied voltage + 20 kV, injection pressure/time 50 mbar/3 sec, sample concetration 10 µg/ml.

In order to find the suitable conditions for the chiral separation of indapamide, a series of preliminary experiments were conducted at different pH and buffer compositions. In the preliminary analysis we used 25 mM phosphoric acid (pH – 2.1), 25 mM disodium hydrogenophosphate – 25 mM sodium didydrogenophosphate (pH – 7) and 25 mM sodium tetraborate (pH – 9.3) BGEs respectively and we modified the pH of the buffer by adding a 0.1M sodium hydroxide solution. Indapamide was detectable in an achiral environment over a pH range 5 to 10.

The type and concentration of CD added to BGE is of primary importance in achieving chiral resolution. Initial concentration of 10 mM neutral CDs were added to the buffer solution, while for charged CDs we added a concentration of 5 mM in order to limit the increase of ionic strength which generated high currents.

The most important rule for chiral recognition is that the chiral selector must be compatible in size and structure to the analyte; a minimum of three molecular interactions has to occur. The size of the hydrophobic cavity is such that, in general, the α-CD can accommodate a single phenyl ring, while β-CD and the γ-CD can accommodate substituted single- and multiple ring systems. This inclusion alone is not enough for chiral recognition: interaction between substituents on the asymmetric center of the analyte and the hydroxyl groups on the CD-rim are also responsible for chiral recognition.

When using a phosphate buffer (pH – 5-8) no chiral separation was observed using native neutral CDs (α-CD, β-CD, γ-CD) or derivatized neutral CDs (HP-β-CD, RAMEB), as we observed only an increase in migration times. The only CD, which exhibited obvious chiral interactions, was the anionic ionized SBE-β-CD.

When using a borate buffer (pH – 8-11) no chiral separation was observed using α-CD, γ-CD and RAMEB, a slight peak splitting was observed for β-CD and HP-β-CD, and the best results were obtained again by using SBE-β-CD.

Consequently we can conclude that SBE-β-CD proved to be the optimum chiral selector for the separation of indapamide enantiomers.

Optimization of the analytical method
Stereoselectivity of the separation is influenced by several experimental parameters, such as CD type and concentration, ionic strength, pH of the BGE, capillary temperature, applied voltage, capillary length, addition of organic solvents and electro-osmotic flow (EOF).

The use of a charged CD derivative (SBE-β-CD) can play a more profound role in the chiral resolution mechanism; the electrostatic interactions with the analyte, the movement of the chiral selector in the opposite direction of the enantiomers and the possibility of separating uncharged compounds representing the main advantages.[13,14]

SBE-β-CD contains four modified primary hydroxyl groups with a butyl chain and sulfonic groups; and due to its chemical poperties is negatively charged and can be commonly used in CE over a wide pH range (2-11).

Compared with neutral selectors, the effect of the concentration of the charged chiral selectors on the selectivity of enantioseparation can be more pronounced; a slight increase/decrease of the concentration of SBE-β-CD led to major overhauls of the migration times and chiral resolutions. In this work optimization of the concentration of the chiral selector was investigated experimentally for SBE- β -CD concentrations from 1 to 10 mM, we selected a concentration of 5 mM as higher concentration generated high currents and instability of the electrophoretic system.

An increase of the buffer concentration led to an increase of the migration times, but had no marked effect on the separation resolution.

Buffer pH is an important condition in CE separations, as the degree of dissociation of the charged selector, analyte charge, and the EOF are all affected by buffer pH. Indapamide is a basic drug with a pKa of 8.8; its net charge at pH between 3 to 5 is not significantly different, showing that analyte charge is insensitive to pH. It is, nevertheless, well known that the EOF is sensitive to pH in the range between 3.0 and 7.0; as it decreases considerably with decreasing pH. Indapamide was detectable at pH above 5.0 but did not elute toward the cathode when buffer pH was reduced to 3.0; this is indicative of a significant decrease in the EOF, and even reversal of the apparent mobility vector. It can also be seen that migration times decreased as the pH was increased from 5 to 11, while chiral resolution increased in the pH range 5 to 7 and deteriorated in the pH range 9 to 11 (Figure 2). A neutral 25 mM disodium hydrogenophosphate – 25 mM sodium

didydrogenophosphate at a pH – 7 was elected as the optimum BGE.

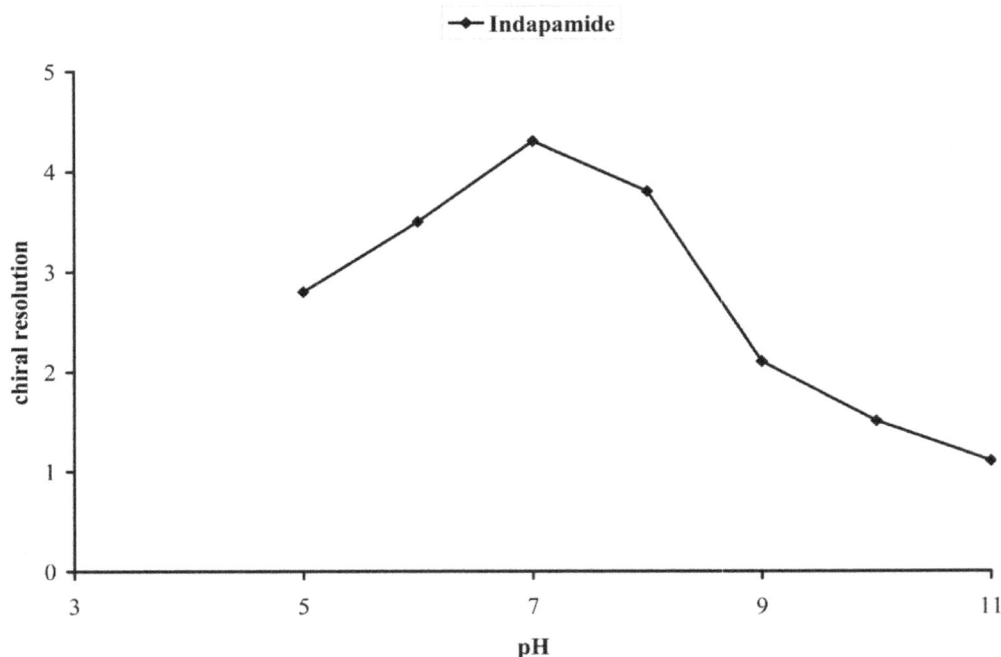

Figure 2. Effect of buffer pH on the indapamide chiral resolution

While the applied voltage had only a slight influence on the chiral resolution, temperature influenced strongly the separation efficiency and the enantiomeric resolution, as a decrease in temperature led to longer migration times but also to an increased chiral resolution. In order to obtain a satisfactory migration times and a high chiral resolution we combined the effects of these two secondary electrophoretic parameters, choosing an applied voltage of + 25 kV at a temperature of 15°C.

A high injection pressure and a short injection time will increase chiral resolution; in order to obtain a quantifiable electrophoretic response and improve enantiomeric resolution we selected an injection pressure of 50 mbar for 1 second.

Taking in consideration all these aspects we can conclude that the optimum electrophoretic conditions for the indapamide enantioseparation are: 25 mM disodium hydrogenophosphate – 25 mM sodium didydrogenophosphate BGE, 5 mM SBE- β -CD chiral selector, buffer pH - 7, applied voltage + 25 kV, temperature 15°C, injection pressure/time 50 mbar/1 sec, UV detection at 242 nm. Applying the optimized electrophoretic conditions we succeeded in the separation of the two enantiomers in approximately 6 minutes, with a resolution of 4.30 and a separation factor of 1.08 (Figure 3).

Because we didn't have at our disposal pure indapamide enantiomers, we couldn't establish the migration order, consequently the two enantiomers

were called taking in consideration their migration order: enantiomer 1 and enantiomer 2.

Analytical performance
The analytical performances of the method were evaluated using the optimized electrophoretic conditions.

The RSD (relative standard deviation) for the migration times and peak areas was calculated by injecting consecutively (n = 6) a sample of 10 μg/ml (Table 1).

Calibration plots were constructed by preparing standard solutions (n = 3) at six concentrations in a specific concentration range (concentration range: 2.5 - 50 μg/ml). The regression equation and correlation coefficient are presented in Table 2.

The limits of detection (LOD) and quantification (LOQ) were estimated as: standard deviation of regression equation/slope of the regression equation multiplied by 3.3 and 10, respectively (Table 2).

The peaks obtained from tablets were similar to those from indapamide standard, no interference from the matrix had been observed. The content of a tablet was found to be 2.5 ± 0.06 mg (mean ± SD, n = 6). Recovery was between 97.2 and 100.7%.

Conclusion
The development of new analytical methods for the separation and determination of enantiomers has attracted great interest in last twenty-five years, since it became evident that that the biological and

pharmacological activity of enantiomers can differ and is mostly restricted to one of the enantiomers. Therefore, there is considerable pressure to develop new analytical methods for enantiomer separation, for enantiomeric purity control, pharmacological studies, pharmacodynamic investigations, clinical studies etc.

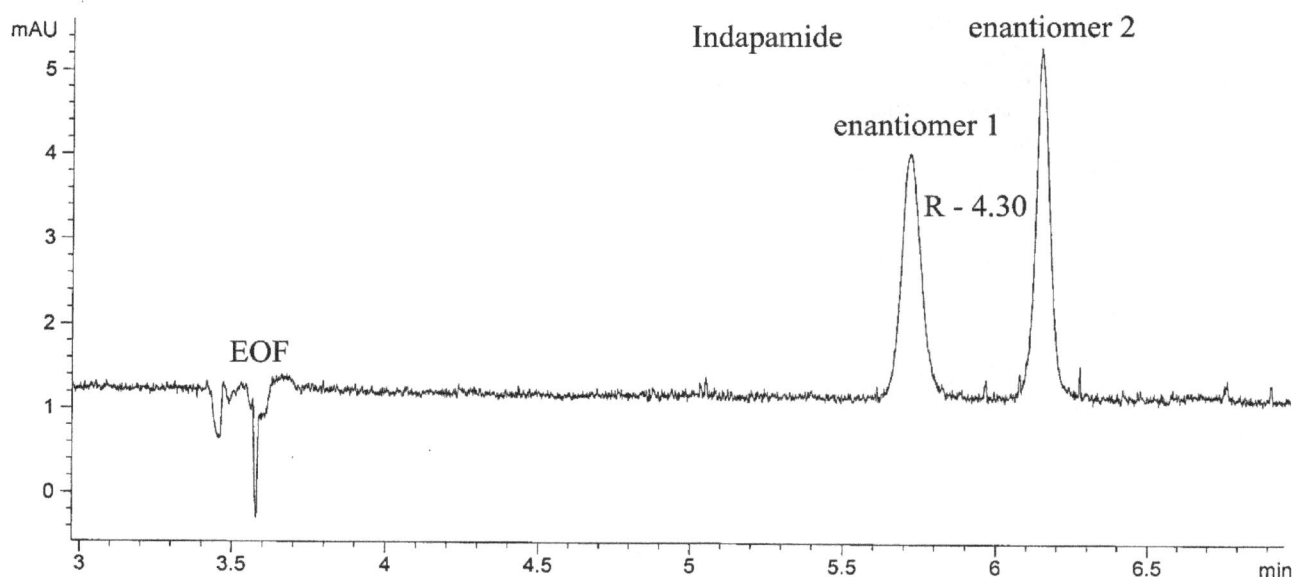

Figure 3. Capillary electrophoretic separation of indapamide enantiomers using SBE- β -CD as chiral selector (experimental conditions: BGE: 25 mM disodium hydrogenophosphate – 25 mM sodium didydrogenophosphate, chiral selector: 5 mM SBE- β -CD, pH - 7, voltage + 25 kV, temperature 15°C, hydrodinamic injection 50 mbar/1 sec., sample concentration 10 µg/ml, UV detection 242 nm)

Table 1. Analytical parameters of the indapamide chiral separation

Indapamide enantiomers	Migration time (min)	RSD migration time (%)	RSD peak area (%)	Electrohoretic mobility (cm^2/kV min)
enantiomer 1	5.70	0.25	0.82	- 8.27
enantiomer 2	6.25	0.23	0.79	- 8.44

Table 2. Calibration data and LOD/LOQ values for indapamide chiral separation (calibration range: 2.5 - 50 µg/ml)

Indapamide enantiomers	Regression equation	Correlation coefficient	LOD (µg/ml)	LOQ (µg/ml)
enantiomer 1	y = 0.462 x + 0.849	0.992	1.85	5.25
enantiomer 2	y = 0.446 x + 0.818	0.997	1.62	4.85

A simple, rapid, reproducible and accurate CZE method has been successfully developed for the enantioseparation of indapamide and applied for the determination of indapamide from tablets. The method uses a simple phosphate buffer and an anionic charged CD, SBE-β-CD, as chiral selector, producing the baseline separation of the two enantiomers with excellent chiral resolution with sharp peaks and relatively short analysis time. Highly satisfactory results were obtained from analysis of tablets, indicating the method is specific, accurate, and suitable for routine analysis of indapamide in pharmaceutical preparations.

Acknowledgments
Our work was supported with a project funded through Internal Research Grants by the University of Medicine and Pharmacy of Târgu Mureş, Romania (grant contract for execution of research projects nr. 22)

Conflict of Interest
The authors report no conflicts of interest.

References
1. Sweetman SC. Martindale: The Complete Drug Reference. 37th ed. London: Pharmaceutical Press; 2011.

2. European Pharmacopoeia. 7th ed. Strasbourg: Council of Europe; 2010.

3. Du B, Pang L, Li H, Ma S, Li Y, Jia X, et al. Chiral liquid chromatography resolution and stereoselective pharmacokinetic study of indapamide enantiomers in rats. *J Chromatogr B Analyt Technol Biomed Life Sci* 2013;932:88-91.

4. Stringham RW, Ye YK. Chiral separation of amines by high-performance liquid chromatography using polysaccharide stationary phases and acidic additives. *J Chromatogr A* 2006;1101(1-2):86-93.

5. Albu F, Georgita C, David V, Medvedovici A. Liquid chromatography-electrospray tandem mass spectrometry method for determination of indapamide in serum for single/multiple dose bioequivalence studies of sustained release formulations. *J Chromatogr B Analyt Technol Biomed Life Sci* 2005;816(1-2):35-40.

6. Girod M, Chankvetadze B, Blaschke G. Enantioseparations in non-aqueous capillary electrochromatography using polysaccharide type chiral stationary phases. *J Chromatogr A* 2000;887(1-2):439-55.

7. Kawamura K, Otsuka K, Terabe S. Capillary electrochromatographic enantioseparations using a packed capillary with a 3 microm OD-type chiral packing. *J Chromatogr A* 2001;924(1-2):251-7.

8. Kato M, Toyo'oka T. Enantiosepation by CEC using chiral stationary phases. *Chromatography* 2001;22(3):159-70.

9. Gübitz G, Schmid MG. *Chiral Separations: Methods and Protocols.* Totowa, New Jersey: Humana Press; 2004.

10. Scriba G. *Chiral Separations: Methods and Protocols*, 2nd ed. New York: Springer Science and Business Media; 2013. p. 271-392.

11. Gübitz G, Schmid MG. Chiral separation principles in capillary electrophoresis. *J Chromatogr A* 1997;792:179-225.

12. Blanco M, Valverde I. Choice of chiral selector for enantioseparation by capillary electrophoresis. *Trend Anal Chem* 2003;22:428-39.

13. Ren X, Dong Y, Liu J, Huang A, Liu H, Sun Y, et al. Separation of chiral basic drugs with sulfobutyl-β -cyclodextrin in capillary electrophoresis. *Chromatographia* 1999;50:363-8.

14. Schmitt T, Engelhardt H. Charged and uncharged cyclodextrins as chiral selectors in capillary electrophoresis. *Chromatographia* 1993;37:475-81.

29

Development and Validation of UV-Visible Spectrophotometric Method for Simultaneous Determination of Eperisone and Paracetamol in Solid Dosage Form

Shantaram Gajanan Khanage*, Popat Baban Mohite, Sandeep Jadhav

Department of Pharmaceutical Chemistry and PG studies, M.E.S. College of Pharmacy, Sonai, Ahmednagar, Maharashtra, India.

A R T I C L E I N F O

Keywords:
Eperisone Hydrochloride
Paracetamol
Iso-absorptive point
Absorption ratio method
Spectrophotometric method
ICH

A B S T R A C T

Purpose: Eperisone Hydrochloride (EPE) is a potent new generation antispasmodic drug which is used in the treatment of moderate to severe pain in combination with Paracetamol (PAR). Both drugs are available in tablet dosage form in combination with a dose of 50 mg for EPE and 325 mg PAR respectively. *Methods*: The method is based upon Q-absorption ratio method for the simultaneous determination of the EPE and PAR. Absorption ratio method is used for the ratio of the absorption at two selected wavelength one of which is the iso-absorptive point and other being the λmax of one of the two components. EPE and PAR shows their iso-absorptive point at 260 nm in methanol, the second wavelength used is 249 nm which is the λmax of PAR in methanol. *Results*: The linearity was obtained in the concentration range of 5-25 μg/mL for EPE and 2-10 μg/mL for PAR. The proposed method was effectively applied to tablet dosage form for estimation of both drugs. The accuracy and reproducibility results are close to 100% with 2% RSD. Results of the analysis were validated statistically and found to be satisfactory. The results of proposed method have been validated as per ICH guidelines. *Conclusion*: A simple, precise and economical spectrophotometric method has been developed for the estimation of EPE and PAR in pharmaceutical formulation.

Introduction

EPE is a chemically (2RS)-1-(4-Ethylphenyl)-2-methyl-3-piperidin-1-ylpropan-1-one monohydrochloride (1:1) (Figure 1). EPE is a new generation antispasmodic drug.[1] It exhibits both skeletal muscle relaxant and vasodilator properties because of its actions within the central nervous system and on vascular smooth muscles and demonstrates a variety of pharmacological effects such as cervical spondylosis, headache and low back pain.[2] EPE is official in Japanese Pharmacopeia and described potentiometric method for its estimation.[3] Literature survey divulge that ESI-MS method for estimation of EPE in human plasma,[4] HPLC/MS, GC/MS, NMR, UV and IR analytical techniques to identify a degradation product of EPE in the tablets dosage form[5] are available. More recently spectrophotometric method for simultaneous estimation of EPE and Diclofenac sodium in synthetic mixture has been reported.[6]

PAR is a chemically N-(4-Hydroxyphenyl) acetamide (Figure 1). PAR is a non-opioid, non-salicylate analgesic with an unclear mechanism of action. PAR is official in IP,[7] BP[8] and USP.[9] Literature survey reveals U.V. and chromatographic methods are available for estimation of PAR in single and combined dosage forms.[10-17] Literature survey also reveals LC-MS, GC-MS, IR[18] and HPTLC[19] methods are reported for estimation of PAR with other drugs in combination.

EPE is a potent new generation antispasmodic drug which is used in the treatment of moderate to severe pain in combination with PAR. Literature survey reveals that no method has been reported for estimation of EPE and PAR in combination. The objective of the present work is to develop new spectrophotometric method for estimation of EPE and PAR in tablet formulation with good accuracy, simplicity, precision and economy over other chromatographic methods and which can be used for routine analysis.

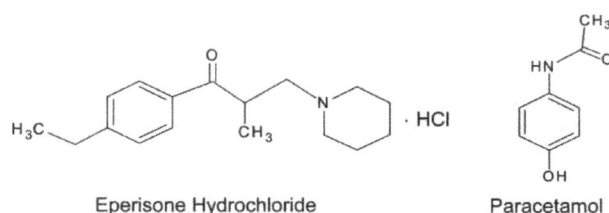

Figure 1. Structure of EPE and PAR

*Corresponding author: Shantaram Gajanan Khanage, M.E.S. College of Pharmacy, Sonai, Ahmednagar, Maharashtra-414105, India.
E-mail: shantaram1982@gmail.com

Materials and Methods

The instrument used in the present study was JASCO double beam UV/Visible Spectrophotometer (Model V-630) with spectral bandwidth of 1 nm and 10 mm a matched quartz cell was used. All weighing was done on electronic balance (Model Shimadzu BL 320-H).

Reagents and Chemicals

Analytically pure sample of EPE and PAR were obtained as a gift sample from Abbott Healthcare pvt. Ltd., Mumbai, India and Wockhardt Ltd., Aurangabad, India respectively. The analytical reagent grade methanol acquired from Loba Chemie, Mumbai, India and used as solvent. Marketed preparation of EPE and PAR was procured from local market.

Preparation of Stock Standard Solutions

Stock standard solutions of EPE and PAR were prepared separately by dissolving 10 mg in 100 mL methanol to obtain concentration 100 μg/mL of each. From these stock solutions, working standard solutions having concentration 10 μg/mL of EPE and 10 μg/mL of PAR were prepared by proper dilutions. They were scanned in the UV region i.e. 400-200 nm. The overlain spectrum (Figure 2) was obtained to determine the maximum absorbance (λ max) and iso-absorptive point.

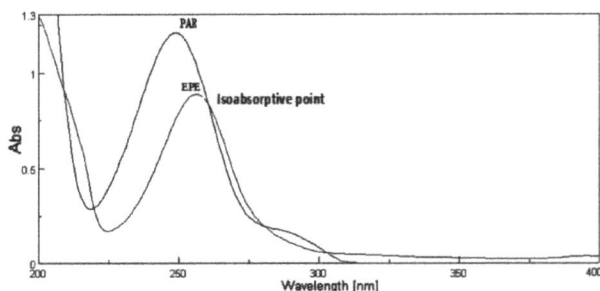

Figure 2. Overlain absorption spectra of EPE (10 μg/mL) and PAR (10 μg/mL) in methanol.

Estimation of EPE and PAR from Pharmaceutical Formulation by Q-Absorbance Ratio Method[20]

Q-Absorbance method uses the ratio of absorbance at two selected wavelengths, one at iso-absorptive point and other being the λ max of one of the two drugs. The content of twenty tablets were accurately weighed and crushed into fine powdered. A quantity of powder equivalent to 5 mg of EPE and 32.5 mg of PAR was transferred to 100 mL volumetric flask containing 60 mL methanol, shaken manually for 20 min and the volume was made up to the mark and filtered through whatmann filter paper (no.41). The solution was further diluted with methanol to give the concentration within Beer's Law range. Absorbance of this solution was measured at 249 nm and 260 nm and concentrations of these two drugs in the tablet formulation were calculated using equation (1) and equation (2).

The concentration of two drugs in mixture was calculated by using following equations:

$$C_{EPE} = \frac{Qm - Qy}{Qx - Qy} \times \frac{A}{ax1} \qquad (1)$$

$$C_{PAR} = \frac{Qm - Qx}{Qy - Qx} \times \frac{A}{ay1} \qquad (2)$$

Where,

$$Qm = \frac{\text{Absorbance of sample at 249 nm}}{\text{Absorbance of sample at 260 nm}}$$

$$Qx = \frac{E\ (1\ \%\ 1cm)\ of\ EPE\ at\ 249\ nm}{E\ (1\ \%\ 1cm)\ of\ EPE\ at\ 260\ nm}$$

$$Qy = \frac{E\ (1\ \%\ 1cm)\ of\ PAR\ at\ 249\ nm}{E\ (1\ \%\ 1cm)\ of\ PAR\ at\ 260\ nm}$$

'A', is the absorbance of mixture at 260 nm and ax1, ax2 and ay1, ay2 are E (1%, 1 cm) of EPE and PAR at 260 nm and 249 nm and Qm= A2/A1, Qy = ay2/ay1 and Qx = ax2/ax1.

Method Validation

Validation of proposed method was done as per ICH guidelines[21] by means of the following parameters.

Linearity

As per ICH guidelines the linearity of an analytical procedure is its ability (within a given range) to obtain test results which are directly proportional to the concentration (amount) of analyte in the sample.[21] An appropriate volume of EPE and PAR in the range of 0.5-2.5 mL and 0.2-1.0 mL respectively were transferred into series of separate 10 mL volumetric flasks and volume was made up to mark with methanol to get concentrations in the range of 5–25 μg/mL and 2-10 μg/mL respectively.

Accuracy and Precision

The accuracy of an analytical procedure expresses the closeness of agreement between the value which is accepted either as a conventional true value or an accepted reference value and the value found. The precision of an analytical procedure expresses the closeness of agreement (degree of scatter) between a series of measurements obtained from multiple sampling of the same homogeneous sample under the prescribed conditions.[21] The accuracy of the proposed methods was checked by recovery studies, by addition of standard drug solution to reanalyzed sample solution at three different concentration levels within the range of linearity for both the drugs. The precision of the analytical method was checked by repeated scanning and measurement of absorbance of solutions (n=5) for EPE and PAR (5 μg/mL for both drugs) without changing the parameter of the proposed spectrophotometry method.

Specificity

Specificity is the ability to assess unequivocally the analyte in the presence of components which may be expected to be present.[21] Typically these might include impurities, degradants, matrix, etc.

Limit of Detection

According to ICH guidelines the detection limit of an individual analytical procedure is the lowest amount of analyte in a sample which can be detected but not necessarily quantitated as an exact value.[21] Limit of detection can be calculated using following equation as per ICH guidelines.

$$LOD = 3.3 \times N/S$$

Where, N is the standard deviation of the peak areas of the drug and S is the slope of the corresponding calibration curve.

Limit of Quantification

The quantitation limit of an individual analytical procedure is the lowest amount of analyte in a sample which can be quantitatively determined with suitable precision and accuracy. The quantitation limit is a parameter of quantitative assays for low levels of compounds in sample matrices, and is used particularly for the determination of impurities and/or degradation products[21]. Limit of quantification can be calculated using following equation as per ICH guidelines.

$$LOQ = 10 \times N/S$$

Where, N is the standard deviation of the peak areas of the drug and S is the slope of the corresponding calibration curve.

Results

The absorbance of the EPE and PAR was measured at 255 nm and 249 nm (Figure 3) respectively and calibration curves were plotted as concentrations *versus* absorbance. The Relative Standard Deviation (RSD) for intra-day analysis of EPE was found in the range of 0.58- 1.14 % (249 nm) and 0.69-1.44 % (260 nm), RSD for Inter-day analysis of EPE was found to be 0.47-1.37% (249 nm) and 0.46-1.03% (260 nm). The RSD for intra-day analysis of PAR was found in the range of 0.39-1.08% (249 nm) and 0.37-1.24% (260 nm), RSD for Inter-day analysis of PAR was found to be 0.64-1.23% (249 nm) and 0.68-1.10% (260 nm). The accuracy and reproducibility is evident from the data as results are close to 100 % and the value of standard deviation and % R.S.D. were found to be < 2 %; shows the high precision of the method. The proposed method is simple, economical, rapid, precise and accurate. Hence it can be used for routine analysis of EPE and PAR in pharmaceutical formulation. The proposed method was found to be specific as there is no interference from other excipients. The LOD for EPE and PAR was found to be 0.12 µg/mL and 0.10 µg/mL respectively at 249 nm, LOD for EPE and PAR was found to be 0.13 µg/mL and 0.11 µg/mL respectively at

260 nm. The LOQ for EPE and PAR was found to be 0.41 µg/mL and 0.32 µg/mL respectively at 249 nm, LOQ for EPE and PAR was found to be 0.38 µg/mL and 0.34 µg/mL respectively at 260 nm. Marketed brand of tablet (Myosone plus) was analyzed, the amounts of EPE and PAR determined by proposed method were found to be 100.28% and 99.89% respectively.

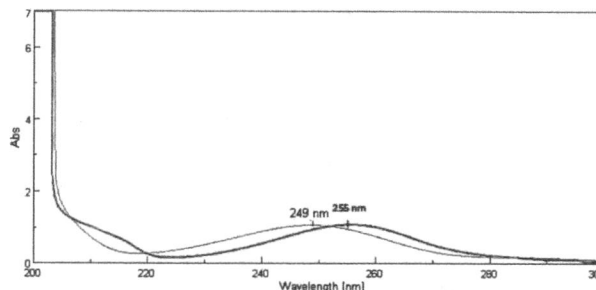

Figure 3. Absorption spectra of standard PAR at 10 µg/mL (Top) and EPE at 25 µg/mL (bottom).

Discussion

In absorbance ratio method (Q-analysis), the primary requirement for developing a method for analysis is that the entire spectra should follow the Beer's law at all the wavelength, which was fulfilled in case of both these drugs. The two wavelengths were used for the analysis of the drugs were 260 nm (iso-absorptive point) and 249 nm (λ-max of PAR) at which the calibration curves were prepared for both the drugs. In methanol, EPE and PAR obeyed linearity in the concentration range of 5-25 µg/mL and 2-10 µg/mL respectively at their respective λmax with correlation coefficient ($r^2 > 0.99$) in both the case. In proposed method precision was studied as repeatability (%RSD<2) and inter and intra-day variations (%RSD<2) for both drugs; shows the high precision of the method (Table 1). The accuracy of method was determined by calculating mean percentage recovery. It was determined at 50, 100 and 150 % level and data are presented in Table 2. The ruggedness of the methods was studied by two different analysts using the same operational and environmental conditions. The developed method for estimation of EPE and PAR in tablet dosage form was found to be simple, accurate, reproducible, sensitive and economic. For projected method we used easily available and cheap solvent like methanol (AR grade), Q analysis method of simultaneous estimation not required any expensive and satisfactory apparatus in contrast to reported chromatographic and hyphenated techniques. So it shows proposed method is simple, economic and rapid for estimation of EPE and PAR in combined dosage forms. Hence the developed method for estimation of EPE and PAR can be constructive in the routine analysis.

Table 1. Optical, Regression characteristics and validation parameters of Q-Absorbance ratio method for analysis of EPE and PAR.

Parameters		EPE		PAR	
		249	260	249	260
Beer's Law Limit (µg/mL)		5-25	5-25	2-10	2-10
Molar Absorptivity (1mole^{-1}cm^{-1})		0.08044	0.085254	0.11036	0.078079
Regression equation (y= mx + c)	Slope (m)	0.097	0.093	0.067	0.039
	Intercept (c)	0.005	0.052	0.042	0.061
Correlation Coefficient (r^2)		0.994	0.991	0.994	0.992
Standard Deviation (S.D)		0.0027	0.0036	0.0047	0.0077
Relative Standard Deviation (RSD or % CV)		0.7461	0.9145	0.6124	0.8345
LOD (µg/mL)		0.12	0.13	0.10	0.11
LOQ (µg/mL)		0.41	0.38	0.32	0.34
Precision (%RSD) (n=5)	Intraday	0.58-1.14	0.69-1.44	0.39-1.08	0.37-1.24
	Interday	0.47-1.37	0.46-1.03	0.64-1.23	0.68-1.10

Conclusion

The developed and validated UV estimation method reported here is rapid, simple, accurate, sensitive and specific. The method was also successfully used for quantitative estimation and analysis of EPE and PAR in combined dosage form. Thus the reported method is of substantial importance and has great industrial applicability for quality control and analysis of EPE and PAR in combined dosage forms. By observing validation parameter and statistical data, the proposed method was found to be satisfactory over other reported chromatographic methods.

Table 2. Recovery studies of EPE and PAR.

Drug	Conc. of drug added		%Recovery ±S.D.*
	µg/mL	%Level	
EPE	5	50	100.55±0.65
	10	100	99.76±0.56
	15	150	101.43±0.26
PAR	5	50	99.37±0.34
	10	100	100.72±0.65
	15	150	99.46±0.49
*Mean of three determinations			

Acknowledgements

The authors are thankful to Principal, M.E.S. College of Pharmacy and secretary, Honorable Prashant Patil Gadakh, Mula Education Society, Sonai, for encouragement and availing of the necessary facilities during the course of investigation. Authors are also gratified to Abbott Healthcare pvt. Ltd., Mumbai, India and Wockhardt Ltd., Aurangabad, India for providing gift sample of Eperisone Hydrochloride and Paracetamol respectively.

Conflict of Interest

The authors report no conflicts of interest.

References

1. Maryadele JN. *The Merck Index: An encyclopedia of chemicals, drugs and biological.* 14th ed. New Jersey: Merck INC., Whitehouse Station; 2006.

2. Cabitza P, Randelli P. Efficacy and safety of eperisone in patients with low back pain: A double blind randomized study. *Eur Rev Med Pharmacol Sci* 2008;12:229-35.

3. Society of Japanese Pharmacopoeia. The Japanese Pharmacopoeia. 15th ed. Shibuya Tokyo Japan: The stationery office; 2006.

4. Ding L, Wei X, Zhang S, Sheng J, Zhang Y. Rapid and sensitive liquid chromatography–electrospray ionization-mass spectrometry method for the determination of eperisone in human plasma: method and clinical applications. *J Chromatogr Sci* 2004;42:254-8.

5. Ding L, Wang X, Yang Z, Chen Y. The use of HPLC/MS, GC/MS, NMR, UV and IR to identify a degradation product of eperisone hydrochloride in the tablets. *J Pharm Biomed Anal* 2008;46(2):282-7.

6. Patel P, Patel S, Patel U. Spectophotometric method for simultenous estimation of Eperisone Hydrochloride and Diclofenac sodium in synthetic mixtures. *Int Res J pharm* 2012;3(9):203-6.

7. Government of India. The Indian Pharmacopoeia. 4th ed. New Delhi, India: Controller of Publication; 1996.

8. British pharmacopoeia. London: Her Majesty's stationary office; 2007.

9. United States Pharmacopeia and National Formulary (USP 30/NF 25). Rockville, MD, USA: United States Pharmacopeial Convention; 2007.

10. Ashraful S, Abuzar S, Kumar P. Validation of UV-Spectrophotometric and RP-HPLC methods for the simultaneous analysis of Paracetamol and Aceclofenac in marketed tablets. *Int J Pharm Life Sci* 2011;2(12):1267-75.

11. Patel M, Shah R, Kadikar H, Patani P, Shukla M. Method development and statistical validation of UV spectrophotometric method for estimation of Tolperisone hydrochloride and Paracetamol in synthetic mixture and combined dosage form. *Int J Pharm Res Bio Sci* 2012;1(1):1-19.

12. Parojcic J, Karljikovic-Rajic K, Duric Z, Jovanovic M, Ibric S. Development of the second-order derivative UV spectrophotometric method for direct determination of paracetamol in urine intended for

biopharmaceutical characterization of drug products. *Biopharm Drug Disp* 2003;24(7):309-14.

13. Shrestha B, Pradhananga R. Spectrophotometric method for the determination of paracetamol. *J Nepal Chem Soc* 2009;24:39-44.

14. Khoshayand MR, Abdollahi H, Ghaffari A, Shariatpanahi M, Farzanegan H. Simultaneous spectrophotometric determination of Paracetamol, Phenyleperine and Chlropheniramine in pharmaceuticals using chemometric approaches. *DARU* 2010;18(4):292-7.

15. Ashraful S, Shultana S, Sayeed M, Dewan I. UV-Spectrophotometric and RP-HPLC Methods for the simultaneous estimation of acetaminophen and caffeine: Validation, comparison and application for marketed tablet analysis. *Int J Pharm* 2012:2(1):39-45.

16. Kirtawade R, salve P, Seervi C, Kulkarni A, Dhabale P. Simultaneous UV Spectrophotometric Method for Estimation of Paracetamol and Nimesulide in Tablet Dosage Form. *Int J Chem Technol Res* 2010;2(2):818-21.

17. Suryan A, Bhusari V, Rasal K, Dhaneshwar S. Simultaneous Quantitation and Validation of Paracetamol, Phenylpropanolamine Hydrochloride and Cetirizine Hydrochloride by RP-HPLC in Bulk Drug and Formulation. *Int J Pharm Sci Drug Res* 2011;3(4):303-8.

18. Trafford AD, Jee RD, Moffat AC, Graham P. A rapid quantitative assay of intact Paracetamol tablets by reflectance near-infrared spectroscopy. *Analyst* 1999;124(2):163-7.

19. Baheti K, Shaikh S, Shah N, Dehghan M. Validated Simultaneous Estimation of Paracetamol and Etoricoxib in Bulk and Tablet by HPTLC Method. *Int J Res Pharm Biomed Sci* 2011;2(2):672-5.

20. Stenlake J, Backett A. *Practical Pharmaceutical chemistry*. 4th ed. New Delhi: C.B.S. Publishers; 2007.

21. International Conference on Harmonization (ICH), Draft guidelines on validation of Analytical Procedure, Definition and Terminology. Geneva: Federal Register; 1995. p. 11260-62.

Influence of Foreign DNA Introduction and Periplasmic Expression of Recombinant Human Interleukin-2 on Hydrogen Peroxide Quantity and Catalase Activity in *Escherichia coli*

Lena Mahmoudi Azar[1], Elnaz Mehdizadeh Aghdam[1], Farrokh Karimi[1,2], Babak Haghshenas[1,3], Abolfazl Barzegari[4], Parichehr Yaghmaei[5], Mohammad Saeid Hejazi[1,6]*

[1] *Department of Pharmaceutical Biotechnology, Faculty of Pharmacy, Tabriz University of Medical Sciences, Tabriz, Iran.*

[2] *Department of Biotechnology, Faculty of Science, Maragheh University, Maragheh, Iran.*

[3] *Institute of Bioscience, University of Putra Malaysia, Kualalumpur, Malaysia.*

[4] *Research Center of Pharmaceutical Nanotechnology, Tabriz University of Medical Sciences, Tabriz, Iran.*

[5] *Islamic Azad University, Science and Research Branch of Tehran, Iran.*

[6] *Faculty of Advanced Biomedical Sciences, Tabriz University of Medical Sciences, Tabriz, Iran.*

ARTICLE INFO

Keywords:
Hydrogen peroxide
Catalase activity
Periplasmic expression
Escherichia coli
Recombinant protein

ABSTRACT

Purpose: Oxidative stress is generated through imbalance between composing and decomposing of reactive oxygen species (ROS). This kind of stress was rarely discussed in connection with foreign protein production in *Escherichia coli*. Effect of cytoplasmic recombinant protein expression on Hydrogen peroxide concentration and catalase activity was previously reported. In comparison with cytoplasm, periplasmic space has different oxidative environment. Therefore, in present study we describe the effect of periplasmic expression of recombinant human interleukin-2 (hIL-2) on H_2O_2 concentration and catalase activity in *Escherichia coli* and their correlation with cell growth. *Methods:* Having constructed pET2hIL2 vector, periplasmic expression of hIL-2 was confirmed. Then, H_2O_2 concentration and catalase activity were determined at various ODs. Wild type and empty vector transformed cells were used as negative controls. *Results:* It was shown that H_2O_2 concentration in hIL-2 expressing cells was significantly higher than its concentration in wild type and empty vector transformed cells. Catalase activity and growth rate reduced significantly in hIL-2 expressing cells compared to empty vector transformed and wild type cells. Variation of H_2O_2 concentration and catalase activity is intensive in periplasmic hIL-2 expressing cells than empty vector containing cells. Correlation between H_2O_2 concentration elevation and catalase activity reduction with cell growth depletion are also demonstrated. *Conclusion:* Periplasmic expression of recombinant hIL-2 elevates the host cell's hydrogen peroxide concentration possibly due to reduced catalase activity which has consequent suppressive effect on growth rate.

Introduction

Prokaryotic expression systems such as *Escherichia coli* have been greatly utilized for production of recombinant proteins; however, they have not been constructed as a foreign protein producer, naturally.[1-3] The physiology of the host cell impeded by plasmid presence and the expression of recombinant genes and consequently cellular stress reactions are imposed.[4,5] Metabolic load is considered as the main reason for cell growth depletion in recombinant cells.[2] The presence of plasmid and its replication as well as overexpression of recombinant genes are causative factors to metabolic load.[6,7] In these conditions, cell growth can be restricted due to the low accessibility of energy and nutrient resources, a condition identified as starvation. Accordingly, expression of many genes for amino acid biosynthesis is repressed. This starvation-like effect seems to be the chief cause for the decreased expression of the foreign gene products in high cell-density cultures.[8]

There are several approaches to improve recombinant protein production, such as selecting high level expression systems, optimizing expression conditions

---

*Corresponding author: Mohammad Saeid Hejazi, Department of Pharmaceutical Biotechnology, Faculty of Pharmacy, Tabriz University of Medical Sciences, Tabriz, Iran. Email: saeidhejazi@tbzmed.ac.ir, msaeidhejazi@yahoo.com

for improving protein solubility[9] and optimization of media formulation.[10,11] Additionally, in order to control protein production induced stresses, some gene manipulations such as metabolic genes[12-15] and stress responsive genes[16-18] have been applied in several cases. In the other side, determination of unknown inhibiting factors during foreign protein production and resolving their inhibitory effects could improve the yield of the production theoretically.

Reactive oxygen species (ROS) such as superoxide $(O_2^{\cdot})$ and hydrogen peroxide (H_2O_2) are produced as normal by-products of aerobic life. Imbalance between generation and elimination of ROS promotes oxidative stress which causes lethal cell damages.[19-23] Oxidation of various cell constituents as DNA,[24] lipids and proteins,[25] induces fundamental changes responsible for death.[26,27] It is established that specific oxidation of thiol groups of proteins involved in detoxification of H_2O_2 and biosynthesis pathway such as cobalamin-independent methionine synthase (MetE) is caused by H_2O_2-induced oxidative stress. MetE is inactivated by H_2O_2 in *E. coli* which is associated with methionine limitation imposed by oxidative stress.[28,29]

The respiratory chain can be the source of as much as 87% of the total H_2O_2 production in *E. coli*.[30] Most of the H_2O_2 in exponentially growing *E. coli* cultures is generated from superoxide ion $(2O_2^{-} + 2e^{-} + 4H^{+} \rightarrow H_2O_2 + O_2)$ and the generation of superoxide anion and hydrogen peroxide depends on the stage of culture development.[30] In *E. coli*, H_2O_2 is removed by two kinds of catalases producing H_2O and O_2. These enzymes include hydroperoxidase I (HPI), existing during aerobic growth and transcriptionally controlled at various levels,[31] and hydroperoxidase II (HPII),[32,33] which is induced during stationary phase.

Having synthesized in the cytoplasm, some of recombinant proteins are sent into the extracytoplasmic spaces chiefly the periplasm.[34,35] Besides, in order to increase cell productivity and product quality, it is a common strategy to export recombinant products to the periplasm. As its oxidative environment leads to appropriate disulfide bond formation and consequent correct folding,[36] less degradation due to presence of fewer proteases[37] and the easy extraction of final proteins.[38] The presence of superoxide dismutases containing copper plus zinc ions (Cu, Zn-SOD)[39,40] and KatG (HPI) enzymes metabolizing superoxide anion and hydrogen peroxide in the periplasmic space of *E. coli*, respectively, protects the environment from oxidative damage.[20]

Reportedly, one of the impacts of starvation on *E. coli* cells is the increasing of some defense proteins responding to oxidative stress. These proteins prevent accumulation of oxidative damage in growth arrested cells.[41] In addition, although, an aerobic environment seems to be preferable for *E. coli* cultivation, oxygen can easily become limited in aerobic fast-growing cultures which influence cell physiology through the accumulation of acetate.[42] In the other side, the presence of oxygen can oxidize electron carriers to generate hydrogen peroxide or superoxide anion, resulting in oxidative stress.[43] In spite of these known associations, relation of metabolic burden and oxidative stress in foreign protein producing cells has not been investigated inclusively. Recently, we studied H_2O_2 concentration and catalase activity following introduction of foreign DNA and recombinant protein expression. Our results showed a significant elevation in hydrogen peroxide concentration as the most stable component of ROS and reduction of catalase activity as an important H_2O_2 decomposer.[44,45] This could be considered as a limiting factor in production of recombinant protein. Following our previous reports and considering the benefits of periplasmic expression of foreign proteins and consequently the high interest in production of recombinant proteins in periplasmic space, we aimed to investigate H_2O_2 concentration and catalase activity following periplasmic expression of recombinant human IL-2 as a non-enzymatic and nontoxic as well as non-functional protein for *E. coli* in the recombinant cells. Moreover, correlation between H_2O_2 concentration and catalase activity following recombinant protein expression with cell growth was studied. The special emphasis is given to the comparison of the alteration in H_2O_2 concentration and catalase activity among recombinant protein expressing, foreign DNA introduced and wild type cells.

Materials and Methods

Bacterial strains and culture media

E. coli DH5α and BL21(DE3) strains were used as host cells for plasmid amplification and recombinant protein expression, respectively. pET-22b(+) expression vector was used for cloning of hIL-2 coding DNA. Bacteria were grown in LB (Bacto-tryptone 10 g/l, yeast extract 5 g/l, and NaCl 10 g/l) or LB agar media supplemented with ampicillin (100 μg/ml) in shaker incubator overnight at 37 °C.

PCR amplification of hIL-2 DNA and construction of pET2hIL2 plasmid

Plasmid r-PWhIL-2B7.MA (a kind gift from Dr. Joop Gäken King's College London, London) was used as the template DNA for mature IL-2 encoding DNA amplification using polymerase chain reaction (PCR) technique. Therefore, a pair of specific forward [5′-CGC GGA TCC TGC ACC TAC TTC AAG T-3′] and reverse [5′-ACT AAG CTT TTA AGT CAG TGT TGA G-3′] primers creating *Bam*HI and *Hind*III restriction sites at 5′ and 3′ ends of the amplified DNA fragment, respectively, were designed based on human interleukin-2 gene sequence. The primers were supplied from Eurofins MWG Operon Company. The PCR reaction was performed to amplify DNA fragments.

The amplified DNA was isolated by gel electrophoresis, extracted using Qiagen gel extraction and cloned into pTZ57R/T cloning vector. *E. coli* DH5α cells were transformed with the cloning solution and were cultured on LB medium containing ampicillin, IPTG and X-gal. Treatment of the clones with *Bam*HI and *Hin*dIII enzymes resulted in the release of hIL-2 coding DNA with sticky ends. The released fragment was extracted from the gel and ligated in pET-22b(+) expression vector resulting in construction of pET2hIL2 vector (Figure 1)

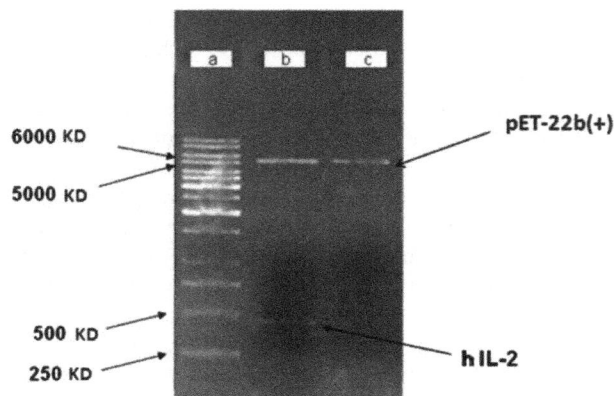

Figure 1. Agarose gel electrophoresis of pET-22b(+) and pET2hIL2 plasmids after digestion with *Bam*HI and *Hin*dIII restriction enzymes. a) 1kb DNA ladder, b) digested pET2hIL2 containing of hIL-2 and c) digested empty vector pET-22b(+).

Evaluation of hIL-2 expression

Having treated with IPTG (0.5 mM), cultures were incubated and then cells harvested by centrifugation at 4000 rpm. Pellets resuspended in 50 μl of loading buffer (2X SDS gel-loading buffer) and 50 μl of 10 mM phosphate buffer (pH 7.0) containing lysozyme. In order to extract periplasmic proteins, the solution was sonicated for 10 minutes and total proteins were isolated after the pellet resuspention in 50 μl of loading buffer and 50 μl of H_2O and boiled for 15 minutes. Then, SDS-PAGE electrophoresis gel (12% separating gel and 5% stacking gel) was used for evaluation of recombinant hIL-2 expression.

Growth curve

In order to draw the growth curve of the cells, optical density (OD) of the cultures was measured spectrophotometrically at 600 nm every half hour. Having adjusted the OD of overnight grown cultures at 1, the samples were diluted 1/100 (v/v) and incubated. As a means to investigate the consequence of recombinant protein expression on the growth rate, the media were treated with IPTG with final concentration of 0.5 mM at OD 0.5. As all following studies, wild type untransformed and pET-22b(+) transformed cells were used as negative controls.

Measurement of H_2O_2 concentration
Sample preparation
1.5 ml of bacterial culture was collected at ODs 0.6, 0.7, 0.8 and 1.2 by centrifugation at 13000 rpm for 10 min. The pellet was homogenized in 1.5 ml of 0.1%

(w/v) trichloroacetic acid by sonication at 22 KHz for 10 min. After centrifugation again at 14000 rpm for 10 min, the final supernatant was used for H_2O_2 assay.

H_2O_2 measurement
The protocol described by Velikova and colleagues[46] was used for H_2O_2 assay. 0.5 ml of the supernatant was added to the mixture of 0.5 ml of 10 mM phosphate buffer (pH 7.0) and 1 ml of 1M potassium iodide and kept in dark place for 10 min. Then, the absorbance of solution was read at 390 nm and H_2O_2 concentration was calculated using the standard curve. The blank sample was made of 1 ml of 10 mM phosphate buffer (pH 7.0) and 1 ml of 1M potassium iodide.

Catalase activity assay
Sample preparation for catalase activity and protein estimation
In order to measure catalase activity, suspended cells in 1 ml of buffer (50 mM phosphate buffer (pH 7.0) and 0.5 mM EDTA) were lysed in sonicator at 22 kHz in an ice bath for 10 min. After removing the pellet by centrifuging at 14000 rpm for 10 min at 4 °C, the supernatant was used to determine catalase activity.

Measurement of catalase activity
Catalase activity measurement was based on H_2O_2 decomposition assay spectrophotometrically. H_2O_2 decomposition was measured according to the absorbance difference between 0 and 5 min at 240 nm in 2 ml reaction mixture and quantified based on standard curve. The reaction mixture contained 200 μl cell extract, 50 mM phosphate potassium buffer (pH 7.0), 0.5 mM EDTA and 10 mM hydrogen peroxide 30%. One catalase activity unit is the amount of enzyme decomposing 1.0 μmole of hydrogen peroxide per minute at pH 7.0 and 25 °C.

Total protein measurement
Total protein concentration was determined according to Bradford method[47] using bovine serum albumin as the standard. 200 μl of cell extract was added to the solution containing 1400 μl of 50 mM K-phosphate buffer, 0.5 mM EDTA and 400 μl of Bradford reagent and the absorbance of reaction was measured at 595 nm between 5 to 30 min.

Statistical analyses
All data were represented as means ± S.E.M of three or four replicates. Statistical analyses were performed using one-way analysis of variance (ANOVA). Statistical assessment of difference between mean values was performed by least significance difference (LSD) test at $p < 0.05$ using SPSS (16 version) software.

Results
Evaluation of recombinant hIL-2 expression
SDS-PAGE analysis was carried out to confirm the expression of recombinant hIL-2 protein.

Bacterial cells were induced with 0.5 mM IPTG at OD 0.5 after and incubation for 2.5 hours in shaker at 37°C. Following the total and periplasmic protein extraction and SDS- PAGE analysis, the existence of a protein band with molecular weight of about 14.5 KDa is corresponding to hIL-2 expression in the cells (Figure 2). Expression of hIL-2 protein was not observed in empty vector transformed and non-induced cells used as negative controls.

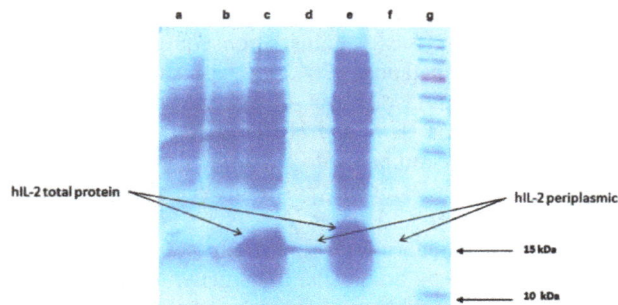

Figure 2. SDS-PAGE analysis of total and periplasmic expression of human interleukin-2. Total protein extracted from non induced pET2hIL2 transformed cells (lane a) and empty pET-22b(+) vector transformed (lane b) as negative controls. Total protein extracted from pET2hIL2 transformed cells after inducing with IPTG 0.5 mM (lane c and lane e), and periplasmic protein extraction pET2hIL2 transformed cells after inducing with IPTG 0.5 mM (lane d and lane f). Lane g is protein ladder.

Growth curve

As shown Figure 3, among three types of bacteria, wild type cells displayed faster growth than recombinant cells. It passes the lag phase and enters exponential phase faster than recombinant bacteria. pET2hIL2 as expressing cells show lower growth than others. It grew slower and passes lag phase and exponential phase later than others and also enters stationary phase earlier than pET-22b(+) and wild type cells. pET-22b(+) as empty vector transformed cells, displayed growth between wild type and expressing cells. It enters exponential phase before hIL-2 expressing cells and after wild type cells. The entrance of empty vector transformed cells into stationary phase was observed after recombinant pET2hIL2 transformed cells, but before wild type.

Measurement of H_2O_2 concentration

H_2O_2 concentration variations are represented in Figure 4. Comparison of bacterial cells H_2O_2 content indicates a significant increase at the amount of H_2O_2 between wild type and hIL-2 expressing cells at each OD. According to Figure 4 increase of H_2O_2 content was observed from OD: 0.6 to OD: 0.7 at all cell types. A noticeable difference between OD: 0.7 and OD: 0.8 was not existed in H_2O_2 quantities, but decrease of H_2O_2 was distinguished at OD: 1.2 in all bacteria. Peak of H_2O_2 amount was 19.43 ± 1 µM at OD: 0.7 related to hIL-2 expressing cells. At the same optical density, pET-22b(+) empty vector transformed cells and wild type cells showed 11.80 ± 0.65 µM and 9.09 ± 1.11 µM

H_2O_2 content respectively. Lowest amount of H_2O_2 was measured as 2.56 ± 0.87 µM and 2.26 ± 0.92 µM at OD: 0.6 and 1.2 in wild type cells. At ODs 0.6, 0.8 and 1.2, the highest amount of H_2O_2 was also measured in recombinant hIL-2 expressing cells as 13.61 ± 0.69 µM, 13.76 ± 1.13 µM and 7.13 ± 0.28 µM respectively. The amounts of H_2O_2 were 8.94 ± 1.13 µM, 11.80 ± 0.65 µM, 8.34 ± 0.66 µM and 3.64 ± 1.02 µM from OD 0.6 to 1.2 in pET-22b(+) empty vector transformed cells, approximately, the quantities between wild type and expressing cells. Finally, comparison of H_2O_2 concentration among different types of bacterial cells at the all ODs showed a significant increase on H_2O_2 amount from wild type to pET2hIL2 expressing cells.

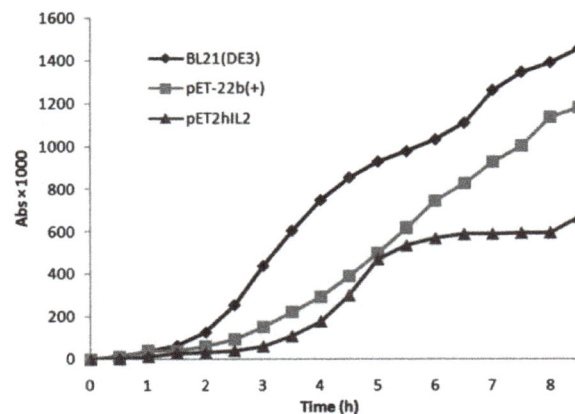

Figure 3. Growth curve of wild type and recombinant E .coli cells (pET-22b(+), pET2hIL2) for 8 hours. Optical density was measured every 30 minutes and induction of the cells was done with IPTG (0.5 mM) at OD: 0.5 by 0.5 mM IPTG.

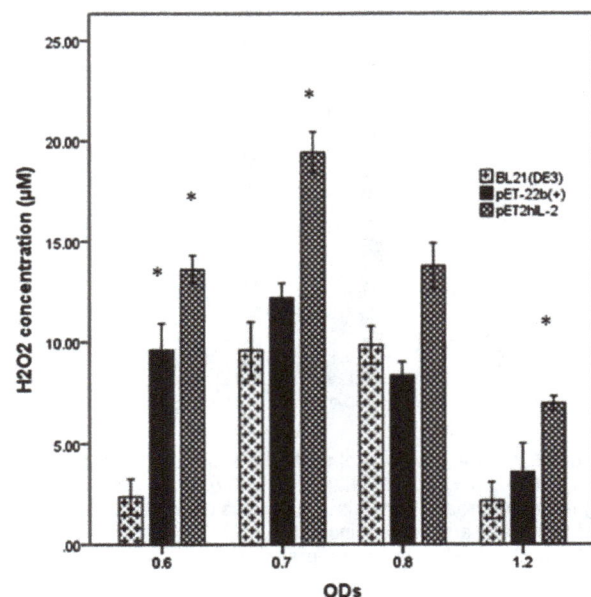

Figure 4. H_2O_2 concentration of wild type (BL21(DE3)) and recombinant E. coli cells (pET-22b(+), pET2hIL2) at OD 0.6, 0.7 0.8 and 1.2. Significant increase in H_2O_2 concentration is observed from BL21(DE3) to recombinant cells which is shown by "*" ($p<0.05$). All data were represented as means ± S.E.M of three or four replicates.

Catalase activity assay

Catalase is an endogenous antioxidant enzyme present in all aerobic cells and removes toxic H_2O_2 molecule from the cell by converting it into H_2O molecule. One catalase unit is the amount of enzyme decomposing 1.0 μmole of hydrogen peroxide per minute at pH 7.0 and 25 °C. As shown in Figure 5, catalase activity was decreased significantly from 11.92 ± 0.72 Umg^{-1}min^{-1} in wild type cells to 9.97 ± 0.61 Umg^{-1}min^{-1} and 5.97 ± 0.78 Umg^{-1}min^{-1} respectively in empty vector transformed cells and expressing cells at OD: 0.6. Wild type cells had maximum catalase activity compared to recombinant bacteria as 16.86 ± 0.66 Umg^{-1}min^{-1} and 17.38 ± 0.76 Umg^{-1}min^{-1} especially at OD: 0.7 and 0.8. Empty vector transformed cells displayed high catalase activity than pET2hIL2 producing cells and low catalase activity than BL21 (DE3) wild type cells at ODs 0.6, 0.7, 0.8 and 1.2 as 9.97 ± 0.61 Umg^{-1}min^{-1}, 12.05 ± 0.59 Umg^{-1}min^{-1}, 12.68 ± 1.04 and 9.85 ± 0.67 Umg^{-1}min^{-1}. The measured catalase activity at all ODs (0.6, 0.7, 0.8 and 1.2) was demonstrated the noticeable decrease from wild type to pET-22b(+) empty vector transformed cells and pET2hIL2 expressing cells. Finally, catalase activity among different types of bacteria at all ODs showed a significant decrease on the level of catalase activity from wild type to pET2hIL2 expressing cells and also, high level of catalase activity was shown at OD: 0.7 and 0.8 related to wild type cells.

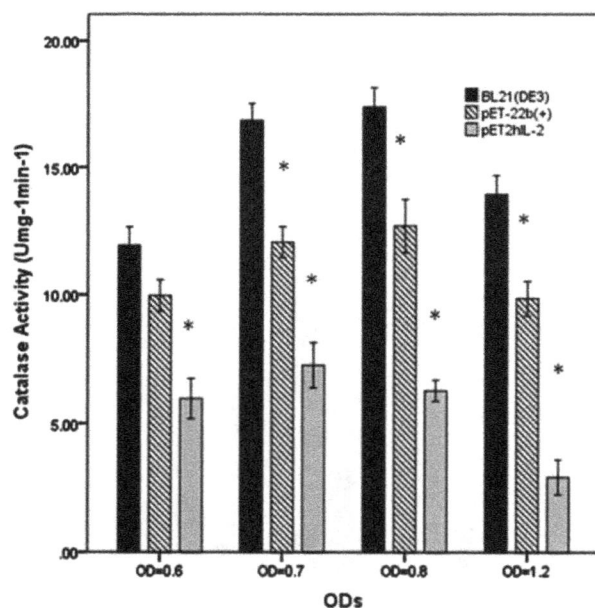

Figure 5. Catalase activity of wild type and recombinant *E. coli* cells (pET-22b(+), pET2hIL2) at OD 0.6, 0.7, 0.8 and 1.2. Significant decrease in catalase activity is distinguished among wild type cells and recombinant *E. coli* cells which are shown by "*" ($p<0.05$). All data were represented as means ± S.E.M of three or four replicates.

Discussion

Reaching high levels of recombinant protein production impairs the metabolism of host cell[48] even if the protein itself is non toxic or has no obvious biological activity on the cell.[2,3] These challenges often occur in the place where recombinant proteins locate. All recombinant proteins are first produced and mostly sited in the cytoplasm.[2] However, in *E. coli*, foreign gene products can be placed in various intracellular compartments, such as the cytoplasm, inner membrane, periplasm, and outer member[49] or can be secreted extracellularly.[50] Aerobic microorganisms are always under the risk of oxidative stress following imbalance between generation and detoxifying of ROS.[51] Nevertheless, *E. coli* and other cells are equipped with several antioxidant enzymes against consequent oxidative damage. For instance, *E. coli* has two forms of superoxide dismutase (MnSOD and FeSOD)[40] and two forms of catalase (HPI and HPII).[33] SOD decomposes the superoxide radical into hydrogen peroxide and oxygen, and catalase catalyses hydrogen peroxide into molecular oxygen and water.[52]

Considering recombinant protein expression as a kind of challenge in the host cells, ROS generation could be one of the causative factors for reduced cell growth and protein production in recombinant cells. This hypothesis was proved in our previous study on cytoplasmic hIL-2 and mouse interleukin-4 (mIL-4) expressing cells. The present study aimed to evaluate ROS generation and cell growth rate following of recombinant protein expression in periplasm, as a location with different aspects of oxidation properties. The best conditions for recombinant protein production such as bacterial hosts, expression systems and products' purification are so important.[53-55] We have already reported H_2O_2 generation following expression of recombinant proteins in *E. coli*.[44,45] In this study the effect of periplasmic expression of hIL-2 on H_2O_2 concentration and catalase activity was investigated. To achieve this goal variation in H_2O_2 concentration and catalase activity were examined in wild type and recombinant cells containing pET-22b(+) and pET2hIL2 vectors. Both transformed cells (pET-22b(+) and pET2hIL2) are ampicillin resistant cells, but pET2hIL2 expressing cells has an extra sequence of hIL-2 gene compared to empty vector pET-22b(+). Assuming that the only difference between pET2hIL2 and pET-22b(+) transformed cells is hIL-2 protein production, the various changes in H_2O_2 concentration and catalase activity in hIL-2 expressing cells and empty vector transformed cells is attributed to absolute effect of the recombinant protein expression. Recombinant cells and wild type cells were also compared in terms of growth rate.

Growth curve analysis (Figure 3) showed the fastest and the highest growth rate for wild type cells. Wild type cells passed lag phase and entered exponential phase faster than recombinant cells. Among recombinant cells, periplasmic protein expressing cells grew slower than wild type cells and empty vector harboring cells. Therefore, empty vector transformed cells had a growth rate between wild type cells and hIL-2 expressing cells. The elevated H_2O_2

concentration was observed in recombinant cells compared to wild type cells. Between transformed cells, H_2O_2 concentration was increased significantly in periplasmic hIL-2 expressing cells compared to empty vector harboring cells (Figure 4). These variations derive from the presence of foreign DNA and recombinant protein expression in recombinant bacterial cells. In contrast to the increase of H_2O_2 concentration, reduction of catalase activity was observed in recombinant cells. Catalase activity was decreased significantly in recombinant cells compared to wild type cells. Maximum catalase activity was observed in wild type cells. Recombinant periplasmic hIL-2 expressing cells had the lowest catalase activity and empty vector pET-22b(+) harboring cells showed quantities between expressing cells and wild type cells, like other comparative instances (Figure 5). The results obtained from the present study show that entrance of foreign DNA in host cells reduces growth rate of recombinant bacteria which is in accordance with H_2O_2 accumulation and catalase activity decline. Variation of H_2O_2 concentration and catalase activity is intensive in periplasmic hIL-2 expressing cells than empty vector containing cells. These results revealed a correlation between expression of recombinant hIL-2 protein and changes in H_2O_2 amount and catalase activity. Our findings suggest complementary studies to elucidate the effect of ROS elimination on the improvement of growth rate and recombinant protein production in recombinant cells.

Conclusion

It is concluded that periplasmic hIL-2 expression affects the host cell's hydrogen peroxide concentration possibly due to reduced catalase activity. These effects results in suppression of the growth rate of the recombinant cells meaning that in addition to metabolic load, "H_2O_2 upshift stress resulted from hIL-2 expression" could be considered as a reason for cell growth repression. Additionally, comparison of recombinant hIL-2 expression and introduction of DNA (empty plasmid) into the cells showed that influence of recombinant hIL-2 expression on the H_2O_2 concentration elevation and catalase activity reduction is more than the effects of empty vector introduction.

Conflict of Interest

The authors report no conflicts of interest.

References

1. Bentley WE, Mirjalili N, Andersen DC, Davis RH, Kompala DS. Plasmid-encoded protein: the principal factor in the "metabolic burden" associated with recombinant bacteria. *Biotechnol Bioeng* 1990;35(7):668-81.
2. Glick BR. Metabolic load and heterologous gene expression. *Biotechnol Adv* 1995;13(2):247-61.
3. Hoffmann F, Rinas U. Stress induced by recombinant protein production in Escherichia coli. *Adv Biochem Eng Biotechnol* 2004;89:73-92.
4. Ron EZ. Bacterial stress response. In: Rosenberg E, DeLong E, Lory S, Stackebrandt E, Thompson F, editors. The prokaryotes. 4th ed. Berlin: Springer; 2013. P. 589-603.
5. Chou CP. Engineering cell physiology to enhance recombinant protein production in Escherichia coli. *Appl Microbiol Biotechnol* 2007;76(3):521-32.
6. Wang Z, Xiang L, Shao J, Wegrzyn A, Wegrzyn G. Effects of the presence of ColE1 plasmid DNA in Escherichia coli on the host cell metabolism. *Microb Cell Fact* 2006;5:34.
7. Grabherr R, Nilsson E, Striedner G, Bayer K. Stabilizing plasmid copy number to improve recombinant protein production. *Biotechnol Bioeng* 2002;77(2):142-7.
8. Yoon SH, Han MJ, Lee SY, Jeong KJ, Yoo JS. Combined transcriptome and proteome analysis of Escherichia coli during high cell density culture. *Biotechnol Bioeng* 2003;81(7):753-67.
9. Doonan S. Protein Purification Protocols. In: Yip TT, Hutchens TW, editors. Methods in Molecular Biology. Totowa, NJ: Humana Press Inc;1996. P. 57-75.
10. Rathore AS, Bilbrey RE, Steinmeyer DE. Optimization of an osmotic shock procedure for isolation of a protein product expressed in E. coli. *Biotechnol Prog* 2003;19(5):1541-6.
11. Broedel SE, Papciak, SM, Jones WR. The selection of optimum media formulations for improved expression of recombinant proteins in *E. coli. Tech Bull* 2001;2:1-7.
12. De Anda R, Lara AR, Hernandez V, Hernandez-Montalvo V, Gosset G, Bolivar F, et al. Replacement of the glucose phosphotransferase transport system by galactose permease reduces acetate accumulation and improves process performance of Escherichia coli for recombinant protein production without impairment of growth rate. *Metab Eng* 2006;8(3):281-90.
13. Vemuri GN, Eiteman MA, Altman E. Increased recombinant protein production in Escherichia coli strains with overexpressed water-forming NADH oxidase and a deleted ArcA regulatory protein. *Biotechnol Bioeng* 2006;94(3):538-42.
14. Picon A, Teixeira De Mattos MJ, Postma PW. Reducing the glucose uptake rate in Escherichia coli affects growth rate but not protein production. *Biotechnol Bioeng* 2005;90(2):191-200.
15. Gosset G. Improvement of Escherichia coli production strains by modification of the phosphoenolpyruvate:sugar phosphotransferase system. *Microb Cell Fact* 2005;4(1):14.
16. Jeong KJ, Choi JH, Yoo WM, Keum KC, Yoo NC, Lee SY, et al. Constitutive production of human leptin by fed-batch culture of recombinant rpoS-

Escherichia coli. *Protein Expr Purif* 2004;36(1):150-6.

17. De Marco A, Vigh L, Diamant S, Goloubinoff P. Native folding of aggregation-prone recombinant proteins in Escherichia coli by osmolytes, plasmid- or benzyl alcohol-overexpressed molecular chaperones. *Cell Stress Chaperones* 2005;10(4):329-39.

18. Lethanh H, Neubauer P, Hoffmann F. The small heat-shock proteins IbpA and IbpB reduce the stress load of recombinant Escherichia coli and delay degradation of inclusion bodies. *Microb Cell Fact* 2005;4(1):6.

19. Cabiscol E, Tamarit J, Ros J. Oxidative stress in bacteria and protein damage by reactive oxygen species. *Int Microbiol* 2000;3(1):3-8.

20. Lushchak VI. Adaptive response to oxidative stress: Bacteria, fungi, plants and animals. *Comp Biochem Physiol C Toxicol Pharmacol* 2011;153(2):175-90.

21. Dong C, Li G, Li Z, Zhu H, Zhou M, Hu Z. Molecular cloning and expression analysis of an Mn-SOD gene from Nelumbo nucifera. *Appl Biochem Biotechnol* 2009;158(3):605-14.

22. Dong C, Zheng X, Li G, Zhu H, Zhou M, Hu Z. Molecular cloning and expression of two cytosolic copper-zinc superoxide dismutases genes from Nelumbo nucifera. *Appl Biochem Biotechnol* 2011;163(5):679-91.

23. Khaket TP, Ahmad R. Biochemical studies on hemoglobin modified with reactive oxygen species (ROS). *Appl Biochem Biotechnol* 2011;164(8):1422-30.

24. Wiseman H, Halliwell B. Damage to DNA by reactive oxygen and nitrogen species: role in inflammatory disease and progression to cancer. *Biochem J* 1996;313 (Pt 1):17-29.

25. Stadtman ER. Metal ion-catalyzed oxidation of proteins: biochemical mechanism and biological consequences. *Free Radic Biol Med* 1990;9(4):315-25.

26. Boonstra J, Post JA. Molecular events associated with reactive oxygen species and cell cycle progression in mammalian cells. *Gene* 2004;337:1-13.

27. Giannattasio S, Guaragnella N, Corte-Real M, Passarella S, Marra E. Acid stress adaptation protects Saccharomyces cerevisiae from acetic acid-induced programmed cell death. *Gene* 2005;354:93-8.

28. Hondorp ER, Matthews RG. Oxidative stress inactivates cobalamin-independent methionine synthase (MetE) in Escherichia coli. *PLoS Biol* 2004;2(11):e336.

29. Leichert LI, Jakob U. Protein thiol modifications visualized in vivo. *PLoS Biol* 2004;2(11):e333.

30. Gonzalez-Flecha B, Demple B. Metabolic sources of hydrogen peroxide in aerobically growing Escherichia coli. *J Biol Chem* 1995;270(23):13681-7.

31. Gonzalez-Flecha B, Demple B. Homeostatic regulation of intracellular hydrogen peroxide concentration in aerobically growing Escherichia coli. *J Bacteriol* 1997;179(2):382-8.

32. Von Ossowski I, Mulvey MR, Leco PA, Borys A, Loewen PC. Nucleotide sequence of Escherichia coli katE, which encodes catalase HPII. *J Bacteriol* 1991;173(2):514-20.

33. Loewen PC, Switala J, Triggs-Raine BL. Catalases HPI and HPII in Escherichia coli are induced independently. *Arch Biochem Biophys* 1985;243(1):144-9.

34. Cornelis P. Expressing genes in different Escherichia coli compartments. *Curr Opin Biotechnol* 2000;11(5):450-4.

35. Baneyx F. Recombinant protein expression in Escherichia coli. *Curr Opin Biotechnol* 1999;10(5):411-21.

36. Messens J, Collet JF. Pathways of disulfide bond formation in Escherichia coli. *Int J Biochem Cell Biol* 2006;38(7):1050-62.

37. Gottesman S. Proteases and their targets in *Escherichia coli*. *Annu Rev Genet* 1996;30:465-506.

38. Anderluh G, Gokce I, Lakey JH. Expression of proteins using the third domain of the Escherichia coli periplasmic-protein TolA as a fusion partner. *Protein Expres Purif* 2003;28(1):173-81.

39. Benov LT, Fridovich I. Escherichia coli expresses a copper- and zinc-containing superoxide dismutase. *J Biol Chem* 1994;269(41):25310-4.

40. Hadji I, Marzouki MN, Ferraro D, Fasano E, Majdoub H, Pani G, et al. Purification and characterization of a Cu,Zn-SOD from garlic (Allium sativum L.). Antioxidant effect on tumoral cell lines. *Appl Biochem Biotechnol* 2007;143(2):129-41.

41. Nystrom T. Starvation, cessation of growth and bacterial aging. *Curr Opin Microbiol* 1999;2(2):214-9.

42. Phue JN, Shiloach J. Impact of dissolved oxygen concentration on acetate accumulation and physiology of E. coli BL21, evaluating transcription levels of key genes at different dissolved oxygen conditions. *Metab Eng* 2005;7(5-6):353-63.

43. Storz G, Imlay JA. Oxidative stress. *Curr Opin Microbiol* 1999;2(2):188-94.

44. Hejazi MS, Karimi F, Mehdizadeh Aghdam E, Barzegari A, Farshdosti Hagh M, Parvizi M, et al. Cytoplasmic expression of recombinant interleukin-2 and interleukin-4 proteins results in hydrogen peroxide accumulation and reduction in catalase activity in *Escherichia coli*. *DARU* 2009;17(2):64-71.

45. Mehdizadeh Aghdam E, Mahmoudi Azar L, Barzegari A, Karimi F, Mesbahfar M, Samadi N, et al. Effect of periplasmic expression of recombinant mouse interleukin-4 on hydrogen peroxide concentration and catalase activity in Escherichia coli. *Gene* 2012;511(2):455-60.

46. Velikova V, Yordanov I, Edreva A. Oxidative stress and some antioxidant systems in acid raintreated bean plants- Protective role of exogenous polyamines. *Plant Sci* 2000;151(1):59-66.

47. Bradford MM. A rapid and sensitive method for the quantitation of microgram quantities of protein utilizing the principle of protein-dye binding. *Anal Biochem* 1976;72:248-54.

48. Boor KJ. Bacterial stress responses: what doesn't kill them can make then stronger. *PLoS Biol* 2006;4(1):e23.

49. Lee HJ, Gu MB. Construction of a sodA::luxCDABE fusion Escherichia coli: comparison with a katG fusion strain through their responses to oxidative stresses. *Appl Microbiol Biotechnol* 2003;60(5):577-80.

50. Georgiou G, Segatori L. Preparative expression of secreted proteins in bacteria: status report and future prospects. *Curr Opin Biotechnol* 2005;16(5):538-45.

51. Paradies G, Petrosillo G, Pistolese M, Ruggiero FM. Reactive oxygen species affect mitochondrial electron transport complex I activity through oxidative cardiolipin damage. *Gene* 2002;286(1):135-41.

52. Lushchak VI. Oxidative stress and mechanisms of protection against it in bacteria. *Biochemistry (Mosc)* 2001;66(5):476-89.

53. Hans PS, Kim Kusk M. Advanced genetic strategies for expression recombinant potein in *Escherichia coli. J Biotechnol* 2004;14:113-28

54. Makrides SC. Strategies for achieving high-level expression of genes in Escherichia coli. *Microbiol Rev* 1996;60(3):512-38.

55. Studier FW, Moffatt BA. Use of bacteriophage T7 RNA polymerase to direct selective high-level expression of cloned genes. *J Mol Biol* 1986;189(1):113-30.

Design Expert Assisted Formulation of Topical Bioadhesive Gel of Sertaconazole Nitrate

Vishal Pande*, Samir Patel, Vijay Patil, Raju Sonawane

H.R. Patel Institute of Pharmaceutical Education and Research, Shirpur, Dhule, Maharashtra, 425405 India.

ARTICLE INFO

Keywords:
Topical bioadhesive gel
Sertaconazole nitrate
Three-level factorial design
Carbapol
NaCMC

ABSTRACT

Purpose: The objective of this work was to develop a bioadhesive topical gel of sertaconazole nitrate with the help of response-surface approach.

Methods: Experiments were performed according to a 3-level factorial design to evaluate the effects of two independent variables [amount of Carbapol 934 = X1) and Sodium carboxymethylcellulose (NaCMC) = X2)] on the bioadhesive character of gel, rheological property of gel (consistency index), and *in-vitro* drug release. The best model was selected to fit the data.

Results: Mathematical equation was generated by Design Expert® software for the model which assists in determining the effect of independent variables. Response surface plots were also generated by the software for analyzing effect of the independent variables on the response. The effect of formulation variables on the product characteristics can be easily predicted and precisely interpreted by using a 3-level factorial design and generated quadratic mathematical equations.

Conclusion: On the basis of product characteristics viscosity, bioadhesiveness, permeation study, in-vitro release, in-vivo studies, TPA and spreadability it can be concluded that the best batch of topical bioadhesive gel of Sertaconazole nitrate would be with 1% Carbopol 934 and 1% NaCMC.

Introduction

Sertaconazole Nitrate is an imidazole derivative antifungal agent. It has several actions like fungistatic, fungicidal, anti-bacterial, anti-inflammatory, antitrichomonal and antipruritic.[1-3] Sertaconazole blocks the synthesis of ergosterol by inhibiting the 14α-demethylase enzyme Ergosterol is a critical component of the fungal cell membrane.[4,5] Inhibition of ergosterol synthesis prevents fungal cells from multiplying and impairs hyphae growth. Chemically, Sertaconazole contains a benzothiophene ring which makes is unique from other imidazole antifungals.[1-6]

Percutaneous drug delivery has some advantages of providing the controlled delivery of drugs. In case of their application such as ointments, creams, it is difficult to expect their effects, because wetting, movement and contacting easily remove them.[7-10] There is a need to develop the new formulations that have suitable bioadhesion. The percutaneous administration of bioadhesive gels has good accessibility and can be applied, localized and removed easily. Because of its excellent accessibility, self-placement of a dosage form is possible.[11,12]

Oleic acid use as penetration enhancer in order to promote absorption of drug, it disrupts the skin barrier, fluidized the lipid channels between corneocytes, alter the partitioning of drug into skin structure or otherwise enhances the delivery into skin.

The mechanism of bioadhesion may include wetting and swelling of polymer, Interpenetration of bioadhesive polymer chain and entanglement of polymer and mucin chain and Formation of weak chemical bond between entangled chains. Carbopols are excellent bioadhesive polymers but they have very low pH in the range of 2.5-3.0 (1% aqueous solution). If they used alone, may cause irritation following topical application due to their low pH.[13-19] Its irritant properties can be reduced by combining it with other non-irritant bioadhesive polymers. Therefore, it was proposed to develop a topical bioadhesive gel systems of Sertaconazole nitrate.

As a result, the aim of the present study was to formulate and evaluate the bioadhesive Sertaconazole nitrate gel by using the combination of Carbopol 934 and Sodium carboxymethylcellulose. In the development of pharmaceutical dosage form with appropriate characteristics, an important issue is to design an optimized pharmaceutical formulation in a short time of period with minimum trials. For that now a day's response surface methodology (RSM) gaining attention to identify and quantify the effect of different formulation variables on the important characteristics.

---

*Corresponding author: Vishal Pande, H. R. Patel Institute of Pharmaceutical Education and Research, Shirpur, Dhule, Maharashtra, 425405 India. Email: vishalpande1376@gmail.com

Factorial design (full factorial) is orthogonal experimental design. It also addresses the interaction between two variables and determines the effect on independent variables such as amount of NaCMC and Carbopol 934 on the formulation characteristics such as bioadhesion, viscosity, permeation study and in-vitro release studies .[20,21]

Materials and Methods
Materials
Sertaconazole nitrate was gifted from Glenmark pharmaceuticals, Carbopol 934 was obtained from Vishal Chem, Mumbai and Sodium CMC was obtained from Loba Chemie, Mumbai, oleic acid was obtained from Loba Chemie, Mumbai. All chemicals were used of analytical grade.

Experimental design
A 3-level factorial design was used to study the effect of two variables on characteristics of topical gel such as bioadhesiveness, viscosity, permeation study and % of drug release in 8 h. Dependent and in dependent variables along with their levels are listed in Table 1. Experimental design of different batches of bioadhesive topical gel is summarized.[21,22]

Table 1. Factors (independent variables), factor levels and responses (dependent variables) used in 3-level full factorial experimental design.

Factors	Type of factors	Factor level used			Response	
		-1	0	1		
X_1	Carbopol 934 (%W/W)	0.5	1	1.5	Y_1	Bioadhesiveness (gf)
X_2	NaCMC (%W/W)	0.5	1	1.5	Y_2	Viscosity (cp)
	-				Y_3	Permeation study (%)
	-				Y_4	In-vitro studies (%)

Preparation of Sertaconazole Gel
The required amount of gelling polymer NaCMC and CB934P was weighed. Weighed polymers were added slowly in the beaker containing distilled water (40 ml) with continuous stirring at 400-600 rpm. The mixture was stirred continuously for 1 h until it forms a clear gel. Accurately weighed Sertaconazole nitrate was dissolved in 30 ml of ethanol and the ethanolic solution of drug was added slowly with stirring (400-600 rpm) in the previously prepared polymer gel. Oleic acid was added as a penetration enhancer (0.03 ml) was added with stirring. The final quantity was made up to 100 g with distilled water. The prepared gel was kept for 24 h for complete polymer desolvation .[17-19]

Viscosity Measurements
The samples were placed in beaker and were allowed to equilibrate for 30 min before measuring the viscosity. Viscosities of formulations before and after gelation were measured by using Brookfield DV-E viscometer using Spindle number-3 at 100 rpm shear rate at room temperature. The average of the reading was used to calculate the viscosity.[15-18]

Drug Content Uniformity
All prepared gels were analyzed for the desired range of Sertaconazole nitrate content and the samples which come within the range of 100 ± 10 were taken for in-vitro release studies. A 100 mg of gel was taken in 10 mL of water and mixed for 15 min. After filtration, 0.5 mL of solution was diluted to 5 mL by means of water and the absorbance of the solution was measured at 260 nm spectrophotometrically. The experiments were done in triplicate.[19]

Bioadhesive testing
The method developed by Singh was slightly modified for studying the bioadhesive character of the prepared gels. The apparatus used for study comprised of two arm balance, one side of which contains two glass plates and other side contains a container. One of the two glass plates were attached permanently with the base of the stage and other one attached with the arm of the balance by a thick strong thread. The membrane used for bioadhesive testing was fresh rat intestinal membrane. Fresh rat intestine was glued to the upper side of the lower plate and another was glued to the lower side of the upper plate by using cyanoacrylate adhesive. The weighed gel (0.5 g) was placed on the rat intestine glued to the upper side of the lower plate. Then upper plate was placed over the lower plate and 50 g preload force (or contact pressure) was applied for 5 min (preload time). After removal of the preload force, the water kept in a bottle at some height was siphoned in the container at the rate of 10 ml per min till the plates were detached from each other. The rate of dropping of water was controlled with on-off switch same as in infusion bottle. The weight of water required for detachment of glass plates was considered as the bioadhesion force of the applied gel.[18,19]

In vitro diffusion studies
In-vitro diffusion study of formulated bioadhesive gels was carried out on Franz diffusion cell having (Diameter of 1.5 cm with a diffusional area of 1.76 cm2). Rat abdominal skin was used as diffusion membrane. Pieces of rat abdominal skin membrane were soaked in phosphate buffer (PB) pH 6.8 for 8 hrs prior to experiment. Diffusion cell was filled with phosphate buffer pH 6.8; Rat abdominal membrane was

mounted on cell. The temperature was maintained at 37±0.5 °C. After a pre-incubation time of 20 minutes, pure drug solution and formulation equivalent to 2.0 mg of Sertaconazole was placed in the donor chamber. At predetermined time points, 0.5 mL samples were withdrawn from the acceptor compartment, replacing the sampled volume with PBS pH 6.8 after each sampling, for a period of 8 hrs. The samples withdrawn were filtered and used for analysis. Blank samples (without Drug) were run simultaneously throughout the experiment to check for any interference. The amount of permeated drug was determined using a UV-spectrophotometer at 260 nm.[19-21]

In vivo study
The digital plethysmometer (Ugo Basile, 7140), which was used for determination of % of inhibition edema. The rats of either sex (150-200 g) were divided into four groups containing six animals in each. The rats were fasted for 12 hours prior to induction of edema however water was available *ad libitum*. Inflammation of hind paw was induced by injecting 0.1 ml of 1% carrageenan in normal saline into the subplantar region of right hind paw. The negative control group was received gel formulation without active drug, the positive control group was received standard marketed gel formulation (standard group), third group was treated with novel formulation (test group) and fourth group was normal. The gel formulations or the reference was applied to the plantar surface of the left hind paw by gently rubbing 0.5 g of the formulation 50 times with the index finger 1 hr before the carrageenan injection. The paw volume was measured with a digital plethysmometer before and 1, 3, 6 hrs after carrageenan injection.
The % inhibition will be calculated by following formula:

% inhibition of edema=100 (1-Vt/Vc)

Where Vt: volume of test; Vc: volume of control

Ex-vivo permeation studies
The percutaneous permeation studies were done by using modified Franz diffusion cell (Diameter of 1.5 cm with a diffusional area of 1.76 cm2) and membranes used was rat abdominal skin. Prepared skin samples (rat skin) was mounted on the receptor compartment of the permeation cell with the stratum corneum facing upward and the dermis side facing downward.
The donor compartment was kept on the receptor compartment and secured tightly with the help of clamps. The receptor compartment was then filled with 30 ml of pH 6.8\ phosphate buffer. The temperature of media was maintained at 37 ± 0.5 °C with the help of temperature controlled water jacket. Weighed bioadhesive gel (2 g equivalent to 50 mg of SN) was then placed in the donor compartment. The receptor compartment containing pH 6.8 phosphate buffer was stirred at 200 ± 5 rpm to maintain the hydrodynamics of the receptor fluid. Sampling (0.5 ml) was carried out at the different intervals up to 8 h. The volume of

release media was maintained by adding equal volume of the fresh media after every sampling. The concentration of SN in the sample was measured spectrophotometrically at 260 nm.[18,19-21]

Texture Profile Analysis
Texture profile analysis (TPA) was performed using a CT3 Texture Analyzer in TPA mode. Formulations (35 g) were transferred into 50-ml bottles, taking care to avoid the introduction of air into the samples. A cylindrical analytical probe (35 mm diameter) was forced down into each sample at a defined rate (1 mm/s) and to a defined depth (10 mm). At least five replicate analyses of each sample were performed at temperatures of 25 °C and 35 °C. From the resulting force–time plots, the hardness (the force required to attain a given deformation), compressibility (the work required to deform the product during the first pass of the probe) and adhesiveness (the work necessary to overcome the attractive forces between the surface of the sample and the surface of the probe) were derived.[27]

Spreadability test
Spreadability test was performed by using CT3 Texture Analyzer in Compression mode. A cone analytical probe (60°) was forced down into each sample at a defined rate (1 mm/s) and to a defined depth (10 mm). The test was performed and results were observed.[27] When a trigger force of 10 g has been achieved, the probe proceeds to penetrate the sample at a test speed of 2 mm/s to a depth of 25 mm. During this time, the force to penetrate the sample increases. When the specified penetration distance has been reached, the probe withdraws from the sample at the post-test speed of 2 mm/s. The maximum force value on the graph is a measure of the firmness of the sample at the specified depth. The area under the positive curve is a measure of the energy required to deform the sample to the defined distance (Hardness Work Done). Research has shown that the firmness and energy required deforming a sample to a defined depth grades samples in order of spreadability. A higher peak load (firmness) and hardness work done value indicate a less spreadable sample. Conversely, a lower peak load (firmness) value coupled with a lower hardness work done value indicates a more spreadable sample.

Statistical analysis of the data
Various RSM computations for the current study were performed employing 45 days Trial Version of Design-Expert software (Version 8.0.6., Stat-Ease Inc., and Minneapolis, MN). Polynomial models including interaction and quadratic terms were generated for all response variables using multiple linear regression analysis. Equations were calculated to determine the effect of each variable on the formulation characteristics. Statistical validity of the model was established on the basis of Analysis of variance

(ANOVA) and the 3D response graphs were constructed using Design-Export software.[20, 21]

Results and Discussion

An ideal formulation for local delivery should exhibit ease of drug release, a good retention at application site and controlled release of drug. The application of bioadhesive gel provides a long stay, adequate drug penetration, high efficiency and acceptability. The NaCMC and carbopol 934 biocompatible and biodegradable polymer has been widely used for pharmaceutical and medical application

Viscosity Measurements

From this study we can observe that as the concentration of polymer increases the viscosity of the formulation increases consequently. From the results at the high concentration of polymer i. e 1% carbopol and 1% NaCMC the viscosity found highest

Bioadhesive testing

In this case we have observed that as the concentration of polymer increases the viscosity and bioadhesion property of the formulation also increases simultaneously. From the results we can conclude that at the high concentration of polymer i.e. 1% carbopol and 1% NaCMC the viscosity and bioadhesion was highest amongst all batches.

In vitro diffusion studies

The Figure 1 shows comparative in vitro performance of various batches of bioadhesive gel . In vitro diffusion study was performed by using dialysis membrane. The % Cumulative drug release from bioadhesive gel in 8 hrs was found to be 95.32% respectively. The result indicates that, the bioadhesive gel having higher conc. of polymer i.e. 1% carbopol and 1% NaCMC has given the highest drug release.

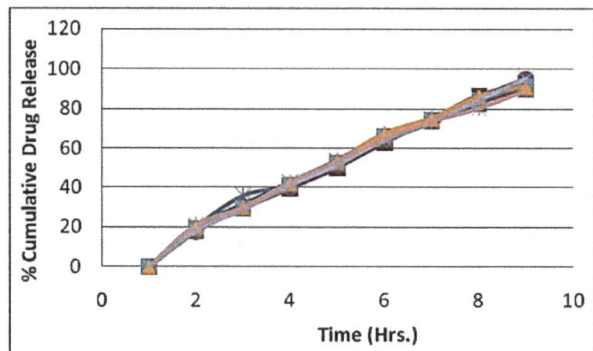

Figure 1. In vitro diffusion study

In vivo anti-inflammatory study

Carrageenan induced paw edema

The Anti-inflammatory effect of developed Bioadhesive gel formulation was compared with marketed volini gel. The results of these studies are given in Table 2. The Figure 2 shows that the mean percent edema value after 6 h application was found to be highest for bioadhesive gel as compared to marketed volini gel. This difference was extremely significant at 5% level of significance ($p<0.05$). Initially the mean percent (%) edema value was high for bioadhesive gel formulation but after 3 h there was a marked decrease in this value which indicates the increase in inflammation. The anti-inflammatory effect of marketed volini gel was up to 6 h significantly increases the percent inhibition of rat paw edema volume then that of prepared bioadhesive gel formulation. So formulated bioadhesive gel indicates that it can be used for local as well as for transdermal drug delivery system. An increase in systemic anti-inflammatory effect of sertaconazole leads to complete inhibition of the inflammation process.

Table 2. Effect of Sertaconazole bioadhesive gel on carrageenan induced paw edema

Group	Formulation	N	Mean wt.(g)	Time (h)	Mean %Edema	%inhibition
1	Control	6	230	1	29.2	-
				3	73.9	-
				6	57.8	-
2	Bioadhesive gel	6	245	1	28.1	3.91%
				3	51.2	30.71 %
				6	25.9	55.19 %
3	Marketed gel	6	235	1	27.6	5.47 %
				3	48.2	34.77 %
				6	22.5	61.07 %

N: Number of rats in each group

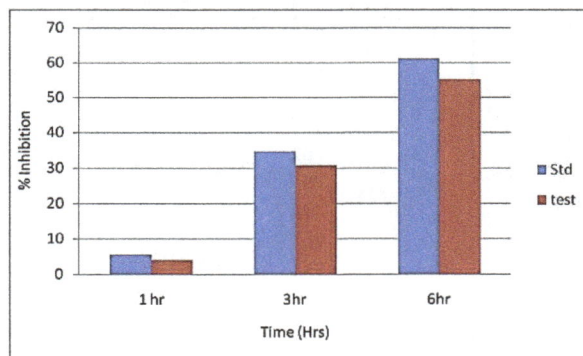

Figure 2. Percent inhibition of rat paw edema volume

Ex-vivo permeation studies

The *Ex-vivo* study was carried out by using rat abdominal skin. The % Cumulative drug release from bioadhesive gel in 8 hrs was found to be 97.23% respectively. The graphical presentation of Ex-vivo permeation study is shown in Figure 3. The result indicates that, the bioadhesive gel having higher conc. of polymer i.e. 1% carbopol and 1% NaCMC found the highest drug release.

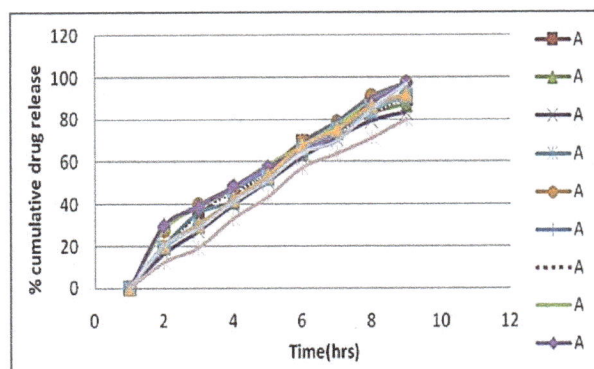

Figure 3. Ex vivo permeation study by using rat abdominal skin

Experiments of 3-level factorial design
Response data for all the 13 experimental runs of 3-level factorial design, performed in accordance with Table 2, are presented in Table 3.

Mathematical modeling
Mathematical relationship was generated between the factors (independent variables) and responses (dependent variables) using the statistical package Design-Expert. First step in mathematical modeling was fitting the experimental data to appropriate model. A suitable model was selected by software on the basis of different parameter obtained from regression analysis such as p-value, adjusted R2, predicted R2 and Predicted Residual Sum of Square (PRESS) value (Tables 4 and 5). Table 3 lists the values of various response parameters of the prepared batches. ANOVA

was applied for estimating the significance of model, at 5% significance level. If more than one model was significant ($p < 0.05$) for the response, the adjusted R2 and PRESS value of the model were compared to select the best mathematical model for that response. Focus on maximizing the value of adjusted R2 and predicted R2. Low PRESS value indicated adequate fitting of model . General quadratic equation for two independent variables is as follow:

$$Y=\beta_0+ \beta_1X_1+ \beta_2X_2+ \beta_3X_1X_2 + \beta_4X_1^2+ \beta_5X_2^2$$

Where: $\beta 0$ is the intercept representing the arithmetic averages of all the quantitative outcomes of 13 runs. $\beta 1$ to $\beta 5$ are all coefficients calculated from the observed experimental values of Y. $X1$ and $X2$ are the coded levels of factors. The terms $X1X2$ and $Xi2$ (i ϵ {1, 2}) represent the interaction and quadratic terms, respectively. Coefficients with one factor represent the effect of that particular factor while the coefficients with more than one factor and those with second order terms represent the interaction between those factors and the quadratic nature of the phenomena, respectively. Synergistic effect and antagonistic effect of factor were indicated by positive sign and negative sign in front of that factor term, respectively.

Drug Content Uniformity
The drug content of the formulated batches was ranging from 92.2% to 99.12%.

Table 3. Results for bioadhesion, viscosity, permeation and in-vitro studies of prepared topical bioadhesive gel with 3-level factorial experimental design.

Run	Viscosity (cp)	Bioadhesiveness (gf)	Permeation (%)	In vitro drug release (%)
1	799	94	90.12	91.23
2	789	91	87.12	90.18
3	891	92	83.24	92.34
4	512	82	90.46	93.2
5	751	98	97.23	95.32
6	751	98	97.23	95.32
7	678	90	91.12	90.12
8	751	98	97.23	95.32
9	751	98	97.23	95.32
10	647	92	91.12	91.22
11	643	91	92.09	91.23
12	751	98	97	95.32
13	544	70	80.23	89.33

Table 4. Fit summary of model for the measured responses Y1 (Viscosity in cp), Y2 (Bioadhesion in gf), Y3 (Permeation study in %) and Y4 (Cumulative percentage release at 8 h in %).

Source	Y1		Y2		Y3		Y4	
	f-value	p-value	f-value	p-value	f-value	p-value	f-value	p-value
Linear vs Mean	23.75	0.0002	2.56	0.1266	2,617E-0.003	0.9974	0.24	0.7899
Quadratic vs 2FI	8.25	0.0144	28.78	0.0004	44.06	0.00001	12.67	0.0047

Viscosity Measurements

From the p-values presented in Table 4, linear model and quadratic model was found to be significant for viscosity. Quadratic model was selected on the basis of maximum value of adj.R^2 and low PRESS value indicating adequate fitting of model mentioned in Table 5. Quadratic model was significant with model f-value of 29.73 (p-value<0.0001). The quadratic equation generated by software is as follows:

$$Y1 = 741.41 + 78.67X_1 + 109.17X_2 + 27.50X_1X_2 + 3.55X_1^2 - 66.95X_2^2$$

Equation reveals that both factors (X1 and X2) affect viscosity characteristics of gel significantly. Equations also indicated that the effect of the change in NaCMC concentration seems to be more pronounced in comparison with that of the change in Carbopol 934 concentration since the coefficient of factor X2 has a larger value than that of factor X1. The combined effect of factors X1 and X2 can further be elucidated with the help of response surface plots (Figure 4A), which demonstrated that Y1 varies in a linear fashion with the amount of both the polymers. However, the steeper ascent in the response surface with NaCMC (X2) – instead of Carbopol (X1) – is clearly discernible from response surface plots, indicating that the effect of NaCMC is comparatively more pronounced than that of Carbopol. From this discussion, one can conclude that the bioadhesion may be changed by appropriate selection of the levels of X1 and X2. (Figure 4B) shows a linear relationship between the observed response values and the predicted values indicating the correctness of the model. The details of Analysis of variance (ANOVA) table for measured responses is presented in Table 6.

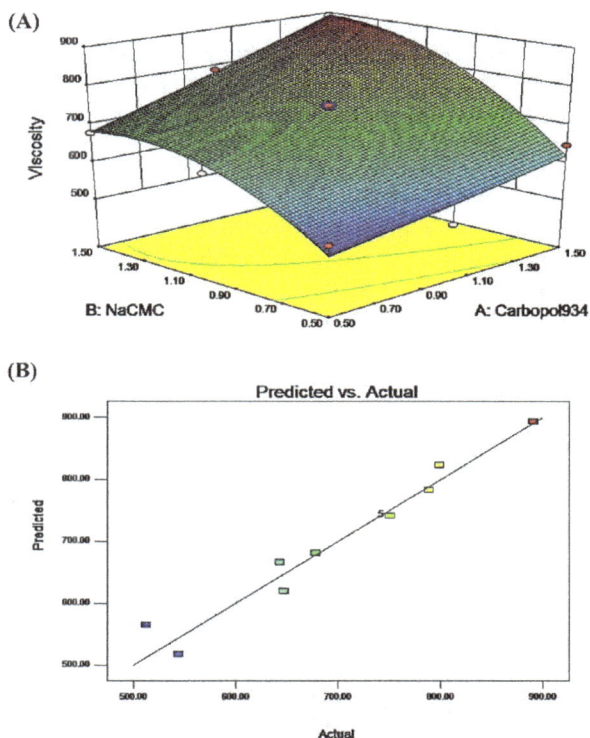

Figure 4. (A) Response surface plot showing the effect of Carbopol 934 and NaCMC on Viscosity (Y1); (B) Linear plot between observed and predicted value of Y1.

Table 5. Model statistical summary of responses for selection suitable model.

Source	Linear			Quadratic		
	Adj. R^2	Pred.R^2	PRESS	Adj. R^2	Pred.R^2	PRESS
Y1	0.7913	0.6788	42242.55	0.9229	0.6274	49000.59
Y2	0.2063	-0.3564	1048.22	0.9011	0.4878	395.81
Y3	-0.1994	-1.1123	801.30	0.9032	0.5706	185.64
Y4	-0.1447	-0.6797	111.14	0.6463	-0.7489	114.67

Table 6. Analysis of variance (ANOVA) table for measured responses.

Model	Y1		Y2		Y3		Y4	
	f-value	p-value	f-value	p-value	f-value	p-value	f-value	p-value
Model	29.73	0.0001	22.87	0.0003	23.40	0.0003	5.39	0.0238
X_1	43.95	0.0003	19.08	0.0033	0.059	0.8152	1.46	0.2602
X_2	84.64	<0.0001	22.01	0.0022	5.932E-0.03	0.9408	0.11	0.7540
X_1X_2	3.58	0.1003	15.70	0.0054	28.79	0.0010	0.014	0.9089
X_1^2	0.041	0.8449	4.13	0.0816	16.57	0.0047	9.43	0.0181
X_2^2	14.65	0.0065	35.81	0.0006	39.32	0.0008	6.35	0.0398

Bioadhesive testing

From the p-values presented in Table 4, linear model and quadratic model was found to be significant for bioadhesion. Quadratic model was selected on the basis of maximum value of adj. R2 and low PRESS value indicating adequate fitting of model (Table 5). Quadratic model was significant with model f-value of

22.87 (p-value<0.0003). The quadratic equation generated by software is as follows:

$$Y1 = 97.31 + 4.50X_1 + 4.53X_2 - 5.00X_1X_2 - 3.07X_1^2 - 9.09X_2^2$$

Equation reveals that both factors (X1 and X2) affect bioadhesion characteristics of gel significantly. Equations also indicated that the effect of the change in

186

NaCMC concentration seems to be more pronounced in comparison with that of the change in Carbopol934 concentration since the coefficient of factor X2 has a larger value than that of factor X1. The combined effect of factors X1 and X2 can further be elucidated with the help of response surface plots (Figure 5A), which demonstrated that Y2 varies in a linear fashion with the amount of both the polymers. However, the steeper ascent in the response surface with NaCMC (X2) – instead of Carbopol 934 (X1) – is clearly discernible from response surface plots, indicating that the effect of NaCMC is comparatively more pronounced than that of Carbopol. From this discussion, one can conclude that the bioadhesion may be changed by appropriate selection of the levels of X1 and X2. (Figure 5B) shows a linear relationship between the observed response values and the predicted values indicating the correctness of the model.

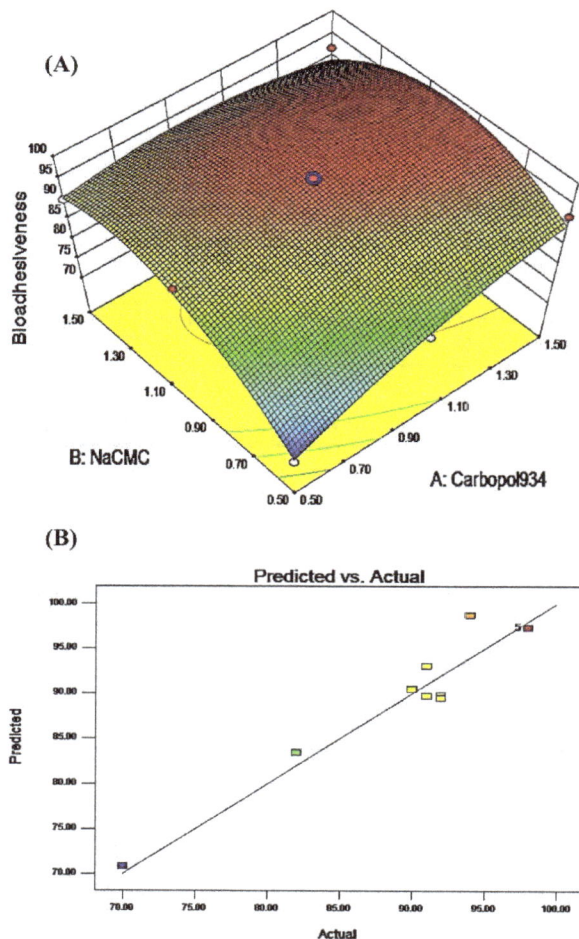

Figure 5. (A) Response surface plot showing the effect of Carbopol 934 and NaCMC on Bioadhesion (Y2); (B) Linear plot between observed and predicted value of Y1.

Permeation studies

From the p-values presented in Table 4, quadratic model was found to be significant for bioadhesion. Quadratic model was selected on the basis of maximum value of adj. R2 and low PRESS value indicating adequate fitting of model (Table 5).

Quadratic model was significant with model f-value of 23.40 (p-value<0.0003). The quadratic equation generated by software is as follows:

$$Y1 = 34.12 + 53.39X_1 + 71.46X_2 - 18.77X_1X_2 - 17.13X_1^2 - 26.40X_2^2$$

Equation reveals that both factors (X1 and X2) affect permeation characteristics of gel significantly. Equations also indicated that the effect of the change in NaCMC concentration seems to be more pronounced in comparison with that of the change in Carbopol934 concentration since the coefficient of factor X2 has a larger value than that of factor X1. The combined effect of factors X1 and X2 can further be elucidated with the help of response surface plots (Figure 6A), which demonstrated that Y3 varies in a linear fashion with the amount of both the polymers. However, the steeper ascent in the response surface with NaCMC (X2) – instead of Carbopol 934 (X1) – is clearly discernible from response surface plots, indicating that the effect of NaCMC is comparatively more pronounced than that of Carbopol. From this discussion, one can conclude that the bioadhesion may be changed by appropriate selection of the levels of X1 and X2. (Figure 6B) shows a linear relationship between the observed response values and the predicted values indicating the correctness of the model.

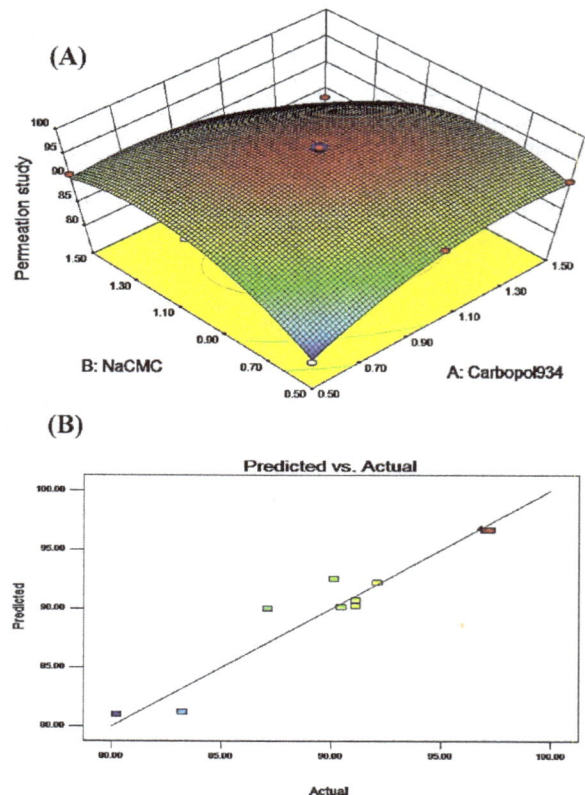

Figure 6. (A) Response surface plot showing the effect of Carbopol 934 and NaCMC on permeation (Y3); (B) Linear plot between observed and predicted value of Y1.

In vitro diffusion studies

From the p-values presented in Table 4, quadratic contribution were found to be significant since p-value is less than 0.05 for both sources. In this case, A, B, AB, A2 and B2 are significant model terms. PRESS value for quadratic model (114.67) was found as indicating in Table 5. Therefore, quadratic model was selected to fit the data of this response. Quadratic model was significant with model f-value of 5.39 (p-value<0.0238). The quadratic equation generated by software is as follows:

$$Y1 = 94.89 + 0.68X_1 - 0.18X_2 + 0.083X_1X_2 - 2.57X_1^2 - 2.11X_2^2$$

In this case, all the model terms (X1, X2, X1X2, X12 and X22) were found to be significant (Table 6). The equation reveals that both factors have antagonistic effect on the drug release. CPR of the drug in 8 h with highest polymer content (1.5% Carbopol 934 and 1.5% NaCMC) was found to be lowest. However, in this equation, it was clearly indicating that the retarding effect of NaCMC was more prominent than Carbopol 934. Coefficient of interactions shown in above equation was also significant which confirms the formation of rigid gel structure of carbopol 934 with NaCMC. At high concentration of NaCMC and Carbopol 934, a very thick gel (highest consistency index value) was formed which provide a very slow release of drug. (Figure 7A) represented the response surface indicating the more pronounced effect of NACMC than Carbopol 934 on Y4. (Figure 7B) represented the observed response value compared with that of predicted values indicating the correctness of model.

Texture profile analysis (TPA) and Spreadability testing

TPA is a method to determine mechanical properties of gel in which an analytical probe is twice depression into the sample at a defined rate to a desired depth, allowing a predefined necessary period between the end of the first and the beginning of second compression shows in Figure 8 (A).

The peak / maximum force is taken as a measurement of firmness; higher the value the thicker is the consistency of the sample. The negative region of the graph produced on probe return is an a result of the weight of sample which is lifted primarily on the upper surface of the disc on return i.e. due to the back extrusion and hence gives again an indication of consistency or resistance to flow off the disc. The maximum negative force is taken as an indication of the stickiness / cohesiveness of the sample. The more negative the value the more stuff the sample.

The observations for spreadability of all formulations are shown in Figure 8 (B). The spreadability of the formulations is a characteristic derived from its more basic property i.e. viscosity. The greater the viscosity the longer will be the time taken for spreading. The gels are expected to spread easily on the skin areas when applied. The spreadability also depends on the polymer in formulation, possessing typical physicochemical properties which create surface tension between slide and product.

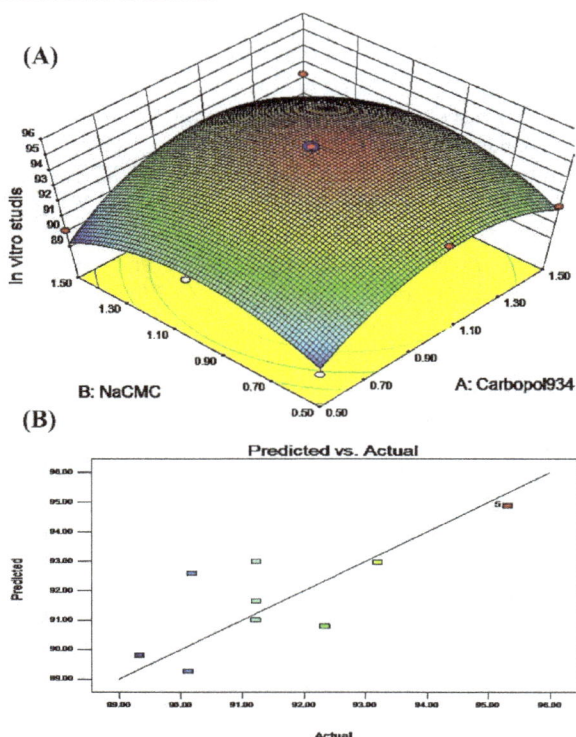

(A)

(B)

Figure 7. (A) Response surface plot showing the effect of Carbopol 934 and NaCMC on In-vitro studies (Y4); (B) Linear plot between observed and predicted value of Y1.

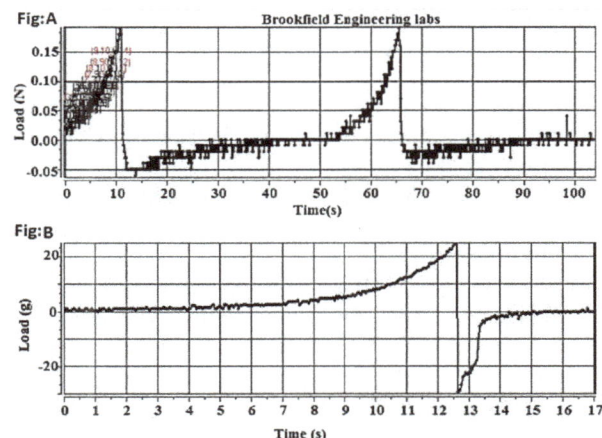

Figure 8. A] Texture profile analysis (TPA) spectra of bioadhesive gel. B] Spreadability pattern of bioadhesive gel.

Conclusion

The present study concludes that topical bioadhesive gel of Sertaconazole nitrate can be formulated by using combination of Carbopol 934 and NaCMC employing the response surface approach. The effect of formulation variables on the product characteristics can be easily predicted and precisely interpreted by using a 3-level factorial design and generated quadratic mathematical equations. On the basis of product characteristics viscosity, bioadhesiveness, permeation study, in-vitro release, TPA and spreadability it can be concluded that the best batch of topical bioadhesive gel of Sertaconazole nitrate would be with 1% Carbopol 934 and 1% NaCMC.

In case of TPA of the bioadhesive gel, as the probe of texture analyzer returns to its starting position, the initial lifting of the weight of the sample on the upper surface of the disc produces the negative part of the graph. This gives an indication of the cohesiveness and resistance of the sample to separate (flow off) from the disc. The maximum negative force on the graph indicates sample adhesive force; the more negative the value the more "sticky" the sample. The area under the negative part of the graph is known as the adhesiveness (the energy required to break probe sample contact) and can give an indication of the cohesive forces of the molecules within the sample. The sertaconazole bioadhesive gel is more adhesive or "sticky" and therefore it is more cohesive than other batches.

Research has shown that the firmness and energy required deforming a sample to a defined depth grades samples in order of spreadability. A higher peak load (firmness) and hardness work done value indicate a less spreadable sample. Conversely, a lower peak load (firmness) value coupled with a lower hardness work done value indicates a more spreadable sample. From Figure 8, Sample of bioadhesive gel is significantly much firmer and has a higher hardness work done (area under the positive curve). This indicates that sertaconazole bioadhesive gel is more spreadable than the other batches prepared.

Conflict of Interest

The authors report no conflicts of interest.

References

1. European pharmacopeia. 6th ed. Strasbourg: Council of Europe; 2008.
2. United States Pharmacopeia 28, National Formulary 23. Rockville: United States Pharmacopoeial Convention; 2005.
3. Wang L, Tang X. A novel ketoconazole bioadhesive effervescent tablet for vaginal delivery: Design in vitro and in vivo evaluation. *Int J Pharm* 2008;350(1-2):181-7.
4. Richardson MD, Warnock DW. Fungal infection: diagnosis and management. London: Blackwell Scientific Publications; 1993.
5. Tawfique K, Danesment T, Warnock D. Clinical pharmacokinetics of sertaconazole. *Clin Pharmacol* 1988;14:13-4.
6. Daneshmend T, Warnock D, Turner A, Robert C. Pharmacokinetics of Sertaconazole in normal subjects. *J Antimicrobial Chem* 1981;8:299-304.
7. Shin S, Cho C, Choi H. Structure and function of skin in dermatological and transdermal formulation. *Drug Dev Ind Pharm* 1999;25:273-8.
8. Walters KA, Roberts MS. The Structure and Function of Skin. In: Walters KA editor. Dermatological and Transdermal Formulation. New York: Marcel Dekker Inc; 2002.
9. Elias PM. Lipids and the epidermal permeability barrier. *Arch Dermatol Res* 1981;270(1):95-117.
10. Naik A, Kalia YN, Guy RH. Transdermal drug delivery: overcoming the skin's barrier function. *Pharm Sci Technolo Today* 2000;3(9):318-26.
11. Khar S, Ahuja R, Javed A, Jain N. Mucoadhesive drug delivery in Controlled and Novel Drug Delivery. 3rd ed. New Delhi: CBS publishers and distributors;1997.
12. Mathiowitz E, Chickering D. Definition, Mechanisms and Theories Of Bioadhesion, Bioadhesive drug delivery system : fundamentals, novel approaches and development. New York: Marcel Dekker;1992.
13. Lee JW, Park JH, Robinson JR. Bioadhesive-based dosage forms: the next generation. *J Pharm Sci* 2000;89(7):850-66.
14. Shin SC, Lee JW, Yang KH, Lee CH. Preparation and evaluation of bioadhesive benzocaine gels for enhanced local anesthetic effects. *Int J Pharm* 2003;260(1):77-81.
15. Shin SC, Kim HJ, Oh IJ, Cho CW, Yang KH. Development of tretinoin gels for enhanced transdermal delivery. *Eur J Pharm Biopharm* 2005;60(1):67-71.
16. Shin SC, Cho CW. Enhanced transdermal delivery of pranoprofen from the bioadhesive gels. *Arch Pharm Res* 2006;29(10):928-33.
17. Shin SC, Kim JY, Oh IJ. Mucoadhesive and physicochemical characterization of Carbopol-Poloxamer gels containing triamcinolone acetonide. *Drug Dev Ind Pharm* 2000;26(3):307-12.
18. Swarbrick J, Boylan JC. Encyclopedia of Pharmaceutical Technology. 2 nd ed. New York: Marcel Dekker INC; 2002.
19. Singh S, Gajra B, Rawat M, Muthu MS. Enhanced transdermal delivery of ketoprofen from bioadhesive gels. *Pak J Pharm Sci* 2009;22(2):193-8.
20. Huang YB, Tsai YH, Yang WC, Chang JS, Wu PC. Optimization of sustained-release propranolol dosage form using factorial design and response surface methodology. *Biol Pharm Bull* 2004;27(10):1626-9.
21. Singh S, Parhi R, Garg A. Formulation of topical bioadhesive gel of aceclofenac using 3-level factorial design. *Iran J Pharm Res* 2011;10(3):435-45.
22. Varshosaz J, Tavakoli N, Saidian S. Development and physical characterization of a periodontal bioadhesive gel of metronidazole. *Drug Deliv* 2002;9(2):127-33.
23. El Gendy AM, Jun HW, Kassem AA. In vitro release studies of flurbiprofen from different topical formulations. *Drug Dev Ind Pharm* 2002;28(7):823-31.
24. Rebelo ML, Pina ME. Release kinetics of tretinoin from dermatological formulations. *Drug Dev Ind Pharm* 1997;23(7):727-30.

A Novel Approach using Hydrotropic Solubalization Technique for Quantitative Estimation of Entacapone in Bulk Drug and Dosage Form

Ruchi Jain[1]*, Nilesh Jain[2], Deepak Kumar Jain[2], Surendra Kumar Jain[2]

[1] Suresh Gyan Vihar University, Jaipur, Rajasthan, India-302025.

[2] Sagar Institute of Research & Technology-Pharmacy, Ayodhya Bypass Road Bhopal, Madhya Pradesh, India – 462041.

ARTICLE INFO

Keywords:
Entacapone
Urea
Ecofriendly
Hydrotropic solubilizing agents

ABSTRACT

Purpose: Analysis of drug utilized the organic solvent which are costlier, toxic and causing environment pollution. Hydrotropic solution may be a proper choice to preclude the use of organic solvents so that a simple, accurate, novel, safe and precise method has been developed for estimation of poorly water soluble drug Entacapone (Water Solubility-$7.97e^{-02}$ g/l). *Methods:* Solubility of entacapone is increased by using 8M Urea as hydrotropic agent. There was more than 67 fold solubility enhanced in hydrotropic solution as compare with distilled water. The entacapone (ENT) shows the maximum absorbance at 378 nm. At this wavelength hydrotropic agent and other tablet excipients do not shows any significant interference in the spectrophotometric assay. *Results:* The developed method was found to be linear in the range of 4-20 µg/ml with correlation coefficient (r^2) of 0.9998. The mean percent label claims of tablets of ENT in tablet dosage form estimated by the proposed method were found to be 99.17±0.63. The developed methods were validated according to ICH guidelines and values of accuracy, precision and other statistical analysis were found to be in good accordance with the prescribed values. *Conclusion:* As hydrotropic agent used in the proposed method so this method is Ecofriendly and it can be used in routine quantitative analysis of drug in bulk drug and dosage form in industries.

Introduction

Entacapone (ENT) is chemically (E)-2-cyano-3-(3, 4-dihydroxy-5-nitrophenyl)-N, N-diethyl-2-propenamide (Figure 1), is a drug that functions as a catechol-O-methyl transferase (COMT) inhibitor, used in the treatment of Parkinson's disease. It is a member of the class of nitrocatechols.[1,2] The drug is not official in any pharmacopoeia. Literature survey revealed few HPLC methods[3,4] has been reported for the determination of ENT in biological fluids. The reported methods for the determination of ENT in tablets includes HPLC[5-11] and spectrophotometric methods.[12,13]

As the environmental pollution it is necessary to preclude the use of organic solvents for analysis of drug. Various techniques have been employed to enhance the aqueous solubility and hydrotropy is one of them. Hydrotropic solubilization is the phenomenon by which aqueous solubility of poorly water soluble drugs and insoluble drugs increases. Maheshwari and Jain et al has used sodium salicylate, sodium benzoate, urea, nicotinamide, sodium citrate and sodium acetate as the most common examples of hydrotropic agents utilized to increase the water solubility of drug.[14-19]

Various organic solvents such as methanol, chloroform, dimethyl formamide and acetonitrile have been employed for solubilization of poorly water-soluble drugs to carry out spectrophotometric analysis. Drawbacks of organic solvents include their higher cost, toxicity and pollution. Hydrotropic solution may be a proper choice to preclude the use of organic solvents. Therefore, it was thought worthwhile to employ this hydrotropic solution to extract out the drug from fine powder of tablets to carry out spectrophotometric estimation. Present work emphasizes on the quantitative estimation of ENT in their dosage form by UV Spectroscopic methods.

Materials and Methods
Instrument
UV-Visible double beam spectrophotometer, Shimadzu model-1700 having spectral bandwidth 3 nm and of wavelength accuracy ±1 nm, with 1cm quartz cells was used.

Reagents and chemicals
Analytical pure sample of ENT was supplied as gift sample from Sun Pharmaceuticals Ind. Ltd. Urea obtained from Merck Chemical Division, Mumbai.

Corresponding author: Ruchi Jain, Research Scholar, Suresh Gyan Vihar University, Jagatpura Mahal, Jaipur, Rajasthan, India-302025.
Email: jainruchi02@gmail.com

Reverse Osmosis (R.O.) Water was used throughout the study.

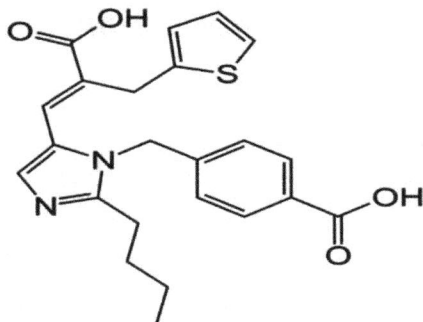

Figure 1. Chemical structure of ENT

Preliminary solubility studies of drugs

An excess amount of drug was added to a screw capped 25 ml of volumetric flask containing different aqueous systems viz. distilled water, different combination of hydrotropic agent. The volumetric flasks were shaken mechanically for 12 hrs at 25±1°C in a mechanical shaker. These solutions were allowed to equilibrate for next 24 hrs and then centrifuged for 5 min at 2000 rpm. The supernatant liquid was taken for appropriate dilution after filtered through whatman filter paper no.41 and analyzed spectrophotometrically against corresponding solvent blank. After analysis, it was found that the enhancement in the solubility of ENT was to be more than and 67 folds in 8 M Urea as compared to solubility studies in other solvents.

Selection of hydrotropic agent

ENT was scanned in hydrotropic agent in the spectrum mode over the UV range (200-400) and 8 M Urea as hydrotropic agent were found to be most appropriate because:

- ENT is soluble in it (67 fold enhancement of solubility)
- ENT is stable in hydrotropic agent (as shown in Figure 2)
- ENT exhibit good spectral characteristics in it.
- Urea solution has no interference with the λ_{max} of ENT i.e 378nm.

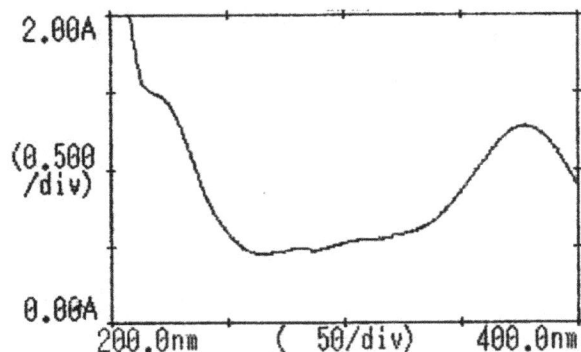

Figure 2. Spectra of ENT in 8 M Urea as Hydrotropic Agent

Establishment of stability profile

Stability of ENT was observed by dissolving in 8 M Urea as hydrotropic agent. Solution of ENT was prepared in the conc. of 12 µg/ml and scanned under time scan for 30 min. Spectra of drug under time scan shows that drug are stable in hydrotropic solution.

Linearity range and calibration graph
Preparation of Standard Stock Solution (Stock-A)

Accurately weighed 100 mg of the ENT was transferred in to 100 ml volumetric flask containing 80 ml of hydrotropic agent and the flask was sonicated for about 10 min to solubilize the drug and the volume was made up to the mark with mixed hydrotropic agent to get a concentration of 1000 µg/ml (Stock-A).

Preparation of Working Standard Solution

The standard solution (1000 µg/ml) was further diluted with distilled water to obtain 4, 8, 12, 16 and 20µg /ml solution and absorbance were noted at 378 nm against distilled water as blank.

Analysis of Marketed Formulation

Marketed formulation Entacom (Intas Pharmaceuticals) was selected for tablet analysis, i. e containing 200 mg ENT. Twenty tablets were accurately weighed, average weight determined and ground to fine powder. An accurately weighed quantity of powder equivalent to 100 mg of ENT was transferred into 100 ml volumetric flask containing 80 ml of hydrotropic solution. The flask was sonicated for about 20 min to solublize the drug; volume was adjusted to mark with hydrotropic agent and filtered through whatman filter paper no. 41. The Absorbance of sample solutions was analyzed on UV spectrophotometer at 378 nm against R.O. water as blank.

Validation Parameters

The developed method was validated as per ICH guidelines (Linearity, Accuracy, Precision and Robustness).[20]

Linearity

Linearity of ENT was established by response ratios of drug. Response ratio of drug was calculated by dividing the absorbance with respective concentration.

Accuracy

To check the degree of accuracy of the method, recovery studies were performed in triplicate by standard addition method at 80%, 100% and 120%. In preanalyzed tablet solution, a definite amount of drug was added and then its recovery was studied. These studies were performed in by adding fixed amount of pure drug solution to the final dilution while varying the concentration of tablet sample solution in the final dilution.

Precision

Precision of the methods was studied at three level as at repeatability, intermediate precision (Day to Day and analyst to analyst) and reproducibility.

Repeatability was performed by analyzing same 5 concentrations of drug for 5 times. Day to Day was performed by analyzing 5 different concentration of the drug for three days in a week.

Reproducibility was performed by analyzing same concentration of drugs for five times in different lab.

Results and Discussions

Based on the solubility, stability and spectral characteristics of the drug, 8M Urea was selected as hydrotropic agent. There was more than 67 fold solubility enhanced in hydrotropic solution as compare with distilled water. After solubilizing the Entacapone in selected hydrotropic agent, it was scanned in spectrum mode and the working wavelength for the estimation, considering the reproducibility and variability was found to be 378 nm. Spectra of ENT is shown in Figure 2, Calibration curve was plotted between concentrations versus absorbance Figure 3. Observation of linearity data has reported in the Table 1. The Result of their optical characteristics has been reported in Table 2.The developed method was found

to be linear in the range of 4-20 μg/ml with linear equation was Y=0.098X + 0.011 and correlation coefficient (r^2) of 0.9998. Drug content of tablet formulation was calculated using calibration curve and values are reported in Table 3. The mean percent label claims of tablets of ENT in formulation-I estimated by the proposed method were found to be 99.17±0.63. These values are close to 100, indicating the accuracy of the proposed analytical method.

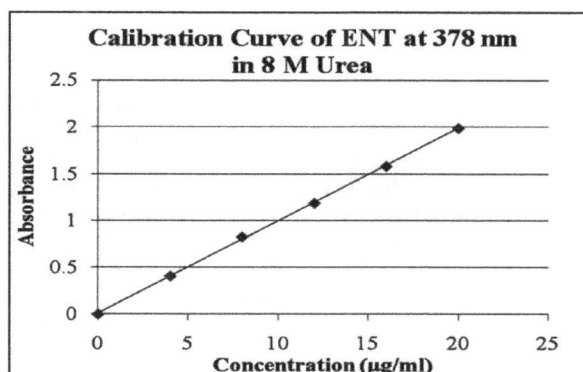

Figure 3. Calibration Curve of ENT at 378 nm in 8 M Urea

Table 1. Linearity ENT at λ_{max} =378 nm in 8 M Urea

Standard Conc. (μg/ml)	Rep-1	Rep-2	Rep-3	Rep-4	Rep-5	Mean
0	0	0	0	0	0	0
4	0.403	0.408	0.41	0.411	0.401	0.4066
8	0.821	0.823	0.812	0.841	0.842	0.8278
12	1.182	1.193	1.195	1.184	1.185	1.1878
16	1.586	1.593	1.554	1.579	1.599	1.5822
20	1.976	1.996	1.99	1.986	1.988	1.9872
Correlation Coefficient (r^2)	-	-	-	-	-	0.9998
Slope (m)	-	-	-	-	-	0.0987
Intercept (c)	-	-	-	-	-	0.0113

Table 2. Optical Characteristic and Linearity Data of ENT in 8 M Urea

S. No.	Parameter	8 M Urea as Hydrotropic Agent
1	Working λ	378 nm
2	Beer's law limit (μg/ml)	4-20
3	Correlation Coefficient (r^2)*	0.9998
4	Slope (m)*	0.098
5	Intercept (c)*	0.011
6	Number of samples (n)	25
*Average of 5 determination of 5 concentrations		

Result of Validation Parameters

Linearity

Linearity was established in the range of 4-20μg/ml and it was reported as response ratio; Table 4. Then a graph was plotted between concentration and response ratio (Figure 4) which assure the linearity of the method.

Accuracy

The values of mean percentage recoveries were also found to show variability in ranging from 97.83±1.03 to 98.92±0.82%. Low values of standard deviation, percent coefficient of variation and standard error further validated the proposed method (Table 5). All these values were very close to 100.

Table 3. Results and Statistical Parameters for Entacom 200 mg Tablet Analysis using 8M Urea

Drug	Label Claim (mg)	Amount Found (mg)	% MEAN*	S.D.*	%COV*	Std. Error*
Entacom200	200	198.67	99.33	0.26	0.262	0.048
Entacom200	200	198.43	99.21	0.73	0.736	0.133
Entacom200	200	197.93	98.96	0.89	0.899	0.163
Mean	-	198.34	99.17	0.63	0.632	0.115

*Average of five in 3 replicates determination

Table 4. Response Ratio of ENT in Hydrotropic Solution

S. No.	8 M Urea as Hydrotropic Agent		
	Conc. (µg/ml)	ABS	Response Ratio
1.	4	0.402	0.10
2.	8	0.81	0.10
3.	12	1.194	0.10
4.	16	1.584	0.10
5.	20	1.99	0.10

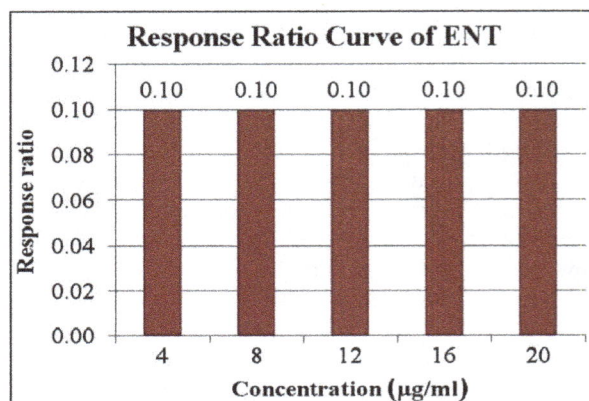

Figure 4. Response Ratio Curve of ENT in 8 M Urea

Table 5. Result of Recovery Studies of Tablet Formulation with Statically Evaluation

Drug	QC Conc. (µg/ml)	Recovery Level % (Amount Drug Added)	Amount of Drug Found (Mean±SD)*	% RSD
ENT	10	80	98.47±1.23	0.332
-	-	100	98.39±1.08	0.447
-	-	120	97.83±1.03	0.40
ENT	12	80	98.86±0.63	0.90
-	-	100	98.92±0.82	0.30
-	-	120	98.29±0.74	0.63

*Average of five determination

Precision

Result of precision at different level were found be within acceptable limits (RSD<2). The results have been reported in Table 6. Presence of hydrotropic agent do not shows any significant interference in the spectrophotometric assay thus further confirming the applicability and reproducibility of the developed method.

Table 6. Result of Precision of ENT

-	Validation Parameter	Percentage Mean ± S.D*. (n=6)	Percentage RSD
With 8 M Urea as Hydrotropic Agent	Repeatability	98.64±1.31	1.33
	Intermediate Precision	-	-
-	Day to Day	98.92±1.42	1.435
-	Analyst to Analyst	98.74±0.86	0.870
-	Reproducibility	98.39±0.70	0.711
-	-	-	-

* Mean of fifteen determinations (3 replicates at 5 concentrations level)

Conclusion

Hence, it is concluded that the proposed methods are new, simple, cost effective, accurate, safe and precise and can be successfully employed in the routine analysis of Entacapone in bulk drug sample and tablet dosage form. Advantage of these methods is that the organic solvent is not essential for the analysis and there was no interference of 8 M urea during the estimation. There is a good scope for other poorly water-soluble drugs which may be tried to get solubilized in 2 M urea solution (as hydrotropic agent) to carry out their spectrophotometric analysis excluding the use of costlier and unsafe organic solvents.

Conflict of Interest

The authors report no conflicts of interest.

References

1. Sweetman SC. Martindale-the complete drug reference. 32nd ed. London: The Pharmaceutical Press; 1999.
2. O'Neil MJ, Smith A, Heckelman PE, Obenchain JR, Gallipeau JR, D'Arecca MA. The Merck Index : An Encyclopedia of Chemicals, Drugs, and Biologicals. 13th ed. Whitehouse Station, NJ: Merck Research Laboratories; 2001.
3. Karlsson M, Wikberg T. Liquid chromatographic determination of a new catechol-O-methyltransferase inhibitor, entacapone, and its Z-isomer in human plasma and urine. *J Pharm Biomed Anal* 1992;10(8):593-600.
4. Bugamelli F, Marcheselli C, Barba E, Raggi MA. Determination of L-dopa, carbidopa, 3-O-methyldopa and entacapone in human plasma by HPLC-ED. *J Pharm Biomed Anal* 2011;54(3):562-7.
5. Sivasubramanian L, Lakshmi KS, Pathuri RR. RP-HPLC estimation of entacapone in bulk and dosage form. *J Pharm Res* 2009;2:1850-1.
6. Zaveri M, Dhru B, Khandhar A. Simultaneous estimation of levodopa, carbidopa and entacapone in pharmaceutical dosage by validated reverse phase high performance liquid chromatography. *Int J Inst Pharm Life Sci* 2012;2:10-9.
7. Ramakrishna NV, Vishwottam KN, Wishu S, Koteshwara M, Chidambara J. High-performance liquid chromatography method for the quantification of entacapone in human plasma. *J Chromatogr B Analyt Technol Biomed Life Sci* 2005;823(2):189-94.
8. Sarsambi PS, Gowrisankar D. Reverse phase HPLC method for the analysis of entacapone in pharmaceutical dosage forms. *Pharm Rev* 2009;7(41):111-2.
9. Issa YM, Hassoun MM, Zayed AG. Application of high performance liquid chromatography method for the determination of levodopa, carbidopa and entacapone in tablet dosage forms. *J Liq Chromatogr Related Technol* 2011;34:2433-47.
10. Tekale P, Mhatre VS, Pai NR, Maurya C, Tekale S. Estimation of entacapone tablets by reverse phase high performance liquid chromatographic method. *J Biosci Discov* 2011;2(3):294-8.
11. Mohamed NG, Mohamed MS. Determination of antiparkinsonism drug entacapone. *J Chil Chem Soc* 2010;55:85-9.
12. Koradia SK, Agola AS, Jivani NP, Manek RA, Pandey S. Development and validation of derivative spectrophotometric method for determination of entacapone in pharmaceutical formulation. *Int J Pharm Res Dev* 2009;1:1-8.
13. Shah J, Banerjee SK, Chhabra GS. UV Spectrophotometric method development and validation for entacapone in bulk and formulation. *J Bull Pharm Res* 2011;1:7-9.
14. Maheshwari RK. A novel application of hydrotropic solubilization in the analysis of bulk samples of ketoprofen and salicylic acid. *Asian J Chem* 2006;18:393-6.
15. Maheshwari RK. Analysis of frusemide by application of hydrotropic solubilization phenomenon. *Indian Pharmacist* 2005;4:55-8.
16. Jain N, Jain R, Thakur N, Gupta BP, Banweer J, Jain S. Novel spectrophotometric quantitative estimation of torsemide in tablets using mixed hydrotropic agent. *Der Pharmacia Lettre* 2010;2(3):249-54.
17. Jain N, Jain R, Thakur N, Gupta BP, Banweer J, Jain S. Novel spectrophotometric quantitative estimation of Hydrochlorothiazide in bulk drug and their dosage forms by using hydrotropic agent. *Int J Appl Pharm* 2010;2:11-4.
18. Jain N, Jain R, Kulkarni S, Jain DK, Jain S. Ecofriendly spectrophotometric method development and their validation for quantitative estimation of Pramipexole Dihyrochloride using mixed hydrotropic agent. *J Chem Pharm Res* 2010;3:548-52.
19. Jain N, Jain R, Jain D, Jain A. Spectrophotometric quantitative estimation of amlodipine besylate in bulk drug and their dosage forms by using hydrotropic agent. *Eur J Chem* 2010;5:212-7.
20. International Conference on Harmonization. ICH, Validation of Analytical Procedures: Text and Methodology (Q2(R1)), IFPMA, Geneva. 2005.

Thermal Analysis Study of Antihypertensive Drugs Telmisartan and Cilazapril

Refaat Ahmed Saber[1]*, Ali Kamal Attia[2], Waheed Mohamed Salem[2]

[1] *Faculty of Technology and Development, Zagazig University, Egypt.*

[2] *National Organization for Drug Control and Research, P.O. Box 29, Cairo, Egypt.*

ARTICLE INFO

Keywords:
Telmisartan
Cilazapril
Antihypertensive
Drugs
Quality control
Thermal analysis

ABSTRACT

Purpose: The aim of the present work is to study the thermal analysis of telmisartan and cilazapril.

Methods: Thermogravimetry (TGA), derivative thermogravimetry (DTG) and differential thermal analysis (DTA) were used through the work to achieve the thermal analysis study of some antihypertensive drugs, telmisartan and cilazapril.

Results: The results led to thermal stability data and also to the interpretation concerning the thermal decomposition. Thermogravimetry data allowed determination of the kinetic parameters such as, activation energy and frequency factor.

Conclusion: The simplicity, speed and low operational costs of thermal analysis justify its application in the quality control of pharmaceutical compounds for medications.

Introduction

Thermal analysis technique that delivers extremely sensitive measurements of heat change can be applied on a broad scale with pharmaceutical development. These methods provide unique information relating to thermodynamic data of the system studied. The increasing use of the combined techniques is providing more specific information, and thus facilities more rapid interpretation of the experimental curves obtained.[1,2] The need to measure a range of physical parameters has led to the development of numerous techniques such as thermogravimety (TGA), derivative thermogravimetry (DTG) and differential thermal analysis (DTA). In pharmaceutical sciences thermal methods of analysis have found important applications.[3-10] TGA, in which the change in mass of a sample heated at constant rate is recorded and plotted vs. temperature, is an effective method for studying thermal stability and determination the kinetic parameters of the decomposition of drugs. TGA is an analytical, quantitative and comparative method capable of producing fast and reproducible results. It can be used in the quality control of drugs with a view to improvement of the final product and for the determination of drug quality via the technological parameters. DTA is used for the identification of pharmaceutical and organic compounds.[11-17]

Telmisartan (TMT), 4-[(2-n-propyl-4-methyl-6-(1-methylbenzimidazol-2-yl)-benzimidazol-1-yl) methyl]-biphenyl-2-carboxylic acid (Figure 1), is an angiotensin II type I receptor blocker. It is widely used in treatment of hypertension.[18,19] It inhibits the angiotensin II receptor in a way that the effect of angiotensin II is blocked resulting in a decrease of blood pressure.[20]

Cilazapril (CPL), (1S,9S)-9-[[1(S)-1-(Ethoxycarbonyl)-3-phenylpropyl] amino] octahydro-10-oxo-6H-pyridazino[1.2-a][1,2]diazepine-1- carboxylic acid (Figure 1), is a potent and specific angiotensin converting enzyme (ACE) inhibitor which lowers peripheral vascular resistance without affecting heart rate. It is used in the treatment of hypertension and congestive heart failure.[21,22] It also prevents the reabsorption of sodium and water from renal tubules and decreases the heart flow rate.[23,24]

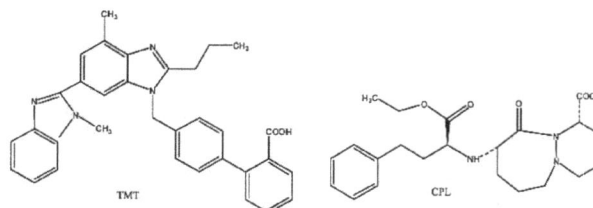

Figure 1. The Structures of TMT and CPL

In the present work two cardiovascular compounds were investigated, Telmisartan and Cilazapril, which

---

*Corresponding author: Refaat Ahmed Saber, Faculty of Technology and Development, Zagazig University, Egypt.
Emails: chem_refaat63@yahoo.com; alikamal1978@hotmail.com

belong to different groups of antihypertensive drugs, were chosen for study.

Materials and Methods
Telmistran and Cilazapril were obtained from reference standard department (NODCAR)., Egypt. The used drugs have high purity (more than 99%).

Methods
The TGA, DTG and DTA Analysis were made using simultaneous TG-DTA apparatus thermal analyzer (Shimadzu DTG-60H).The experiments were performed between ambient and 1000 °C. The temperature program had a heating rate 10 °C/min. Dry nitrogen at a low rate of 30 ML/min was used as the purge gas. The sample mass was kept in the range of 5 mg. α-Al$_2$O$_3$ was used as the reference material.

The thermodynamic parameters of decomposition processes of the used drugs namely activation energy (E*), enthalpy (ΔH*), entropy (ΔS*) and Gibbs free energy change of the decomposition (ΔG*) were evaluated graphically by employing the Horowitz-Metzger and Coats-Redfern relations.

Horowitz-Metzger method[25]
For the first order kinetic process, the Horowitz-Metzger equation can be represented as follow:

$$\log.[\log \frac{W_f}{W_f - W}] = \frac{\theta.E^*}{2.303RT_s^2} - \log 2.303 \quad (1)$$

Where W$_f$ was the mass loss at the completion of the decomposition reaction, W was the mass loss up to temperature T, R was the gas constant, T$_s$ was the DTG peak temperature and θ = T-T$_s$. A plot of log [log W$_f$/(W$_f$ - W)] against θ would give a straight line and E* could be calculated from the slope.

Coats-Redfern Method[26]
For the first order kinetic process, the activation energy (E*) in J.mol^{-1} could be calculated from the following equation:

$$\log\left(\frac{\log\left[W_f / W_f - W\right]}{T^2}\right) = \log\left[\frac{AR}{\phi E^*}\left(1 - \frac{2RT}{E^*}\right)\right] - \frac{E^*}{2.303RT} \quad (2)$$

Where ϕ was the heating rate. Since 1-2RT / E$^*\cong$1, the plot of the left-hand side of equation (2) against 1/T would give a straight line. E* was then calculated from the slope and the Arrhenius constant (A) was obtained from the intercept. The entropy ΔS*, enthalpy ΔH* and free energy ΔG* of activation were calculated using the following equations:

$$\Delta S^* = 2.303 [\log (Ah / kT)] R \quad (3)$$
$$\Delta H^* = E^* - RT \quad (4)$$
$$\Delta G^* = H^* - T_s \Delta S^* \quad (5)$$

Where k and h were the Boltzman and Planck constants, respectively. So the calculated values of E*, ΔS*, ΔH* and ΔG* could be obtained.

Results and Discussion
Figures (2, 3) show the TGA, DTG and DTA curves of the TMT and CPL, respectively. Table 1 presents the data concerning the main thermal reactions of the examined compounds. Table 2 gives the corresponding DTA reactions.

Thermal analysis of Telmisartan
The TGA and DTG curves of TMT (Figure 2a) show that the compound is thermally stable up to 262 °C. Between 262 and 712 °C, the TGA curve shows mass losses in two steps, while the DTG curve shows one sharp peak and other broad peak. The first step between 262 and 493 °C, a fast process with a mass loss 54.17% is probably due to the thermal decomposition of the compound with the elimination of biphenyl carboxlic acid (C$_{13}$H$_9$O$_2$) and C$_5$H$_9$N$_2$ groups. The second step between 493 and 712 °C where the mass loss is 45.83% is ascribed to pyrolysis of the compound and the loss of C$_{15}$H$_{12}$N$_2$ molecule (Table 1).

The DTA curve of TMT (Figure 2b) shows an endothermic flattened peak with its maximum at 456.63 °C. The main thermal decomposition reaction is endothermic peaks followed by exothermic peaks at 569.27 °C and 610.90 °C may be due to the pyrolysis of the compound. In addition the mentioned peaks, the compound has an endothermic reaction which is not accompanied by weight loss, the reaction has its maximum at 265.84 °C. This reaction is endothermic and may be attributed to melting of the compound. Thermal degradation pattern of TMT was presented in Figure 4a

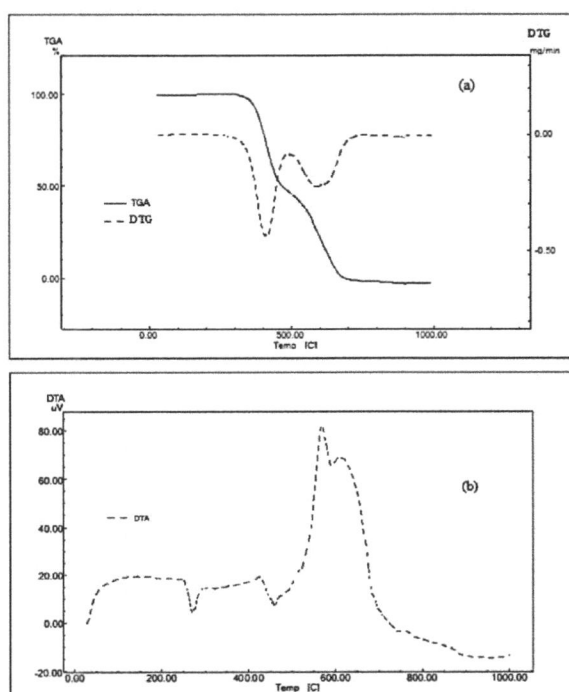

Figure 2. Thermal analysis curves (TGA, DTG and DTA) of TMT

Thermal analysis of Cilazapril

The TGA and DTG curves in (Figure 3a) show that CPL is thermally stable up to 140 °C then the thermal decomposition of CPL occurs. These curves also show that the mass loss up to 663 °C begins with a fast process, followed by slow process. The first step, which involves amass loss of 87.50%, is probably due to the elimination of ethoxycarbonyl, carboxylic, carbonyl, phenylpropyl amino and pyridazino groups. The final loss of 12.50% is ascribed to the pyrolysis of the compound and the loss of C_4H_7 group (Table 1).

The DTA curve of cilazapril (Figure 3b) has a shoulder at the beginning of the first endothermic reaction at 99.65 °C this may be attributed to the partial melting and recrystallization of the compound at 63.21 °C. The endothermic peak at 99.65 °C is due to the melting of the compound. An endothermic peak at 411.19 °C may be due to the decomposition of the compound followed by an exothermic peak at 564.33 °C may be attributed to the pyrolysis of the compound. Thermal degradation pattern of CPL was presented in Figure 4b.

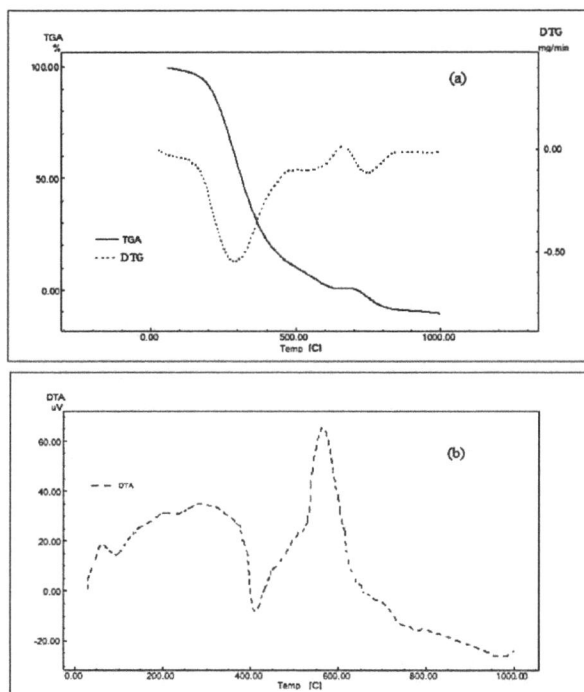

Figure 3. Thermal analysis curves (TGA, DTG and DTA) of CPL

Regarding the thermal stability of the compound, it can be concluded from their decomposition reaction that CPL starts to decompose at lower temperature than TMT. That is, TMT is more thermally stable than CPL. The melting temperatures of the examined compounds are determined by using the melting points of the compounds obtained by using DTA, and the melting point apparatus, the results are compared with the data stated in the literature.[18,21]

It is clear that results obtained from the DTA figures are comparable with the literature, and hence can be used for the determination the melting point of these TMT and CPL (Table 2).

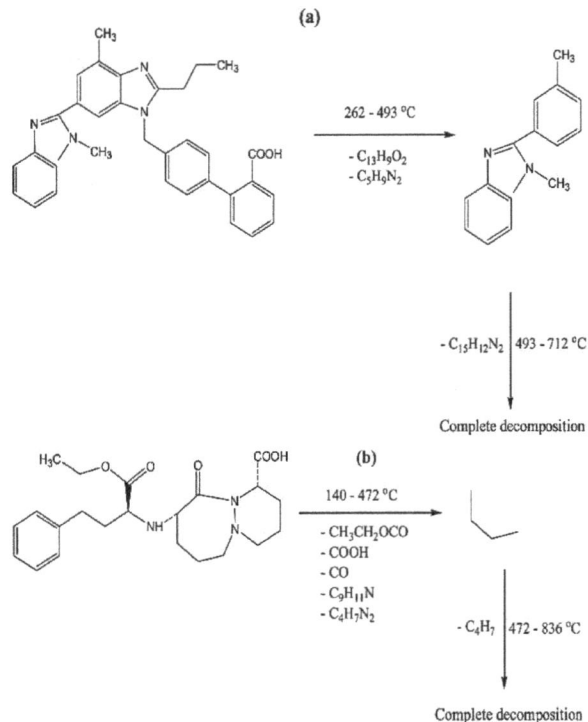

Figure 4. Thermal degradation patterns of TMT (a) and CPL (b)

Table 1. The thermal decomposition reaction of TMT and CPL

Drug	First step			Second step		
	Wt.Loss (%)	Start (°C)	End (°C)	Wt.Loss (%)	Start (°C)	End (°C)
TMT	45.83	262	493	54.17	493	712
CPL	12.50	140	472	87.50	472	836

Table 2. DTA peaks and melting points of TMT and CPL

Drug	Endothermic Peaks (°C)	Exothermic Peaks (°C)	DTA Method(°C)	MeltingPoint Apparatus (°C)
TMT	265.84,456.63	569.27,610.90	265.84	263
CPL	99.65,411.19	564.33	99.65	98

Kinetics and thermodynamic parameters

There were many methods used for the determination of the kinetic parameters. From these, Horowitz and Metzger and Coats and Redfern were applied (Figure 5).

Table 3 shows that the activation energy values (E^*) of TMT are higher than that of CPL. This conclusion is in accordance with previous conclusion for the thermal decomposition reaction of the compounds. The first reaction of CPL needs lower activation energy and hence the compound is the less stable and starts to decompose first.

Table 3. Thermodynamic parameters of the thermal decomposition of TMT and CPL

Drug	Temperature range (°C)	Thermodynamic parameters				
		E^* (kJ/mol) HM (CR)	A (S^{-1}) HM (CR)	ΔS^* (kJ/mol. K) HM (CR)	ΔH^* (kJ/mol) HM (CR)	ΔG^* (kJ/mol) HM (CR)
TMT	262-493	86.50 (99.27)	1.06×10^5 (1.71×10^6)	-110.49 (-128.23)	90.60 (95.87)	132.14 (148.17)
CPL	140-472	50.82 (63.65)	4.88×10^2 (6.97×10^3)	-154.1 (-171.08)	52.63 (61.26)	92.53 (110.50)

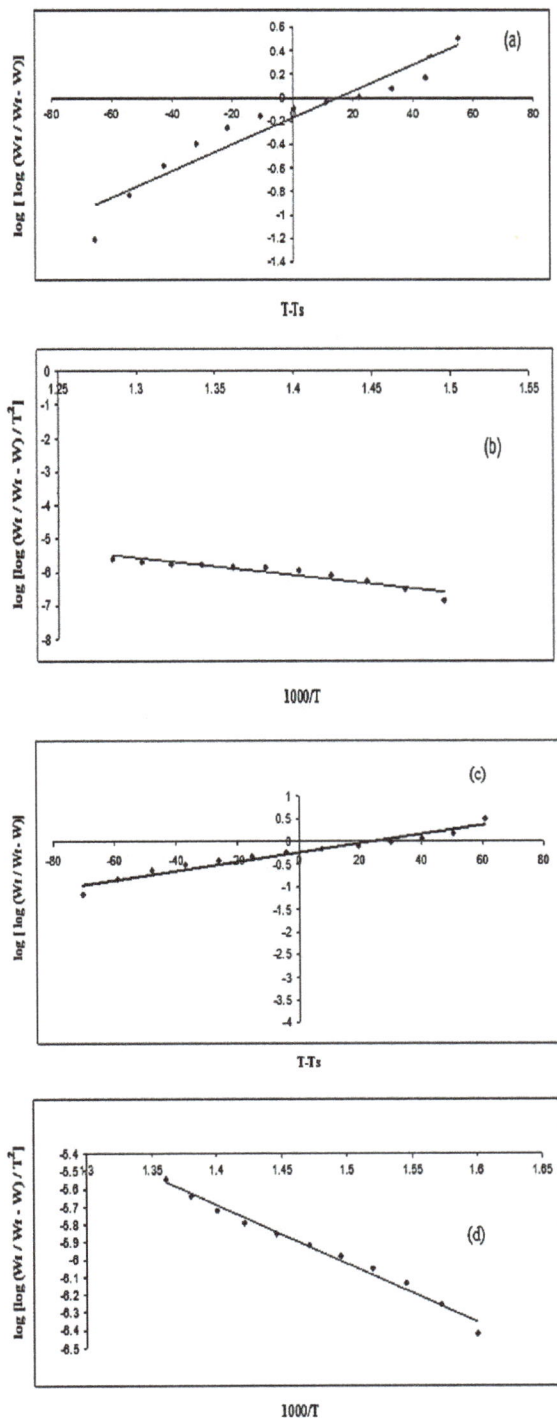

Figure 5. Horowitz-Metzger and Coats-Redfern plots of the decomposition of TMT (a, b) and CPL (c, d), respectively.

Conclusion

The studied compounds TMT and CPL are characterized by having main decomposition reaction and consist of two stages. Besides stability studies, thermal analysis is of value for determining melting temperatures, and water content. The use of clean techniques, and the speed and the simplicity of the analytical methods applied to obtain the results are the reasons behind the even growing importance of thermal analysis in the quality control of active ingredients for medication.

Acknowledgements

The authors extend their appreciation to the National Organization for Drug Control and Research for enabled the possibilities and devices to accomplish this work. Also our greetings to the soul of our Professor doctor Mohamed Elries.

Conflict of Interest

The authors declare that they have no conflict of interest.

References

1. Fifield FW, Kealey D. Principles and practice of analytical chemistry. 4th ed. London: Blackie Academic & Professional; 1995.
2. Ford JL, Timmings P. Pharmaceutical thermal analysis techniques and applications. Chichister UK: Ellis Harwood; 1989.
3. Giron D. Applications of thermal analysis and coupled techniques in pharmaceutical industry. *J Therm Anal Calorim* 2002;68:335-57.
4. Bruno FP, Caira MR, Monti GA, Kassuha DE, Sperandeo NR. Spectroscopic, thermal and X-ray structural study of the antiparasitic and antiviral drug nitazoxanide. *J Mol Struct* 2010;984(1-3):51-7.
5. Zayed MA, Fahmey MA, Hawash MF. Investigation of diazepam drug using thermal analyses, mass spectrometry and semi-empirical MO calculation. *Spectrochim Acta A Mol Biomol Spectrosc* 2005;61(5):799-805.
6. Wassel AA, El-Ries MA, Hawash MF. Structural investigation of captopril drug, using thermal analysis, mass spectral fragmentation and semi-empirical MO-calculations. *J Pharm Res* 2010;3(3):618-23.
7. Radha S, Gutch PK, Ganesan K, Vijayaraghavan R, Suman J, Subodh D. Thermal analysis of interactions between an oxime and excipients in

some binary mixtures by differential scanning calorimetry and thermagravimetric analysis. *J Pharm Res* 2010;3(3):590-5.

8. Oliveira GGG, Ferraz HG, Matos JSR. Thermoanalytical study of glibenclamide and excipients. *J Therm Anal Calorim* 2005;79(2):267-70.

9. Attia AK, Ibrahim MM, El-Ries MA. Thermal analysis of some antidiabetic pharmaceutical compounds. *Adv Pharm Bull* 2013;3(2):419-24.

10. Attia AK, Mohamed Abdel-Moety M. Thermoanalytical investigation of terazosin hydrochloride. *Adv Pharm Bull* 2013;3(1):147-52.

11. Tita B, Fulias A, Stefanescu M, Marian E, Tita D. Kinetic study of decomposition of ibuprofen under isothermal conditions. *Rev Chim-Bucharest* 2011;62(2):216-21.

12. Tomassetti M, Catalani A, Rossi V, Vecchio S. Thermal analysis study of the interactions between acetaminophen and excipients in solid dosage forms and in some binary mixtures. *J Pharm Biomed Anal* 2005;37(5):949-55.

13. El-Ries MA, Abo-Attia FM, El-Bayoumi A, Eman GS. Thermal characterization of leflunomide. *Insight Pharm Sci* 2011;1(2):18-23.

14. Attia AK, Hassan NY, El-Bayoumi A, Abdel-Hamid SG. Thermoanalytical study of alfuzosin HCl. *Int J Curr Pharm Res* 2012;4(3):101-5.

15. Abdel-Razeq SA, Salama NN, Abdel-Atty Sh, El-Kosy N. Thermoanalytical study and purity determination of azelastine Hydrochloride and emedastine difumarate. *Pharm Anal Acta* 2012;3(8):2153-435.

16. Haung Y, Ycheng K, Dalimore AD. The thermal analysis study of the drug captopril. *Thermochim Acta* 2001;367:43-58.

17. Elries MA, Ahmed IS, Salem WM. The Thermal analysis study of the tenoxicam. *J Drug Res Egypt* 2010;31(1):89-92.

18. Neil MJO. The Merck index, an encyclopedia of chemicals, drugs and biologicals, 14th ed. New Jersey: Merck research laboratories, Whitehouse station; 2006.

19. Wexler RR, Greenlee WJ, Irvin JD, Goldberg MR, Prendergast K, Smith RD, et al. Nonpeptide angiotensin II receptor antagonists: the next generation in antihypertensive therapy. *J Med Chem* 1996;39(3):625-56.

20. Willenheimer R, Dahlof B, Rydberg E, Erhardt L. AT1-receptor blockers in hypertension and heart failure: clinical experience and future directions. *Eur Heart J* 1999;20(14):997-1008.

21. Szucs T. Cilazapril. *Drugs* 1991;41 Suppl 1: 18-24.

22. Natoff IL, Nixon JS, Francis RJ, Klevans LR, Brewster M, Budd J, et al. Biological properties of the angiotensin-converting enzyme inhibitor cilazapril. *J Cardiovasc Pharmacol* 1985;7(3):569-80.

23. Foye OW. Principles of medicinal chemistry. 3rd ed. Philadelphia: Lea & Jebliger;1989.

24. Gilman GA, Rall TW, Nies AS, Taylor P. The pharmacological basis of therapeutics. 8th ed. New York: Pergamon press; 1990.

25. Horowitz HH, Metzger G. A new analysis of thermogravimetric traces. *Anal Chem* 1963;35(10):1464-8.

26. Coats AW, Redfern JP. Kinetic parameters from thermogravimetric data. *Nature* 1964;201(4914):68-9.

Permissions

List of Contributors

Gabriel Hancu, Brigitta Simon, Aura Rusu and Árpád Gyéresi
Department of Pharmaceutical Chemistry, Faculty of Pharmacy, University of Medicine and Pharmacy, Târgu Mureş, Romania

Eleonora Mircia
Department of Organic Chemistry, Faculty of Pharmacy, University of Medicine and Pharmacy, Târgu Mureş, Romania

Jalal Abdolalizadeh, Ali Aghebati Maleki and Koushan Sineh sepehr
Immunology Research Center, Tabriz University of Medical Sciences, Tabriz, Iran

Leili Aghebati Maleki
Immunology Research Center, Tabriz University of Medical Sciences, Tabriz, Iran
Tabriz International University of Medical Sciences, Tabriz University of Medical Sciences, Tabriz, Iran
Department of Immunology, Faculty of Medicine, Tabriz University of Medical Sciences, Tabriz, Iran

Jafar Majidi, Behzad Baradaran and Tohid Kazemi
Immunology Research Center, Tabriz University of Medical Sciences, Tabriz, Iran
Department of Immunology, Faculty of Medicine, Tabriz University of Medical Sciences, Tabriz, Iran

Radhika Bhaskar, Rahul Bhaskar, Mahendra K. Sagar and Vipin Saini
Department of Pharmacy, Mahatma Jyoti Rao Phoole University, Jaipur, India

Mohammad Ahangarzadeh Rezaee, Mohammad Reza Nahaei, Mohammad Hossein Soroush, Tahereh Pirzadeh, Mostafa Davodi, Mona Ghazi and Reza Bigverdi
Tabriz Research Center of Infectious and Tropical Diseases, Tabriz University of Medical Sciences, Tabriz, Iran

Zoya Hojabri and Mohammad Aghazadeh
Tabriz Research Center of Infectious and Tropical Diseases, Tabriz University of Medical Sciences, Tabriz, Iran

Morteza Ghojazadeh
Physiology department, Faculty of Medicine, Tabriz University of Medical Sciences, Tabriz, Iran

Omid Pajand
Student Research Committee, Tabriz University of Medical Sciences, Tabriz, Iran

Petikam lavudu and Chepuri Divya
Department of Pharmaceutical Biotechnology, Vishnu Institute of Pharmaceutical Education and Research, Narsapur, Andhra Pradesh-500072

Avula Prameela Rani
University College of Pharmaceutical Sciences, Acharya Nagarjuna University, Guntur, Andhra Pradesh-522510

Chandra Bala Sekaran
Department of Biotechnology, Jagarlamudi Kuppuswamy Choudary College, Guntur, Andhra Pradesh-522006

Jalal Abdolalizadeh
Research Center for Pharmaceutical Nanotechnology, Tabriz University of Medical Sciences, Tabriz, Iran
Student' Research Committee, Tabriz University of Medical Sciences, Tabriz, Iran

Yadollah Omidi
Research Center for Pharmaceutical Nanotechnology, Tabriz University of Medical Sciences, Tabriz, Iran
Ovarian Cancer Research Center, Translational Research Center, University of Pennsylvania, Philadelphia, PA 19104, USA

Jafar Majidi Zolbanin
Drug Applied Research Center, Tabriz University of Medical Sciences, Tabriz, Iran
Immunology Research Center, Tabriz University of Medical Sciences, Tabriz, Iran

Behzad Baradaran
Immunology Research Center, Tabriz University of Medical Sciences, Tabriz, Iran

Mohammad Nouri
Biochemistry Department, Medicine Faculty, Tabriz University of Medical Sciences, Tabriz, Iran

AliAkbar Movassaghpour
Hematology and Oncology Research Center, Tabriz University of Medical Sciences, Tabriz, Iran

Safar Farajnia
Biotechnology Research Center, Tabriz University of Medical Sciences, Tabriz, Iran

Meesaraganda Sreedevi, Yadati Narasimha Spoorthy and Lakshmana Rao Krishna Rao Ravindranath
Sri Krishnadevaraya Univerisity, Anantapur, Andhra Pradesh, India

Aluru Raghavendra Guru Prasad
ICFAI Foundation for Higher Education, Hyderabad, Andhra Pradesh, India

Ali Kamal Attia and Mona Mohamed Abdel-Moety
National Organization for Drug Control and Research, Cairo, Egypt

Namasani Santhosh Kumar, Avula Prameela Rani and Telu Visalakshi
University College of Pharmaceutical Sciences, Acharya Nagarjuna University, Nagarjuna nagar, India-522 510

Chandra Bala Sekaran
Department of Biotechnology, Jagarlamudi Kuppuswamy Choudary College, Guntur, India - 522 006

Mohammad Aziz Dollah and Mohamad Hafanizam Bin Hassan
Biomedical Department, Faculty of Medicine and Health Sciences, University Putra Malaysia, Selangor, Malaysia

Saadat Parhizkar
Medicinal Plants Research Centre, Yasuj University of Medical Sciences (YUMS), Yasuj, Iran

Latiffah Abdul Latiff
Community Health Department, Faculty of Medicine and Health Sciences, University Putra Malaysia, Selangor, Malaysia

Shantaram Gajanan Khanage
Research scholar, Department of Pharmacy, Vinayaka Missions University, Salem, Sankari main road, NH-47, Tamilnadu, India-636308

Appala Raju
Department of Pharmaceutical chemistry, H.K.E.'S College of Pharmacy, Sedam road, Gulbarga, Karnataka, India-585105

Popat Baban Mohite
Department of Pharmaceutical chemistry, M.E.S. College of Pharmacy, Sonai, Tq Newasa, Dist.-Ahmednagar, Maharashtra, India-414105

Ramdas Bhanudas Pandhare
Department of Pharmacology, M.E.S. College of Pharmacy, Sonai, Tq-Newasa, Dist.-Ahmednagar, Maharashtra, India-414105

Abolfazl Aslani and Hajar Jahangiri
Department of Pharmaceutics, School of Pharmacy and Novel Drug Delivery Systems Research Center, Isfahan University of Medical Sciences, Isfahan, Iran

Koushan Sineh Sepehr, Behzad Baradaran and Fatemeh Zare Shahneh
Drug Applied Research Center, Tabriz University of Medical Sciences, Tabriz, Iran

Jafar Majidi, Jalal Abdolalizadeh and Leili Aghebati
Immunology Research Center, Tabriz University of Medical Sciences, Tabriz, Iran

Eskandar Moghimipour and Anayatollah Salimi
Nanotechnology Research Center, Jundishapur University of Medical Sciences, Ahvaz, Iran

Soroosh Eftekhari
Department of Pharmaceutics, Faculty of Pharmacy, Jundishapur University of Medical Sciences, Ahvaz, Iran

Davoud Asgari, Hadi Valizadeh, Mohammad Reza Rashidi, Vala Kafil and Javid Shahbazi
Research Center for Pharmaceutical Nanotechnology, Faculty of Pharmacy, Tabriz University of Medical Sciences, Tabriz, Iran

Mostafa Heidari Majd
Research Center for Pharmaceutical Nanotechnology, Faculty of Pharmacy, Tabriz University of Medical Sciences, Tabriz, Iran
Faculty of Pharmacy, Zabol University of Medical Sciences, Zabol, Iran
Student Research Committee, Tabriz University of Medical Sciences, Tabriz, Iran

Jaleh Barar and Yadollah Omidi
Research Center for Pharmaceutical Nanotechnology, Faculty of Pharmacy, Tabriz University of Medical Sciences, Tabriz, Iran
Ovarian Cancer Research Center, University of Pennsylvania, Philadelphia, USA

Saeed Ghasemi and Ali Abdollahi
Department of Medicinal Chemistry, Faculty of Pharmacy, Tabriz University of Medical Sciences, Tabriz, Iran

Soodabeh Davaran and Davoud Asgari
Department of Medicinal Chemistry, Faculty of Pharmacy, Tabriz University of Medical Sciences, Tabriz, Iran
Research Center for Pharmaceutical Nanotechnology, Tabriz University of Medical Sciences, Tabriz, Iran

Javid Shahbazi Mojarrad
Department of Medicinal Chemistry, Faculty of Pharmacy, Tabriz University of Medical Sciences, Tabriz, Iran
Tuberculosis and Lung Disease Research Center, Tabriz University of Medical Sciences, Tabriz, Iran

Simin Sharifi
Research Center for Pharmaceutical Nanotechnology, Tabriz University of Medical Sciences, Tabriz, Iran

Leili Aghebati Maleki, Behzad Baradaran, Jalal Abdolalizadeh and Jafar Majidi
Immunology Research Center, Tabriz University of Medical Sciences, Tabriz, Iran
Tabriz Pharmaceutical Technology Incubator (TPTI)

Fatemeh Ezzatifar
Immunology Research Center, Tabriz University of Medical Sciences, Tabriz, Iran

Gabriel Hancu, Camelia Câmpian, Aura Rusu and Hajnal Kelemen
Department of Pharmaceutical Chemistry, Faculty of Pharmacy, University of Medicine and Pharmacy, Târgu Mureş, Romania

Eleonora Mircia
Department of Organic Chemistry, Faculty of Pharmacy, University of Medicine and Pharmacy, Târgu Mureş, Romania

Ali Kamal Attia, Magda Mohamed Ibrahim and Mohamed Abdel Nabi El-Ries
National Organization for Drug Control and Research, Cairo, Egypt

Bohlool Habibi Asl
Department of Pharmacology, Faculty of Pharmacy, Tabriz University of Medical Sciences, Tabriz, Iran

Haleh Vaez
Department of Pharmacology, Faculty of Pharmacy, Tabriz University of Medical Sciences, Tabriz, Iran
Student Research Committee, Faculty of Pharmacy, Tabriz University of Medical Sciences, Tabriz, Iran

Samin Hamidi
Student Research Committee, Faculty of Pharmacy, Tabriz University of Medical Sciences, Tabriz, Iran

Faculty of Pharmacy, Tabriz University of Medical Sciences, Tabriz, Iran

Turan Imankhah
Faculty of Pharmacy, Tabriz University of Medical Sciences, Tabriz, Iran

Shantaram Gajanan Khanage and Popat Baban Mohite
Department of Pharmaceutical Chemistry and PG studies, M.E.S. College of Pharmacy, Sonai, Ahmednagar, Maharashtra, India-414105

Ramdas Bhanudas Pandhare
Department of Pharmacology, M.E.S. College of Pharmacy, Sonai, Tq-Newasa, Dist.-Ahmednagar, Maharashtra, India-414105

S. Appala Raju
Department of Pharmaceutical chemistry, H.K.E.'S College of Pharmacy, Sedam road, Gulbarga, Karnataka, India-585105

Gabriel Hancu, Brigitta Simon, Hajnal Kelemen, Aura Rusu and Árpád Gyéresi
Department of Pharmaceutical Chemistry, Faculty of Pharmacy, University of Medicine and Pharmacy, Târgu Mureş, Romania

Eleonora Mircia
Department of Organic Chemistry, Faculty of Pharmacy, University of Medicine and Pharmacy, Târgu Mureş, Romania

Pavan Ram Kamble, Karimunnisa Sameer Shaikh and Pravin Digambar Chaudhari
Department of Pharmaceutics, Modern College of Pharmacy, Nigdi, Pune, Maharashtra, India-411044

Jafar Ezzati Nazhad Dolatabadi and Seyed Morteza Ghareghoran
Research Center for Pharmaceutical Nanotechnology, Tabriz University of Medical Sciences, Tabriz, Iran

Ahad Mokhtarzadeh
Faculty of Pharmacy, Mashhad University of Medical Sciences, Mashhad, Iran

Gholamreza Dehghan
Department of Plant Biology, Faculty of Natural Science, University of Tabriz, Tabriz, Iran

Moorthi Chidambaram and Kathiresan Krishnasamy
Department of Pharmacy, Annamalai University, Chidambaram, Tamil Nadu, India

Ali Kamiar
Faculty of Pharmacy, Student Research Committee, Tabriz University of Medical Sciences, Tabriz, Iran

Reza Ghotaslou
Department of Microbiology, School of Medicine, Tabriz University of Medical Sciences, Tabriz, Iran

Hadi Valizadeh
Research Center for Pharmaceutical Nanotechnology and Faculty of Pharmacy, Tabriz University of Medical Sciences, Tabriz, Iran

Manal A. El-Shal
National Organization for Drug Control and Research (NODCAR), Pyramid Ave Cairo, Egypt

Amelia Tero-Vescan
Department of Biochemistry, Faculty of Pharmacy, University of Medicine and Pharmacy, Târgu Mureş, Romania

Gabriel Hancu and Mihaela Oroian
Department of Pharmaceutical Chemistry, Faculty of Pharmacy, University of Medicine and Pharmacy, Târgu Mureş, Romania

Anca Cârje
Department of Drug Analysis and Analytical Chemistry, Faculty of Pharmacy, University of Medicine and Pharmacy, Târgu Mureş, Romania

Shantaram Gajanan Khanage, Popat Baban Mohite and Sandeep Jadhav
Department of Pharmaceutical Chemistry and PG studies, M.E.S. College of Pharmacy, Sonai, Ahmednagar, Maharashtra, India

Lena Mahmoudi Azar and Elnaz Mehdizadeh Aghdam
Department of Pharmaceutical Biotechnology, Faculty of Pharmacy, Tabriz University of Medical Sciences, Tabriz, Iran

Farrokh Karimi
Department of Pharmaceutical Biotechnology, Faculty of Pharmacy, Tabriz University of Medical Sciences, Tabriz, Iran
Department of Biotechnology, Faculty of Science, Maragheh University, Maragheh, Iran

Babak Haghshenas
Department of Pharmaceutical Biotechnology, Faculty of Pharmacy, Tabriz University of Medical Sciences, Tabriz, Iran
Institute of Bioscience, University of Putra Malaysia, Kualalumpur, Malaysia

Abolfazl Barzegari
Research Center of Pharmaceutical Nanotechnology, Tabriz University of Medical Sciences, Tabriz, Iran

Parichehr Yaghmaei
Islamic Azad University, Science and Research Branch of Tehran, Iran

Mohammad Saeid Hejazi
Department of Pharmaceutical Biotechnology, Faculty of Pharmacy, Tabriz University of Medical Sciences, Tabriz, Iran
Faculty of Advanced Biomedical Sciences, Tabriz University of Medical Sciences, Tabriz, Iran

Vishal Pande, Samir Patel, Vijay Patil and Raju Sonawane
H.R. Patel Institute of Pharmaceutical Education and Research, Shirpur, Dhule, Maharashtra, 425405 India

Ruchi Jain
Suresh Gyan Vihar University, Jaipur, Rajasthan, India-302025

Nilesh Jain, Deepak Kumar Jain and Surendra Kumar Jain
Sagar Institute of Research & Technology-Pharmacy, Ayodhya Bypass Road Bhopal, Madhya Pradesh, India – 462041

Refaat Ahmed Saber
Faculty of Technology and Development, Zagazig University, Egypt

Ali Kamal Attia and Waheed Mohamed Salem
National Organization for Drug Control and Research, Cairo, Egypt

Index

A

Affinity Purification, 11, 32-33
Alanine Aminotransferase, 53, 55, 57
Almotriptan Malate, 26, 30-31
Ambrisentan, 46, 48-49, 52
Amino Acid, 32, 94, 172
Antihistamines, 104-108, 115
Ascetic Fluid, 9, 11, 73-76, 103
Aspartate Aminotransferase, 53-55, 57

B

Beta-lactam Antibiotics, 130, 133

C

Capillary Chromatography, 1, 8
Capillary Electrophoresis, 1, 7-8, 104-105, 108, 160-162, 166
Catalase Activity, 172-174, 177-178
Cephalosporins, 6, 8, 130-134
Cetirizine, 104-105, 113, 171
Chalcones, 61, 122-123, 127
Chiral Separation, 4-5, 8, 161-162, 165-166
Cyclic Voltammetry, 155, 158, 160
Cystic Fibrosis, 21, 24-25

D

Desloratadine, 104-105, 108
Differential Scanning Calorimetry, 41, 78-79, 135, 137, 139
Direct Compression Method, 65, 69, 71
Dissolution Rate, 135, 138-142
Doripenem, 21-25
Doxorubicin, 93-97

E

Effervescent Tablet, 65-66, 188
Eperisone Hydrochloride, 167, 170

F

Farnesyltransferase Inhibitor, 94, 97
Flavonoid, 143
Flow Cytometry, 32-35, 76, 88
Fluorescence-activated Cell Sorting, 32-33
Folate Receptor, 87, 91-93
Folic Acid, 87-89, 92-93
Fusion Method, 65, 71

G

Glibenclamide, 45, 109, 114, 198

Gliclazide, 15, 20, 114

H

High Performance Liquid Chromatography, 1, 193
Hot Plate Method, 59-60, 63, 122, 124-125, 127
Human Hematopoietic Stem, 9, 12
Hybridoma Cells, 9-10, 12-13, 73-76, 99-101
Hybridoma Technology, 9, 13, 73, 75, 99, 102
Hydrochloric Acid, 37, 132

I

Imidazole, 37, 39-40, 94-95, 97, 180
Imipenem, 21-25
Indapamide, 161-166
Ion-pair Complex, 46, 48, 50
Isoxazole, 59-60, 64, 129

K

Ketotifen, 115-119, 121

L

Liquid Load Factor, 135-136, 138
Loratadine, 104-105, 108

M

Magnetic Resonance Imaging, 87
Melanoma Cancer Stem Cells, 73, 76
Metformin, 15, 20, 113-114
Methylene Blue, 46-49, 52
Micellar Electrokinetic, 1, 4, 7-8
Monoclonal Antibody, 9-14, 32, 73-77, 99, 101-103

N

Nanoprecipitation Method, 147-150
Naproxen, 78-84, 142

O

Olanzapine, 155-156, 159-160

P

Penicillins, 6, 130-134
Periplasmic Space, 172-173
Pioglitazone, 15, 20, 109, 113-114
Polymeric Nanoparticles, 147, 149
Propylene Glycol, 78-81, 136, 138
Protein A-sepharose, 9
Pseudomonas Aeruginosa, 21, 24-25, 39